Nephrology

THIRD EDITION

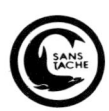

Editor: Charles Mitchell
Project Manager: Linda S. Napora
Copy Editor: Therese J. Grundl
Designer: Dan Pfisterer
Illustration Planner: Ray Lowman
Production Coordinator: Charles E. Zeller

Copyright © 1995
Williams & Wilkins
428 East Preston Street
Baltimore, Maryland 21202, USA

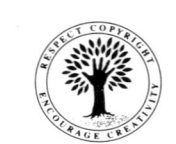

All rights reserved. This book is protected by copyright. No part of this book may be reproduced in any form or by any means, including photocopying, or utilized by any information storage and retrieval system without written permission from the copyright owner.

Accurate indications, adverse reactions, and dosage schedules for drugs are provided in this book, but it is possible that they may change. The reader is urged to review the package information data of the manufacturers of the medications mentioned.

Printed in the United States of America
Library of Congress Cataloging in Publication Data

Nephrology / editors, C. Craig Tisher, Christopher S. Wilcox.—3rd ed.
    p. cm.—(House office series)
  Rev. ed. of: Nephrology for the house officer. 2nd ed. c1993.
  Includes bibliographical references and index.
  ISBN 0-683-08277-9
  1. Nephrology. 2. Kidneys—Diseases. I. Tisher, C. Craig, 1936–
  II. Wilcox, Christopher S. III. Nephrology for the house officer. IV. Series.
  [DNLM: 1. Kidney Diseases—handbooks. WJ 39 N4394 1995]
RC903.N45 1995
616.6'1—dc20
DNLM/DLC
for Library of Congress   94-27308
                                                                                        CIP
                                                           94 95 96 97 98
                                          1 2 3 4 5 6 7 8 9 10

Reprints of chapter(s) may be purchased from Williams & Wilkins in quantities of 100 or more. Call Isabella Wise in the Special Sales Department, (800) 358-3583.

HOUSE OFFICER SERIES

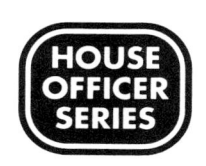

Nephrology

THIRD EDITION

EDITORS

C. Craig Tisher, M.D.

Professor of Medicine and Pathology and Anatomy and Cell Biology
Chief, Division of Nephrology, Hypertension and Transplantation
Associate Chairman for Academic Affairs, Department of Medicine
University of Florida College of Medicine
Gainesville, Florida

Christopher S. Wilcox, M.D., Ph.D.

Professor of Medicine, Pharmacology and Therapeutics
Director, Hypertension Center
University of Florida College of Medicine
Chief, Nephrology and Hypertension Section, Medical Service
Department of Veterans Affairs Medical Center
Gainesville, Florida

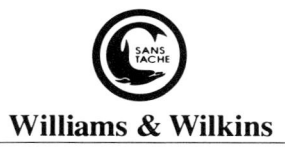

Williams & Wilkins

BALTIMORE • PHILADELPHIA • HONG KONG
LONDON • MUNICH • SYDNEY • TOKYO

A WAVERLY COMPANY

To Audrae Tisher and Linda Wilcox

Preface

This clinical nephrology text has been written to assist both the house officer and the medical student in the care of patients with disorders in which the kidney plays a central or dominant role in the disease process. It should also be a valuable resource for those who are just beginning their subspeciality training in nephrology as well as for physicians whose primary training is in another medical subspeciality.

Nephrology encompasses a wide variety of disciplines that include renal physiology and pathophysiology, renal anatomy and pathology, biochemistry, immunology, metabolism, pharmacology, and molecular biology. Although this handbook is primarily a practical clinical manual, out of necessity it must draw on knowledge derived from research in the clinical and basic sciences to present the latest information that is available for proper diagnosis and treatment of kidney disease and kidney dysfunction.

This third edition of *Nephrology* in the House Officer Series contains 26 chapters that are written in a concise yet detailed manner to serve as a primer in clinical nephrology. Chapter 1 provides a brief review of the principal structural and functional features of the kidney. Chapter 2 presents a practical approach to the physiologic and radiologic evaluation of the kidney and includes a section on clinical indications for kidney biopsy. Chapter 3 reviews the clinical significance of hematuria and underscores those clinical situations that require investigation. The etiology, evaluation, and pathophysiology of proteinuria and the nephrotic syndrome are discussed in Chapter 4, and the complications and management of the latter are reviewed.

Chapter 5 discusses specific disease entities that are glomerular in type including focal segmental glomerulosclerosis, minimal change disease, membranous glomerulonephritis, postinfectious proliferative glomerulonephritis, rapidly progressive glomerulonephritis, antiglomerular basement membrane disease (Goodpasture's syndrome), membranoproliferative glomerulonephritis, IgA nephropathy (Berger's disease), and fibrillary glomerulonephritis. Systemic diseases that frequently involve the kidneys are presented in Chapter 6 and include systemic lupus erythematosus, systemic vasculitis, Schönlein-Henoch purpura, hemolytic-uremic syndrome, thrombotic thrombocytopenic purpura, progressive systemic sclerosis, multiple myeloma, and amyloidosis.

In Chapter 7, diabetic nephropathy receives special emphasis because of its prevalence and because of its major role as a cause of end-stage renal failure. Chapters 8 and 9 are devoted to detailed discussions of acute and chronic renal failure, respectively. Both chapters are filled with practical information on the recognition and management of these common entities.

Chapters 10–13 are devoted to extensive discussions of the most common encountered fluid, acid-base, and electrolyte disorders. Emphasis is placed on their recognition and management. Renal stone disease is reviewed in Chapter 14, and a working scheme is presented to aid in identification of the various causes of this poorly understood problem. Chapter 15 focuses on urinary tract infections and outlines the best approach to their diagnosis and treatment. Chapter 16 discusses tubulointerstitial nephritis, a disease process with various etiologies that can lead to acute or chronic renal failure. Chapter 17 reviews the diagnosis and management of those entities that are seen principally in adult renal cystic disease patients. The subject of AIDS and kidney disease is reviewed in Chapter 18, and the recently recognized entity, HIV-associated nephropathy, is discussed. Appropriate guidelines for the management of acute and chronic renal failure in patients with HIV infection are outlined.

Chapters 19–21 provide an extensive discussion regarding diagnosis and treatment of the major forms of primary and secondary hypertension. The use of hemodialysis and peritoneal dialysis in the management of acute and chronic renal failure is described in Chapters 22 and 23. Chapter 24 discusses proper management of the renal transplant patient. Chapter 25 emphasizes the importance of proper nutrition in acute and chronic renal failure. The handbook concludes with Chapter 26, which reviews the use of drugs in renal failure and includes an extensive set of tables to aid in proper drug dosing.

The text was written and reviewed by the faculty and fellows in the Division of Nephrology, Hypertension and Transplantation at the University of Florida. Their collective experience, skill, and knowledge and that of their colleagues have been incorporated into each chapter. The editors have reviewed and revised each chapter extensively to ensure practicality, accuracy, and conciseness. The editorial assistance of Ranee H. Soo Hoo was invaluable. We believe the third edition of *Nephrology* will be extremely useful in the management of patients with kidney disease, hypertension, and related disorders.

Contributors

From the Division of Nephrology, Hypertension and Transplantation at the University of Florida College of Medicine, Gainesville, Florida:

Yousri M. H. Barri, M.D.
Clinical Fellow in Nephrology

Nicolas J. Guzman, M.D.
Assistant Professor of Pharmacology and Therapeutics and Medicine

Bruce C. Kone, M.D.
Assistant Professor of Medicine

Kirsten M. Madsen, M.D., Ph.D.
Associate Professor of Medicine

Donald R. Mars, M.D.
Associate Professor of Medicine

John C. Peterson, M.D.
Associate Professor of Medicine

Eleanor L. Ramos, M.D.
Assistant Professor of Medicine

Edward A. Ross, M.D.
Associate Professor of Medicine

Geraldine S. Shaw, M.D.
Clinical Fellow in Nephrology

C. Craig Tisher, M.D.
Professor of Medicine and Pathology and Anatomy and Cell Biology

I. David Weiner, M.D.
Assistant Professor of Medicine

Christopher S. Wilcox, M.D., Ph.D.
Professor of Medicine and Pharmacology and Therapeutics

Charles S. Wingo, M.D.
Professor of Medicine and Physiology

Contents

Preface	*vii*
Contributors	*xi*
1. Anatomy of the Kidney KIRSTEN M. MADSEN	1
2. Evaluation of Kidney Structure and Function C. CRAIG TISHER and CHRISTOPHER S. WILCOX	13
3. Hematuria NICOLAS J. GUZMAN	25
4. Proteinuria and the Nephrotic Syndrome DONALD R. MARs	30
5. Glomerulonephritis C. CRAIG TISHER	36
6. Renal Involvement in Systemic Diseases GERALDINE S. SHAW and C. CRAIG TISHER	46
7. Diabetic Nephropathy C. CRAIG TISHER	62
8. Acute Renal Failure NICOLAS J. GUZMAN and JOHN C. PETERSON	69
9. Chronic Renal Failure JOHN C. PETERSON	83
10. Disorders of Water Balance BRUCE C. KONE and CHARLES S. WINGO	94
11. Potassium Disorders CHARLES S. WINGO	108
12. Acid-Base Disorders CHARLES S. WINGO	121

13. Calcium, Phosphorus, and Magnesium Disorders 138
JOHN C. PETERSON

14. Renal Stone Disease 152
I. DAVID WEINER

15. Urinary Tract Infection 161
JOHN C. PETERSON

16. Tubulointerstitial Nephritis 168
NICOLAS J. GUZMAN

17. Renal Cystic Disease 176
CHISTOPHER S. WILCOX

18. AIDS and Kidney Disease 183
C. CRAIG TISHER

19. Approach to the Hypertensive Patient 189
CHRISTOPHER S. WILCOX

20. Secondary Forms of Hypertension 198
CHRISTOPHER S. WILCOX

21. Treatment of Hypertension 209
YOUSRI M. H. BARRI and CHRISTOPHER S. WILCOX

22. Hemodialysis 228
EDWARD A. ROSS and YOUSRI M. H. BARRI

23. Peritoneal Dialysis 241
DONALD R. MARS and EDWARD A. ROSS

24. Renal Transplant Patients 254
ELEANOR L. RAMOS

25. Nutrition in Renal Failure 267
EDWARD A. ROSS

26. Use of Drugs in Renal Failure 277
NICOLAS J. GUZMAN

Index 291

Chapter 1

Anatomy of the Kidney

Kirsten M. Madsen

GROSS ANATOMY

The kidneys are located retroperitoneally from the T12 to the L3 vertebra. The right kidney is positioned slightly lower than the left. Each kidney is approximately 11–12 cm long, 5–7.5 cm wide, and 2.5–3 cm thick. Kidney weight in adult men is 125–170 g and in adult women is 115–155 g. On the medial margin is a cleft, the hilus, through which the renal pelvis, the renal artery and vein, lymphatics, and a nerve plexus pass into the sinus of the kidney (Fig. 1.1). The renal pelvis, an expansion of the upper end of the ureter, continues into funnel-shaped tubes called the calyces that connect with the renal papillae. The kidney is covered by a tough fibrous capsule that is normally smooth and easily removable.

The kidney can be divided into cortex and medulla. In humans, the medulla forms 8–18 renal pyramids, the bases of which are located at the corticomedullary junction (Fig. 1.1). The apices of the pyramids extend toward the renal pelvis, each forming a papilla. From the base of the pyramids, medullary rays consisting of collecting ducts and the straight portions of proximal and distal tubules extend into the cortex. Based on segmentation of the nephron (Fig. 1.2), the medulla can be divided into an outer medulla, which in turn can be subdivided into an outer and inner stripe, and an inner medulla, which includes the renal papilla. The functional unit of the kidney is the nephron, which consists of a renal corpuscle or glomerulus and its associated tubule (Fig. 1.2). The tubular portion of the nephron is composed of three major subdivisions: the proximal

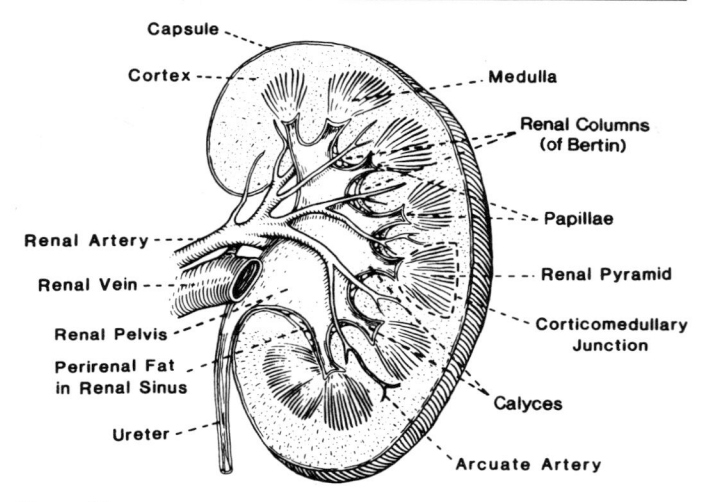

Figure 1.1. Cut surface of a bisected kidney.

convoluted tubule (PCT), the loop of Henle, and the distal convoluted tubule (DCT). The latter continues into the collecting duct system, which is derived from the ureteric bud and, strictly speaking, is not part of the nephron. The loop of Henle includes the proximal straight tubule (pars recta of the proximal tubule), the thin limb segments, and the thick ascending limb (TAL) (pars recta of the distal tubule).

Each human kidney contains approximately 1.2 million nephrons. Those originating from outer and midcortical glomeruli have short loops of Henle that bend in the inner stripe of the outer medulla. Juxtamedullary nephrons originating from glomeruli located near the corticomedullary junction have long loops of Henle that reach into the inner medulla. In the human kidney 10–15% of the glomeruli belong to long-looped nephrons.

MICROSCOPIC ANATOMY

Glomerulus

The glomeruli are located in the cortex. The human glomerulus measures approximately 200 µm in diameter, and it includes a capillary tuft and the surrounding parietal epithelium of Bow-

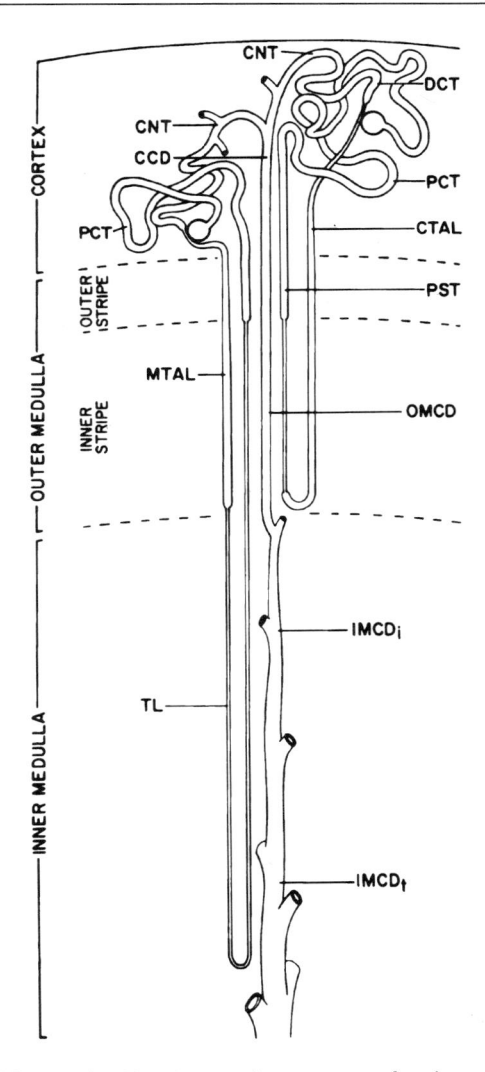

Figure 1.2. Relationships among various segments of nephron and zones of kidney. *CCD*, cortical collecting duct; *CNT*, connecting segment; *CTAL*, cortical thick ascending limb; *DCT*, distal convoluted tubule; *IMCD$_i$*, initial inner medullary collecting duct; *IMCD$_t$*, terminal inner medullary collecting duct; *MTAL*, medullary thick ascending limb; *OMCD*, outer medullary collecting duct; *PCT*, proximal convoluted tubule; *PST*, proximal straight tubule; *TL*, thin limb of Henle's loop.

man's capsule. The glomerulus is responsible for the formation of an ultrafiltrate of plasma. It consists of a capillary network lined by a thin fenestrated endothelium, a central mesangial region, and the visceral epithelium with its associated basement membrane (Fig. 1.3A). The filtration barrier between the blood and the urinary space is composed of the fenestrated endothelium, the peripheral glomerular basement membrane, and the slit pores between the foot processes of the visceral epithelial cells (Fig. 1.3B). The thin *endothelium* is perforated by pores or fenestrae measuring approximately 70–100 nm in diameter. It constitutes the initial barrier to the passage of blood constituents but is not believed to represent a significant barrier to the passage of macromolecules.

The glomerular basement membrane is located between the endothelium and the visceral epithelium and is approximately 300 nm thick. It is composed of three layers: a central dense layer, the lamina densa, and two electronlucent layers, the lamina rara externa and lamina rara interna. The glomerular basement membrane is believed to constitute a size-selective as well as a charge-selective barrier to the passage of macromolecules. It is composed of various glycoproteins, including type IV and type V collagen, laminin, fibronectin, and negatively charged glycosaminoglycans rich in heparan sulfate. These anionic sites appear to be important in establishing the charge-selective characteristics of the filtration barrier.

The *visceral epithelial cells* (or podocytes) have long cytoplasmic processes that divide into foot processes or pedicles that are in close contact with the glomerular basement membrane. The space between adjacent foot processes is called the filtration slit or slit pore, and it is closed by a thin membrane, the slit diaphragm. The foot processes possess a negative surface charge that is rich in sialic acid and is important for maintaining the normal structure and function of the filtration barrier. Removal of the anionic surface coat causes the foot processes to disappear and to be replaced by a continuous band of cytoplasm along the glomerular basement membrane. Similar changes called "foot process fusion" or "effacement" are observed in various proteinuric conditions.

The *mesangium* is separated from the capillary lumen by the endothelium and consists of mesangial cells and surrounding mesangial matrix. The mesangial cells provide structural support

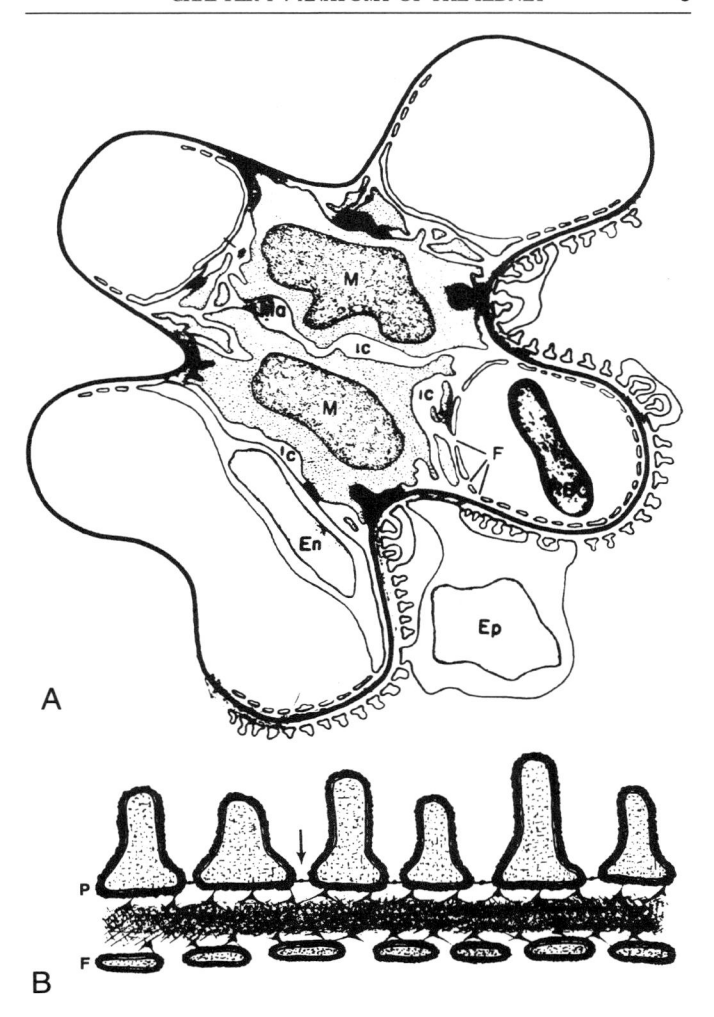

Figure 1.3. **A.** Relationship among endothelial cells (*En*), epithelial cells (*Ep*), and mesangial cells (*M*) of glomerulus. *F*, endothelial fenestrae; *Ma*, mesangial matrix; *IC*, intercellular channels. (From Latta H. Ultrastructure of the glomerulus and juxtaglomerular apparatus. In: Geiger SR, ed. Handbook of physiology. Bethesda: American Physiological Society, 1973:1–30.) **B.** Glomerular basement membrane with adjoining endothelial fenestrae (*F*) and epithelial foot processes (*P*) with slit pores (*arrow*). (From Kanwar YS, Farquhar MG. J Cell Biol 1979;81:137.)

for the capillary loops. They contain numerous filaments and have contractile as well as phagocytic properties. Cell contraction is believed to limit filtration, perhaps by reducing the area of the glomerular filter. It is stimulated to contract by angiotensin II, arginine vasopressin, and thromboxane, a response that is inhibited by prostaglandin E_2. Mesangial cells are phagocytic, and in certain forms of glomerulonephritis they appear to be involved in the sequestration of immune complexes from the glomerular tuft.

The *parietal epithelium* of Bowman's capsule is continuous with the visceral epithelium at the vascular pole. At the urinary pole there is an abrupt transition from the parietal epithelium to the epithelium of the proximal tubule.

Juxtaglomerular Apparatus

The juxtaglomerular apparatus located at the vascular pole of the glomerulus has tubular and vascular components. The vascular components include the terminal portion of the afferent arteriole, the initial portion of the efferent arteriole, and the extraglomerular mesangium between the arterioles. The tubular component is a specialized part of the TAL called the macula densa. Some cells in the vascular portion of the juxtaglomerular apparatus contain numerous granules. These granular cells secrete renin that, through the formation of angiotensin, is involved in regulation of tubuloglomerular feedback and in control of aldosterone-stimulated sodium and potassium transport. Therefore, the juxtaglomerular apparatus is important in the control of renal hemodynamics and salt excretion.

Proximal Tubule

The proximal tubule includes an initial pars convoluta, or PCT, and a pars recta, or proximal straight tubule, that is located in the medullary ray (Fig. 1.2). The PCT has numerous lateral cell processes that extend from the apical to the basal surface of the cell and interdigitate with similar cell processes from adjacent cells (Fig. 1.4). Mitochondria are located in these processes in close proximity to the cell membrane. The presence of these lateral cell processes and interdigitations gives rise to a complex extracellular compartment between the cells. This intercellular space is separated from the tubule lumen by the tight junction or zonula occludens. A prominent endocytic-lysosomal system is

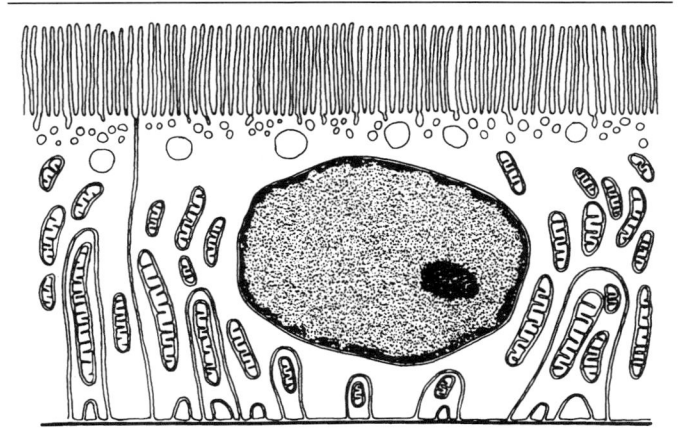

Figure 1.4. Proximal tubule cell.

present in the cells and is important in the reabsorption and catabolism of proteins from the tubule fluid. Based on morphologic differences, the proximal tubule can be subdivided into three distinct segments. The S_1 segment corresponds to the initial PCT; the S_2 segment corresponds to the terminal PCT and the initial proximal straight tubule; and the S_3 segment constitutes the remainder of the proximal straight tubule.

The main function of the proximal tubule is the reabsorption of sodium, chloride, bicarbonate, potassium, phosphate, water, and organic solutes, such as glucose and amino acids, and the secretion of organic acids and bases, including common drugs such as salicylates, barbiturates, penicillin, and many diuretics. Much of the sodium reabsorption is an active process mediated by the Na^+-K^+-ATPase or sodium pump located in the basolateral plasma membrane. The transport of the various anions and organic solutes across the luminal membrane is coupled to the reabsorption of sodium down its concentration gradient. Fluid reabsorption is accomplished primarily by isosmotic water flow through the cell and the intercellular spaces.

Thin Limb of Henle's Loop

The thin limb of Henle's loop extends from the proximal tubule to the TAL (Fig. 1.2). Short-looped nephrons have only a short descending thin limb segment that is located in the inner stripe of the outer medulla. Long-looped nephrons have both a long descending and a long ascending thin limb. Four morphologically distinct segments can be identified in the thin limb. All are lined by a flat epithelium containing few cell organelles.

The thin limb of Henle's loop is important in the countercurrent multiplication mechanism. The descending limb is permeable to water but impermeable to sodium, whereas the ascending limb is almost impermeable to water but highly permeable to sodium and modestly permeable to urea. Accordingly, water diffuses out of the descending limb, and subsequently sodium exits the ascending limb down its concentration gradient. Thus, the countercurrent mechanism is involved in the maintenance of a hypertonic medullary interstitium and in the formation of a dilute tubule fluid.

Distal Tubule

The distal tubule includes the TAL, which can be subdivided into a medullary and a cortical segment, the macula densa, and the DCT (Fig. 1.2). The transition from the TAL to the DCT occurs shortly after the macula densa. Cells of the TAL and the DCT possess extensive invaginations of the basolateral plasma membrane and interdigitations of cell processes between adjacent cells. Numerous elongated mitochondria are located in the lateral cell processes in close proximity to the plasma membrane. In contrast to the proximal tubule, the luminal membrane of the distal tubule does not possess a brush border (Fig. 1.5). The ultrastructural composition of the distal tubule is characteristic of an epithelium involved in active transport. Both the TAL and the DCT are responsible for active reabsorption of sodium chloride, which is important in the countercurrent multiplication process and the urinary concentrating and diluting mechanism. Because the TAL is relatively impermeable to water, the active reabsorption of sodium chloride creates a hypertonic interstitium and ensures the delivery of a hypotonic tubule fluid to the DCT. The TAL is the site of action of the loop diuretics (e.g., furosemide), whereas thiazide diuretics exert their effect mainly on the DCT.

The *connecting segment* is located between the distal tubule and the collecting duct (Fig. 1.2). It is a transition region where a mixture of cells from adjacent regions can be encountered

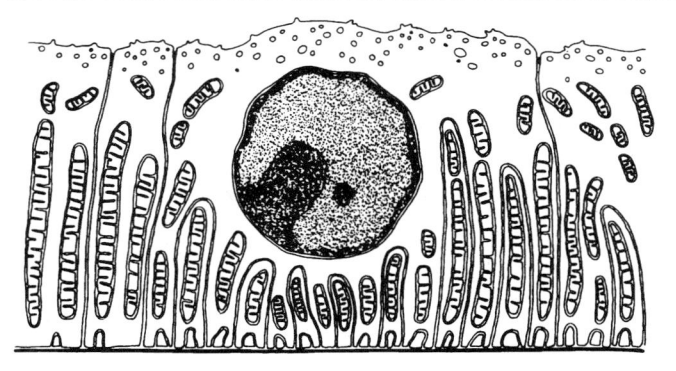

Figure 1.5. Distal tubule cell.

including DCT cells, connecting tubule cells, and collecting duct cells (intercalated and principal cells).

Collecting Duct

The collecting duct system can be divided into the cortical, outer medullary, and inner medullary collecting duct (IMCD) (Fig. 1.2). The cortical collecting duct includes the initial collecting tubule and the segment located in the medullary ray. The epithelium of both the cortical collecting duct and the outer medullary collecting duct is composed of two distinct cell types, principal cells and intercalated cells, the latter constituting approximately one-third of the cells. Principal cells have a light cytoplasm with few cell organelles and a relatively smooth luminal surface (Fig. 1.6), whereas intercalated cells have a dark staining cytoplasm with many mitochondria and numerous small tubulovesicles (Fig. 1.7). The luminal surface of intercalated cells is covered with microprojections that are either microvilli or microplicae. Two different configurations of intercalated cells have been observed, type A cells that are involved in hydrogen ion secretion and type B cells that secrete bicarbonate. A main function of principal cells in the cortical collecting duct is potassium secretion.

Intercalated cells gradually disappear in the early portion of the IMCD and are absent in the papillary portion. Cells in the terminal two-thirds of the IMCD are believed to constitute a distinct cell type that is called the IMCD cell. The IMCD cells

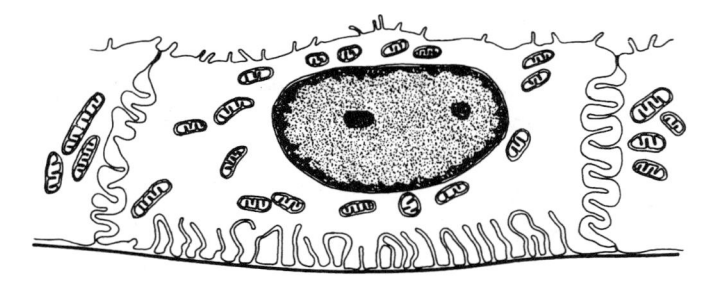

Figure 1.6. Principal cell.

have a very light cytoplasm and few organelles. They increase in height as the collecting duct descends toward the papillary tip. The principal cells and the IMCD cells are responsive to antidiuretic hormone. In the presence of antidiuretic hormone, water is reabsorbed from the collecting duct, which leads to the formation of a hypertonic urine. In the absence of antidiuretic hormone, the collecting duct is relatively impermeable to water, and a hypotonic urine is formed.

Interstitium

The interstitium is composed of interstitial cells and a loose flocculent extracellular material rich in glycosaminoglycans. Interstitial tissue is sparse in the cortex where two types of interstitial cells have been described: one that resembles a fibroblast and another less common mononuclear cell. In the medulla there is a gradual increase in the amount of interstitial tissue from the outer medulla to the papillary tip. Three different types of interstitial cells have been described in the medulla: type I, the typical renomedullary interstitial cell; type II, a mononuclear cell; and type III, a pericyte. The renomedullary (type I) cells are very prominent in the inner medulla where they are arranged in rows between adjacent tubules and vessels resembling rungs on a ladder. These cells have numerous lipid inclusions or droplets whose function is not known with certainty. The renomedullary cells are important sites of prostaglandin E_2 production.

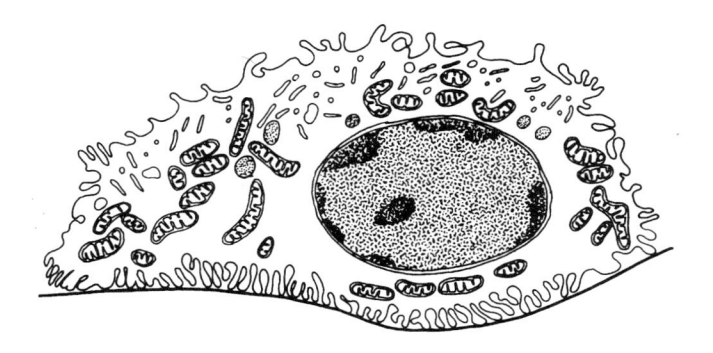

Figure 1.7. Intercalated cell.

Vasculature

The blood flow to the kidneys is large, amounting to approximately 1200 mL/min (20–25% of cardiac output). The renal artery divides into anterior and posterior segmental branches at the hilus of the kidney (Fig. 1.1). From the segmental arteries, lobar arteries run toward the papillae where they divide into interlobar arteries that ascend along the sides of the renal pyramids. At the corticomedullary junction they continue into the arcuate arteries that run parallel to the surface of the kidney. From the arcuate arteries, interlobular arteries ascend into the cortex where they give off afferent arterioles to the glomeruli. Blood leaves the glomeruli through the efferent arterioles that form the peritubular capillary networks in the cortex. The efferent arterioles from juxtamedullary glomeruli descend into the outer medulla where they form vascular bundles containing the vasa recta through which the outer and inner medulla is supplied. Blood from the capillaries drains into the interlobular, arcuate, and interlobar veins, which accompany arteries of the same name, and finally leaves the kidney through the renal vein. Networks of lymphatics are present in the renal cortex and the renal capsule, but lymphatics have not been described in the medulla. In the cortex they follow the arteries and are embedded in the periarterial interstitial tissue.

Innervation

The kidneys are innervated mainly via the celiac plexus and the greater splanchnic nerve. Adrenergic nerve fibers follow the blood vessels throughout the cortex and outer stripe of the outer medulla. Nerve endings have also been described in contact with both proximal and distal tubules in the cortex and with various components of the juxtaglomerular apparatus.

Suggested Readings

Clapp WL, Abrahamson DL. Development and gross anatomy of the kidney. In: Tisher CC, Brenner BM, eds. Renal pathology with clinical and functional correlations, 2nd ed. Philadelphia: Lippincott, 1994:3–59.

Kriz W, Kaissling B. Structural organization of the mammalian kidney. In: Seldin DW, Giebisch G, eds. The kidney: physiology and pathophysiology. New York: Raven, 1992:707–777.

Madsen KM, Brenner BM. Structure and function of the renal tubule and interstitium. In: Tisher CC, Brenner BM, eds. Renal pathology with clinical and functional correlations, 2nd ed. Philadelphia: Lippincott, 1994:661–698.

Tisher CC, Brenner BM. Structure and function of the glomerulus. In: Tisher CC, Brenner BM, eds. Renal pathology with clinical and functional correlations, 2nd ed. Philadelphia: Lippincott, 1994:143–161.

Tisher CC, Madsen KM. Anatomy of the kidney. In: Brenner BM, Rector FC, Jr, eds. The kidney, 5th ed. Philadelphia: Saunders, 1994, in press.

Chapter 2

Evaluation of Kidney Structure and Function

C. Craig Tisher and Christopher S. Wilcox

The patient with kidney disease will often present with nonspecific signs and symptoms including nausea, anorexia, lethargy, edema, dyspnea, and diminished urine output. Consequently, the physician must rely on laboratory studies to assist the evaluation and diagnosis of kidney disease. This chapter will review the basic screening and diagnostic studies used to assess renal function.

URINALYSIS

A urinalysis should be part of the initial evaluation of all patients, especially those with hypertension or suspected renal disease. A fresh urine specimen is obtained by collecting a midstream sample using clean catch techniques. A dipstick is used to check pH, protein, glucose, and hemoglobin. The urine is then centrifuged for 3–5 min at no more than 3000 rpm before examination.

Findings from Specimen

Color

A normal urine appears clear and yellow. Other colors suggest an abnormal constituent reflecting an underlying disorder: dark brown or yellow (bilirubinuria); red (hemoglobinuria, myoglobinuria, porphyria, or drugs such as rifampin and Pyridium); turbid white (pyuria, crystalluria).

Specific Gravity

Often measured by dipstick, the specific gravity, which ranges between 1.001 and 1.030, provides an estimate of urine osmolality. A specific gravity of 1.010 corresponds roughly to a urine osmolality of 285 mOsm/kg H_2O, which is isosmotic with plasma. A markedly elevated specific gravity suggests the presence of hyperosmolar substances such as radiocontrast dyes or extreme volume depletion.

pH

Urine pH is usually determined by dipstick and depends on systemic acid-base balance. It is generally <7.0. A pH of >7.0 may indicate urease producing bacteria or a bicarbonate diuresis.

Glucose

Normally, glucose is not found in the urine. Therefore, its presence suggests hyperglycemia or diminished proximal tubular reabsorption of glucose.

Hemoglobin

Hemoglobin is not present in normal urine samples. Its presence should lead to examination of the sediment for red blood cells. If they are not found, hemoglobinuria or myoglobinuria must be considered.

Leukocyte Esterase

A positive reaction on the dipstick indicates the presence of at least four leukocytes per high-power field.

Nitrite

Although it lacks sensitivity, this dipstick test indicates the presence of bacteria capable of reducing nitrates to nitrites.

Protein

A dipstick can detect a protein concentration as low as 10–15 mg/dL. However, the dipstick method does not differentiate between a positive test from a dilute specimen, which may be significant, and a positive test from a concentrated specimen, which may be insignificant. Consequently, a positive test should be followed by a 24-hr urine collection for measurement of total protein excretion. Proteinuria in excess of 150 mg/24 hr in an adult is considered abnormal and should be investigated further. More than $3.5 \text{ g}/24 \text{ hr}/1.73 \text{ m}^2$ of protein defines proteinuria in the nephrotic range. Another disadvantage of the dipstick method is its failure to detect Bence Jones protein. In such cases, a mixture of 7.5 mL of 3 sulfosalicylic acid and 2.5 mL urine will precipitate any protein that is present. Causes of false-positive dipstick results include contamination with certain antiseptics, the presence of phenazopyridine (Pyridium), a urine pH of >8.0, and gross hematuria.

Examination of Urinary Sediment

The supernatant is first decanted from the centrifuged sediment. Gentle tapping of the centrifuge tube resuspends the sediment. A drop is then transferred to a glass slide, and a coverslip is applied for microscopic examination.

Erythrocytes

Up to three erythrocytes per high-power field may be found in normal urine samples. If more are identified, examination of their shape may indicate their source. A variable shape suggests glomerular origin, whereas a uniform configuration suggests an extraglomerular source.

Leukocytes

Up to two white blood cells per high-power field may be seen in a normal urine sample. Greater numbers suggest the presence of a urinary tract infection or inflammation. However, if urine cultures with pyuria are negative for bacteria, entities such as prostatitis, chronic urethritis, renal tuberculosis, renal stones, or papillary necrosis should be suspected. Interstitial nephritis may be suggested by the identification of eosinophils on Wright's or Hansel's stain of the urine sediment.

Renal Tubular Epithelial Cells

Although not observed in normal urine samples, these large cells with prominent nuclei are often seen with acute tubular necro-

Table 2.1
Urine Casts

Hyaline	Mucoprotein matrix without cellular elements; does not indicate renal disease
Red cell	Indicates glomerular bleeding
Leukocyte	Common in pyelonephritis but observed in interstitial nephritis and glomerulonephritis
Renal tubular epithelial	Observed with acute tubular necrosis, glomerulonephritis, and tubulointerstitial diseases
Granular waxy	Represents degenerative cellular elements
Broad	Characteristic of chronic renal failure

sis, glomerulonephritis, or pyelonephritis. With proteinuria in the nephrotic range, degenerating epithelial cells are seen as "oval fat bodies," and under polarized light display a "Maltese cross" configuration.

Casts

Casts represent a mold of the renal tubular lumen and are composed of protein and cellular elements. There are several types that may be associated with specific conditions (Table 2.1).

ASSESSMENT OF GLOMERULAR FILTRATION

Blood Urea Nitrogen

Blood urea nitrogen (BUN) is freely filtered at the glomerulus, but because up to 50% of the filtered BUN is eventually reabsorbed, it does not provide a reliable estimate of the glomerular filtration rate (GFR). Moreover, many conditions may affect BUN independent of the GFR.

- Increased BUN: high-protein diet, gastrointestinal bleeding, corticosteroids, tissue trauma, tetracyclines;
- Decreased BUN: low protein diet, liver disease, sickle cell anemia;
- Normal range: 7–18 mg/dL or 2.5–6.4 mmol/L.

Serum Creatinine

Unlike BUN, serum creatinine (S_{cr}) provides a reasonable estimate of the GFR because creatinine is primarily filtered with only a small but variable component of tubular secretion. Thus, a rise in S_{cr} from 1.0 to 2.0 mg/dL indicates a decrease in renal function of roughly 50%. Like the BUN, many factors may affect S_{cr} without actually affecting GFR.

- Increased S_{cr}: ketoacidosis, ingestion of cooked meat, drugs that inhibit tubular secretion of creatinine (cimetidine, acetylsalicylic acid, trimethoprim);
- Decreased S_{cr}: diminished muscle mass associated with cachexia, aging, low protein intake.

Estimation of GFR

S_{cr} can be used in the Cockcroft-Gault formula, along with age, gender, and weight, to give an estimation of GFR.

Male $\quad$ GFR $= \dfrac{(140 - \text{age (yr)}) \times \text{lean body weight (kg)}}{S_{cr} \text{ (mg/dL)} \times 72}$

Female $\quad$ GFR $= $ value for male $\times 0.85$

However, a better estimate of GFR is obtained by measuring creatinine clearance (C_{cr}).

$$C_{cr} = \dfrac{\text{urine creatinine (mg/dL)} \times \text{urine volume (mL/24 hr)}}{\text{serum creatinine (mg/dL)} \times 1440 \text{ min}}$$

Normal ranges for C_{cr} follow:

Male $\quad$ 97–137 mL/min/1.73 m^2 or 0.93–1.32 mL/sec/m^2 IU
Female $\quad$ 88–128 mL/min/1.73 m^2 or 0.85–1.23 mL/sec/m^2 IU

An improper urine collection results in an inaccurate C_{cr}. Urine should contain 15–20 mg creatinine/kg body weight/day for males and 10–15 mg creatinine/kg body weight/day for females. These values decline with advancing age. Finally, as C_{cr} approaches 20 mL/min, the proportion of creatinine found in the urine that has been filtered decreases. This is because a larger percentage of creatinine is secreted into the urine by the tubules as the GFR falls. Therefore, a truly low GFR may be overestimated by C_{cr}.

RADIOLOGIC ASSESSMENT

Renogram

The renogram is used to delineate renal shape and to measure renal function. Several radiopharmaceutical preparations are available. Technetium diethylenetriamine pentaacetic acid is freely filtered by the glomerulus and is not reabsorbed. It is used to estimate GFR. Furosemide may be administered during the renogram to assess obstruction. Technetium dimercaptosuccinate is bound to the tubules and delineates the contour of functional renal tissue; it is particularly useful to assess cortical scarring from pyelonephritis or vesicoureteral reflux or to diagnose a renal infarct. Radioiodinated orthoiodohippurate (Hippuran) is secreted into the tubules. Hippuran is used to assess renal plasma flow. A combination of plasma sampling and renal scanning can be used to assess overall and single kidney function. Changes in the diethylenetriamine pentaacetic acid and/or Hippuran scan after captopril provide a valuable index of functionally important renal artery stenosis in patients with hypertension (see Chapter 20). Radionuclide studies are of little benefit when the single kidney GFR is below 15 mL/min (Table 2.2).

Ultrasonography

Ultrasound resolution is 1–2 cm. It can be used to identify the cortex, medulla, renal pyramids, and a distended collecting system or ureter (Table 2.3). A kidney length of <9 cm or a size difference of >1.5 cm between the two kidneys is abnormal in an adult. *Simple cysts* are common and are uniformly benign. They contain no internal echoes, have a sharply defined smooth internal wall, and have increased "through transmission" of sound energy posteriorly. Other hypoechoic renal mass lesions

Table 2.2
Indications for a Renal Scintigram or Renogram

To quantify total renal function and contribution of each kidney
To detect obstruction
To evaluate a suspected scar or infarct
To evaluate renovascular hypertension

Table 2.3
Indications for Renal Ultrasound

To quantify renal size
To screen for hydronephrosis
To characterize renal mass lesions
To evaluate perirenal space for abscess or hematoma
To screen for autosomal dominant polycystic kidney disease
To localize kidney for invasive procedures
To assess residual bladder volume in excess of 100 mL
To evaluate for renal vein thrombosis (Doppler)
To assess renal blood flow (Doppler)

to consider include lymphoma, melanoma, infarct, hematoma, and xanthogranulomatous pyelonephritis. Complex cysts or solid lesions require further investigation with computed tomography (CT), magnetic resonance imaging (MRI), or possibly angiography. Ultrasound has become the procedure of choice in the early diagnosis or screening of autosomal dominant polycystic kidney disease. *Hydronephrosis* appears as a multiloculated fluid collection within the renal sinus. However, ultrasound does not assess the functional importance of obstruction. An apparent obstruction can occur with anatomic variants such as an extrarenal pelvis, vesicoureteric reflux, and pregnancy. Hydronephrosis may persist after obstruction has been relieved. A furosemide renogram may document functional obstruction.

Intravenous Pyelography

The intravenous pyelogram (IVP) provides an overview of the kidneys, ureters, and bladder. The nephrogram is formed by opacification of the renal parenchyma; its density depends on the GFR, rate of tubular fluid reabsorption, dose of radiographic contrast agent, and rate of intravenous injection. The IVP can demonstrate gross differences in function between the kidneys from the nephrogram phase. Renal insufficiency (S_{cr} >2–3 mg/dL) decreases the diagnostic value of the IVP and greatly increases the danger of causing acute renal failure. Normal renal size as measured by pyelography is >11 cm, which exceeds that measured by ultrasound because of a magnification of approximately 10%. The left kidney is normally larger than the right. The IVP should be examined for renal size and position, calcifications, distorting intrinsic or extrinsic mass lesions, adequacy of parenchymal thickness, abnormalities of cortical contour or papillary appearance, dilatation or blunting of calyces, abnormal position or course of the ureters, reflux, congenital variants, and completeness of bladder emptying (Table 2.4).

Computed Tomography

CT is useful for further investigation of abnormalities discovered on ultrasound or IVP. CT is performed with contrast except when limited to demonstrating hemorrhage or calcification. The contrast media are filtered by the glomeruli and concentrated in the tubules, thus allowing parenchymal enhancement and visualization of neoplasms or cysts. The renal vessels and ureters can be identified. CT is useful in the evaluation of mass lesions or fluid collections in the kidney or retroperitoneal space, particularly when ultrasound examination is hindered by intraabdominal gas or by obesity (Table 2.5).

Magnetic Resonance Imaging

The loss of the corticomedullary demarcation on MRI is a nonspecific feature of renal disease. Renal cysts are well visualized, but, unlike CT, foci of calcification cannot be accurately defined by MRI. In the staging of solid renal lesions, MRI may be superior to CT because it can detect tumor thrombus in major vessels and can distinguish hilar collateral vessels from lymph nodes. However, some renal neoplasms appear homogeneous with surrounding normal renal parenchyma and therefore may be missed with currently available noncontrast MRI. MRI can help in differentiating adrenal mass lesions because characteristic images may occur in pheochromocytoma. MRI is useful to diagnose renal vein thrombosis (Table 2.6).

Table 2.4
Indications for an Intravenous Pyelogram

To assess renal size and contour
To investigate recurrent urinary tract infection
To detect and locate calculi
To evaluate suspected urinary tract obstruction
To evaluate cause of hematuria

Table 2.5
Indications for Computed Tomography

To further evaluate a renal mass
To display calcification patterns in a mass
To evaluate a nonfunctioning kidney
To delineate extent of renal trauma
To guide percutaneous needle aspiration or biopsy
To diagnose adrenal causes for hypertension

Table 2.6
Indications for Magnetic Resonance Imaging

To serve as an adjunct to CT in evaluating renal masses
To serve as an alternative to CT in patients who are intolerant of radiographic contrast agents
To evaluate suspected pheochromocytoma
To assess renal vein thrombosis

Arteriography and Venography

Contrast imaging of the arterial and venous vasculature is useful to assess renal artery stenosis, nephrosclerosis, renal vein thrombosis, renal infarction, or a renal mass. It is performed by percutaneous cannulation of femoral vessels, sometimes aided by digital subtraction techniques. *Arteriography* is useful in the evaluation of atherosclerotic or fibrodysplastic stenotic lesions of the renal arteries, aneurysms, arteriovenous fistulae, large vessel vasculitis, and renal mass lesions. It can be combined with selective renal vein renin sampling for evaluation of renovascular hypertension, with percutaneous transluminal balloon angioplasty, or with renal ablation. *Venography* is performed to diagnose renal vein thrombosis.

Summary

Radiologic tests can be very valuable diagnostic tools; however, they are expensive and carry a risk of adverse reactions. Proper patient selection and preparation can increase the value of the procedure and diminish the toxicity. Even the nonionic radiocontrast agents can induce acute renal failure or vascular thrombosis. Prevention and management of radiocontrast-induced renal damage are discussed in Chapter 8. Consultation with the radiologist before selecting the test is often very helpful.

RENAL BIOPSY

Percutaneous needle biopsy of the kidney can be helpful for establishing a diagnosis, assessing prognosis, monitoring disease progression, and selecting a rational therapy.

Indications

Acute Renal Failure

When the underlying cause of acute renal failure is not evident initially or recovery of renal function has not occurred after 3–4 weeks of supportive therapy, biopsy may be necessary to distinguish acute tubular necrosis from a host of other renal diseases that may require alternative management (see Chapter 8).

Nephrotic Syndrome

Renal biopsy is usually performed in the adult nephrotic patient without evidence of systemic disease to diagnose primary glomerular diseases. The most frequently encountered entities include membranous glomerulonephritis, focal segmental glomerulosclerosis, membranoproliferative glomerulonephritis, IgA nephropathy, amyloidosis, and minimal change disease (see Chapters 4 and 5).

Proteinuria

In the setting of persistent proteinuria of 2 g/24 hr/1.73 m^2 or more or when associated with an abnormal urine sediment or with documented functional deterioration, a renal biopsy may detect underlying kidney disease. Patients with orthostatic proteinuria do not require biopsy (see Chapter 4).

Hematuria

Renal biopsy may be helpful in patients with microscopic hematuria persisting longer than 6 months or in those with episodic gross hematuria or a family history of hematuria, particularly when there is an associated abnormal urine sediment or proteinuria. Secondary causes of hematuria must be excluded.

Likely pathologic findings include benign essential hematuria, Alport's syndrome, and IgA nephropathy. Usually biopsy is not helpful in the clinical setting of isolated microscopic hematuria (see Chapter 3).

Systemic Disease

Various systemic disorders may have associated kidney involvement. These include diabetes mellitus, systemic lupus erythematosus, Schönlein-Henoch purpura, polyarteritis nodosa, Goodpasture's syndrome, Wegener's granulomatosis, and certain dysproteinemias. Biopsy is often performed to confirm the diagnosis, to establish the extent of renal involvement, and to guide management (see Chapter 6).

Transplant Allograft

Biopsy of the allograft helps differentiate various forms of rejection from acute tubular necrosis, drug-induced interstitial nephritis or nephrotoxicity, hemorrhagic infarction, and de novo or recurrent glomerulonephritis (see Chapter 24).

Contraindications

Commonly accepted contraindications to percutaneous needle biopsy include a solitary or ectopic kidney (except transplant allografts), a horseshoe kidney, the presence of an uncorrected bleeding disorder, severe uncontrolled hypertension, renal infection, renal neoplasm, or an uncooperative patient.

Patient Preparation and Complications

Percutaneous renal biopsy is an *inpatient* procedure. Routine laboratory tests before biopsy should include a prothrombin time, partial thromboplastin time, complete blood count, platelet count, blood type and antibody screen for possible crossmatching should the need for transfusion arise, and urinalysis to eliminate urinary tract infection. If coagulation parameters are abnormal, a bleeding time should be obtained. The percutaneous biopsy is usually performed with ultrasound or fluoroscopic guidance. After biopsy, the patient should remain at strict bed rest for 24 hr. Frequent vital signs are recorded to monitor evidence of hypovolemia owing to hemorrhage. Hematocrits are obtained 4–6 hr after the biopsy and again the next morning. Aliquots of each voided urine are saved to observe for gross hematuria.

The most frequent complication is bleeding that is usually self-limited. Significant bleeding requiring transfusion, percutaneous arterial embolization of a bleeding vessel, or nephrectomy is uncommon, with an occurrence rate of 2.1%. The mortality rate of 0.07% is comparable with that of percutaneous liver biopsy or coronary angiography. When percutaneous needle biopsy is technically not feasible and a histologic diagnosis is imperative, an open biopsy performed in the operating room under general anesthesia should be considered.

The tissue specimen should be submitted for light microscopy, immunofluorescence microscopy, and electron microscopy and evaluated by a pathologist experienced in interpretation of kidney biopsies.

Suggested Readings

Amis ED. Contemporary uroradiology. Radiol Clin North Am 1991;29: 437–650.

Cockcroft DW, Gault MH. Prediction of creatinine clearance from serum creatinine. Nephron 1976;16:31–41.

Deininger HK, Beil D, Schmidt C, et al. Digital subtraction angiography and other noninvasive methods for evaluation of renal circulation and hypertension. Uremia Invest 1985;9:231–241.

Fine EJ, Axelrod M, Blaufox MD. Physiologic aspects of diagnostic renal imaging. Semin Nephrol 1985;5:188–207.

Levey AS, Perrone RD, Madias NE. Serum creatinine and renal function. Annu Rev Med 1988;39:465–490.

Schoolwerth AC. Hematuria and proteinuria: their causes and consequences. Hosp Pract 1987;22:45–62.

Tisher CC. Clinical indications for kidney biopsy. In: Tisher CC, Brenner BM, eds. Renal pathology with clinical and functional correlations, 2nd ed. Philadelphia: Lippincott, 1994:75–84.

Tisher CC, Croker BP. Indications for and interpretation of the renal biopsy: evaluation by light, electron and immunofluorescence microscopy. In: Schrier RW, Gottschalk CW, eds. Diseases of the kidney, 5th ed. Boston: Little, Brown, 1992:485–510.

Chapter 3

Hematuria

Nicolas J. Guzman

Hematuria is the presence of abnormal quantities of erythrocytes in the urine. Careful examination of the sediment from a freshly voided urine may show up to three erythrocytes per 10–20 high-power fields (or 8000 erythrocytes/mL centrifuged urine). Although this value is commonly accepted as the upper limit of normal, approximately 10% of normal subjects will excrete as many as 10 erythrocytes per high-power field. However, in an otherwise normal subject, the persistent excretion of more than three erythrocytes per high-power field is an indication for evaluation of the genitourinary tract. Table 3.1 lists some important clinical features associated with hematuria.

DETECTION

Gross hematuria is easily detected by visual inspection. Microscopic hematuria can be detected by light microscopic inspection of the urinary sediment or by the use of orthotoluidine-impregnated paper strips that give positive results with urine containing as little as three to five erythrocytes per high-power field. This test, however, also detects hemoglobinuria and myoglobinuria. Occasionally, on microscopic examination, calcium oxalate crystals, yeast, and air bubbles can be mistakenly identified as erythrocytes; however, the paper strip method will be negative. Large numbers of erythrocytes are found in urine samples obtained by urethral catheterization and in voided specimens from menstruating females.

Table 3.1
Relationship between Clinical Findings and Origin of Hematuria

Sign or Symptom	Renal Parenchyma	Urinary Tract
Pain	Dull flank pain	Suprapubic pain with dysuria, colicky flank pain
Blood clots	Absent in glomerular diseases, may occur with trauma and vascular anomalies	Common
Cellular casts	Common in glomerular diseases	Absent
Proteinuria >150 mg/dL	Common	Absent
Red blood cell morphology	Usually distorted	Normal

EVALUATION

Initial laboratory studies should include a urinalysis, coagulation tests, and urine cultures. If pyuria is present, a Gram stain of the urine should be performed. Sterile pyuria coupled with hematuria suggests renal tuberculosis.

Once *infectious* etiologies have been excluded, an intravenous pyelogram should be obtained to exclude renal or pelvic calcifications and masses. If this study is negative, a cystoscopy with biopsy of all suspicious lesions should be performed and the material sent for culture and pathological examination. If the bladder appears normal, selective ureteric urine samples should be inspected for hematuria and sent for culture and cytology. If cystoscopy is nondiagnostic or if the intravenous pyelogram reveals a renal mass or calcifications, a renal ultrasound should be performed to determine if the mass is solid or cystic or to identify renal calculi. Further characterization of structural and vascular lesions usually requires retrograde pyelography, a computed tomography scan, an angiogram, or a combination of these studies.

Glomerular causes of hematuria (see Chapter 5) should be considered in all patients in whom complete evaluation fails to provide a definitive diagnosis. Renal biopsy should be considered early in patients presenting with hematuria associated with proteinuria or red blood cell casts.

Despite extensive investigations, the cause of the hematuria will remain unknown in 10–15% of all patients.

DIFFERENTIAL DIAGNOSIS

Glomerular Causes

Primary glomerulopathies commonly present with hematuria, red blood cell casts, or both. Worldwide, IgA nephropathy is the most common glomerular disease associated with either gross or microscopic hematuria (see Chapter 5).

Renal involvement in systemic diseases, such as systemic lupus erythematosus, Schönlein-Henoch purpura, and vasculitides commonly causes hematuria. The presence of fever, arthralgias, skin rash, or purpura suggests a systemic disorder. Positive serologic tests for *collagen-vascular disease*, or hypocomplementemia and cryoglobulinemia, usually indicate the cause of the hematuria. *Wegener's granulomatosis* and *Goodpasture's syndrome* present commonly with pulmonary involvement and hemoptysis. Antineutrophilic cytoplasmic antibodies help in the diagnosis of Wegener's granulomatosis. Antiglomerular basement membrane antibodies are characteristic of Goodpasture's syndrome.

Poststreptococcal glomerulonephritis is characterized by a history of recent skin or throat infection and elevated titers of antistreptolysin O, antihyaluronidase, or anti-DNase. Fever associated with the appearance of a heart murmur suggests infective endocarditis, particularly in patients with prosthetic heart valves and a history of recent dental procedures or those who are intravenous drug abusers. Blood cultures will usually demonstrate the causative organism. Echocardiography may disclose the presence of vegetations.

Hereditary nephritis or Alport's syndrome very commonly presents with hematuria. The diagnosis is suggested by a family history of kidney disease, kidney failure, deafness, and ocular abnormalities. Audiometry is abnormal in half of these patients. Benign essential hematuria or thin glomerular basement membrane disease also presents as isolated hematuria.

Vascular Causes

Renal vein thrombosis may present with hematuria. These patients will commonly have a history of nephrotic syndrome, and their laboratory evaluation may reveal a hyperchloremic metabolic acidosis, proteinuria, and glycosuria (Fanconi's syndrome). The diagnosis is made by selective renal venography, magnetic resonance imaging, or Doppler ultrasound.

Sudden back pain and hematuria, particularly in a patient with an aortic aneurysm, atrial fibrillation, or a recent myocardial infarction, suggest *renal arterial embolism*. Renal angiography is the procedure of choice to identify this condition.

Arteriovenous malformations can present as asymptomatic hematuria. The diagnosis is usually made by angiography.

Cystic Disease

Patients with *polycystic kidney disease* usually have a family history of kidney failure. Physical examination may disclose an abdominal mass. The diagnosis can be made with renal ultrasound.

Tubulointerstitial Disease

Hypersensitivity interstitial nephritis is suspected when a patient with recent drug exposure presents with hematuria and sterile pyuria. Skin rash may or may not be present. Peripheral eosinophilia is common, and eosinophiluria, when present, is a helpful clue.

Papillary necrosis is usually an acute and dramatic condition. It should be considered whenever hematuria occurs in a patient with analgesic nephropathy, sickle cell disease or trait, or diabetes mellitus complicated by acute pyelonephritis with obstruction.

Acute bacterial pyelonephritis usually presents with fever, back pain, and pyuria with bacteriuria.

Other Causes

Urinary tract infection is a common cause of hematuria and usually presents with dysuria and pyuria. Tumors such as renal cell carcinoma and transitional cell carcinoma frequently present with hematuria. Other common causes include renal calculi, trauma, and prostatic diseases. Systemic coagulation disorders may also present as hematuria.

TREATMENT

Hematuria rarely produces enough blood loss to require volume replacement. The passing of blood clots can, however, cause severe pain and urinary obstruction, which may require urethral catheterization and saline irrigation. In cases of structural lesions causing severe hematuria, surgery may be indicated. Correction of a coagulopathy, if present, is essential. In most patients, the treatment of hematuria is directed toward the primary cause.

Suggested Readings

Benson G, Brewer E. Hematuria: algorithms for diagnosis II. JAMA 1981;246:993–995.

Brewer E, Benson G. Hematuria: algorithms for diagnosis I. JAMA 1981;246:877–880.

Fairley KF. Urinalysis. In: Schrier RW, Gottschalk CW, eds. Diseases of the kidney, 5th ed. Boston: Little, Brown, 1993:335–359.

Glassock RJ. Hematuria and pigmenturia. In: Massry SG, Glassock RJ, eds. Textbook of nephrology, 2nd ed. Baltimore: Williams & Wilkins, 1989:491–500.

Lieberthal W. Hematuria and the acute nephritic syndrome. In: Jacobson HR, Striker GE, Klahr S, eds. The principles and practice of nephrology, 1st ed. Philadelphia: Decker, 1991:244–250.

Llach F. Tests, procedures, and treatments: the urine. In: Papper's clinical nephrology, 3rd ed. Boston: Little, Brown, 1993:521–568.

Chapter 4

Proteinuria and the Nephrotic Syndrome

Donald R. Mars

A healthy adult has <150 mg protein in a 24-hr urine collection; 60% is composed of filtered plasma proteins (20–40 mg albumin), and 40% consists of glyco- and immunoproteins. When the amount excreted is $3.5 g/24 hr, proteinuria is in the "nephrotic range." Cardinal features of the nephrotic syndrome are listed in Table 4.1. Other clinical findings may include periorbital edema, hypertriglyceridemia, and hypercoagulability.

Proteinuria may reflect a serious underlying renal or systemic disorder, or it may be idiopathic (Table 4.2).

PATHOPHYSIOLOGY

In the healthy individual the glomerular capillary wall functions as a barrier to exclude proteins from entering the urinary space by size discrimination and electrical charge. With glomerular injury the size and charge selective barriers may be damaged. Ordinarily, molecules with a molecular radius of <17 Å readily pass the glomerular filter, whereas those with a molecular radius

Table 4.1
Cardinal Features of the Nephrotic Syndrome

Proteinuria $ 3.5 g/24 hr/1.73 m^2
Hypoalbuminemia (serum albumin <3.5 g/dL)
Hypercholesterolemia (>200 mg/dL)
Peripheral edema ± anasarca

Table 4.2
Common Causes of Proteinuria or Nephrotic Syndrome

Primary Glomerular Disorders
  Orthostatic or postural proteinuria (benign)
  Membranous glomerulonephritis
  Idiopathic membranoproliferative glomerulonephritis
  Focal segmental glomerulosclerosis
  IgA nephropathy
  Minimal change disease
  Proliferative glomerulonephritis
Secondary Disorders
  Hereditary-familial: diabetes mellitus, Alport's syndrome, sickle cell disease
  Autoimmune: systemic lupus erythematosus, Goodpasture's syndrome, Wegener's granulomatosis, polyarteritis nodosa, rheumatoid arthritis
  Infectious: postinfectious glomerulonephritis, endocarditis, hepatitis B
  Drug-induced: nonsteroidal antiinflammatory agents, heroin, gold, mercury
  Neoplastic: Hodgkin's disease, lymphomas, leukemia, multiple myeloma
  Miscellaneous: amyloidosis, preeclampsia-eclampsia, renovascular hypertension, interstitial nephritis, fever, exercise

of >44 Å are excluded. Albumin, with a molecular radius of 36 Å, has a fractional clearance of approximately 10% of the glomerular filtration rate.

The glomerular capillary wall has a fixed negative or anionic charge on the endothelial surface, throughout the glomerular basement membrane, and on the epithelial cell layer, which allows the capillary wall to repel negatively charged plasma proteins.

If the glomerulus is intact, only trace amounts of albumin escape in the glomerular filtrate. Proteins smaller than albumin (<68,000 daltons), however, are filtered to varying degrees and are reabsorbed by the proximal tubule. Under normal circumstances, up to 1500 mg of protein/24 hr are filtered. Most is reabsorbed by the proximal tubule where the protein undergoes catabolism. As a result, <150 mg of protein are excreted each day in the urine. "Tubular" proteinuria occurs when the proximal tubule is damaged, thus interfering with protein reabsorption. This form of proteinuria rarely exceeds 1500 mg/24 hr unless there is associated glomerular injury.

Overproduction of low molecular weight paraproteins, as seen in light chain disease and multiple myeloma, saturates the proximal tubular reabsorptive capacity, at times allowing several grams of protein to spill into the urine.

Hypoalbuminemia and Starling Forces

The sequence of events leading from proteinuria to the nephrotic syndrome depends on the development of hypoalbuminemia. Hypoalbuminemia reduces the plasma oncotic pressure and thereby allows intravascular fluid to shift to the interstitial space. This results eventually in peripheral edema, anasarca, and ascites. As effective arterial blood volume falls, counterregulatory measures produce salt and water retention through activation of the renin-angiotensin-aldosterone and sympathetic nervous systems, which return the effective arterial blood volume toward normal. The trade-off for the maintenance of the effective arterial blood volume and stable blood pressure is worsening of the edema, anasarca, and ascites.

Lipid Alterations

Lipid metabolism is also greatly altered in the nephrotic syndrome. Plasma levels of very low density and low density lipoproteins are elevated, whereas high density lipoprotein levels are decreased. Persistence of these abnormalities can result in accelerated atherogenesis.

Hypercoagulable State

Nephrotic patients tend toward a hypercoagulable state because of the loss of clotting factors (e.g., antithrombin III, protein C, protein S) and increased hepatic production of fibrinogen and α_2-globulin. This predisposes to renal vein thrombosis and pulmonary embolus. The former may increase urine protein excretion further.

CLINICAL PRESENTATION

In general, edema occurs when the plasma albumin concentration falls below 3 g/dL. Ascites often leads to dyspnea owing to decreased diaphragmatic excursion, but the sudden onset of dyspnea should increase the suspicion of a pulmonary embolus in this higher risk population.

INVESTIGATIONS

Routine screening for proteinuria is performed with the common urine dipstick test. The test is qualitative only and is of little value unless the urine specific gravity is measured simultaneously, because a small amount of protein in a highly concentrated urine specimen may have no significance.

A 24-hr urine collection is required to quantify protein excretion. The patient should be instructed to void and discard the first morning specimen. All urine passed thereafter for 24 hr is collected and saved, including the first void the next morning. To ensure an adequate urine collection and to gain useful information about kidney function, the 24-hr creatinine clearance should also be determined (see Chapter 2). The 24-hr creatinine excretion should be at least 15–20 mg/kg in a male and 10–15 mg/kg in a female.

Microscopic analysis of a centrifuged urine specimen is an important step in the evaluation. Oval fat bodies are usually observed in the nephrotic syndrome. The presence of hematuria, pyuria, and cellular casts suggests glomerulonephritis.

Blood chemistries can provide valuable information in proteinuric patients. A plasma albumin of <3.5 g/dL is typical of proteinuria in the nephrotic range or the full-blown nephrotic syndrome. However, this can also occur in malnourished patients, in states of increased protein metabolism, including systemic illness or corticosteroid administration, or after surgical stress. Elevations of triglyceride levels (>300 mg/dL) and cholesterol (>200 mg/dL) are a reflection of the nephrotic syndrome. Elevated serum creatinine and blood urea nitrogen levels indicate renal insufficiency.

SPECIAL STUDIES

Renal ultrasound is employed to determine the presence of two kidneys, their size, and the degree of echogenicity and to exclude lower urinary tract obstruction.

The following serologic studies are obtained to diagnose systemic disorders such as systemic lupus erythematosus, rheumatoid arthritis, postinfectious glomerulonephritis, and hepatitis:

- Antinuclear antibody pattern and titer;
- C_3, C_4, and CH_{50};
- Rheumatoid factor;
- Antistreptolysin 0 and antihyaluronidase titers;
- Serum and urine electrophoresis;
- Serum immunoelectrophoresis;
- Hepatitis battery;
- Cryoglobulins.

A glucose tolerance test should be obtained if there is a suspicion of underlying diabetes mellitus. Renal biopsy is performed to identify specific kidney pathology if noninvasive tests are not definitive (see Chapter 2).

MANAGEMENT

In general, of all patients with proteinuria, those with the nephrotic syndrome require the most aggressive management directed at minimizing the complications of excessive urine protein loss including peripheral edema and ascites, the hypercoagulable state, and hyperlipidemia.

Protein loss leads to hypoalbuminemia, thereby facilitating the development of edema, anasarca, and ascites. Loss can be limited by reducing protein intake to 0.5–0.6 g/kg/day and treating the patient with an angiotensin-converting enzyme inhibitor that reduces glomerular capillary pressure and protein excretion. Nonsteroidal antiinflammatory drugs may also help reduce proteinuria. If the daily urine protein loss exceeds 10 g or the serum albumin concentration is <2.0 g/dL, additional protein should be added to the diet to balance daily protein loss.

Peripheral edema and *ascites* are managed by dietary salt restriction and the judicious use of diuretics. The goal should be the control of peripheral edema but not its elimination. Many patients with severe hypoalbuminemia have a contracted intravascular fluid volume. Diuretic therapy in this setting may cause prerenal azotemia and orthostatic hypotension. Gentle diuresis is indicated for severe edema of the lower extremities, especially where there is skin breakdown and weeping, as well as tight ascites with pleural effusions and respiratory distress. The use of an aldosterone antagonist or a potassium-sparing diuretic is rational in this setting. A combination of a loop diuretic and a second agent, such as metolazone or hydrochlorothiazide, that acts more distally may provide a significant diuretic action, although this combined regimen greatly enhances the risk of fluid and electrolyte depletion.

The *hypercoagulable state* in patients with the nephrotic syndrome may lead to *renal vein thrombosis*, which requires immediate hospitalization and anticoagulation with heparin. Patients are later converted to warfarin and treated for an additional 6 months. Recurrent thrombosis requires prolonged anticoagulation.

Hyperlipidemia, including hypercholesterolemia and hypertriglyceridemia, places the nephrotic patient at greater risk for cardiovascular disease. Dietary management should be instituted when the serum cholesterol exceeds 200 mg/dL or the triglycerides exceed 300 mg/dL. Lipid lowering agents may be necessary in selected patients.

Suggested Readings

Bernard DB, Salant DJ. Clinical approach to the patient with proteinuria and the nephrotic syndrome. In: Jacobson HR, Striker GE, Klahr S, eds. The principles and practice of nephrology. Philadelphia: Decker, 1991:250–261.

Groggel GC, Border WA. Nephrotic syndrome. In: Suki WN, Massry SG, eds. Therapy of renal diseases and related disorders. Boston: Kluwer Academic, 1991:317–331.

Schrier RW. Pathogenesis of sodium and water retention in high-output and low-output cardiac failure, nephrotic syndrome, cirrhosis, and pregnancy (parts 1 and 2). N Engl J Med 1988;319:1065–1071, 1127–1134.

Chapter 5

Glomerulonephritis

C. Craig Tisher

Glomerulonephritis results from stimulation of the immune system leading to inflammation of the glomerulus and other components of the renal parenchyma. When limited to the kidney parenchyma, it is termed a "primary" glomerulonephritis. If part of a widely disseminated immune process, it is classified as a "secondary" form of glomerulonephritis (see Chapter 6).

CLINICAL PRESENTATION

Typically, patients present with a "nephritic urinary sediment," characterized by hematuria, pyuria, cellular and granular casts, and varying degrees of proteinuria. However, many types of glomerulonephritis are associated with the nephrotic syndrome (e.g., membranous glomerulonephritis, minimal change disease (MCD), or focal segmental glomerulosclerosis) (see Chapter 4) or with gross hematuria (e.g., IgA nephropathy). When glomerulonephritis is part of a multisystem disease, the clinical presentation will often be characteristic of that disease, and renal involvement may be clinically evident (e.g., Goodpasture's syndrome or systemic lupus erythematosus) (see Chapter 6). Patients who present with red blood cell casts in the urine sediment or with a rapidly rising serum creatinine deserve special consideration. Many will develop irreversible renal failure early in their disease and must be diagnosed and treated aggressively. The laboratory studies listed in the following section should be obtained, but a kidney biopsy should not be delayed while awaiting the results. Often institution of aggressive therapy, such as corticosteroids and a cytotoxic agent, is warranted even before the biopsy results are known.

LABORATORY EVALUATION

Careful examination of the urine sediment is the cornerstone of the evaluation of patients with glomerulonephritis. A 24-hr urine collection for creatinine clearance and total protein should be obtained to quantify residual renal function and urine protein excretion. Renal ultrasound should be performed to exclude reversible causes of renal insufficiency, to measure kidney size, and to prepare for biopsy. Routine studies, such as electrolytes, liver function tests (especially albumin), and cholesterol, should be obtained early in the disease. Adults with significant proteinuria (>1 g/24 hr) need a serum immunoelectrophoresis and urine protein electrophoresis. To further characterize the etiology of glomerulonephritis, the following laboratory studies should be considered:

- Complement components (C_3, C_4, CH_{50});
- Antinuclear antibodies - rheumatoid factor - erythrocyte sedimentation rate;
- Antiglomerular basement membrane (anti-GBM) antibody titer;
- Hepatitis serologies;
- Antineutrophilic cytoplasmic antibodies;
- Streptococcal screen or antistreptolysin O titers;
- Human immunodeficiency virus (HIV) titer.

PATHOGENESIS

The etiology and pathogenesis of many forms of glomerulonephritis are poorly understood. Antigens, including DNA, viruses, bacteria, or proteins of other tissues, can stimulate immune activation and antibody formation in glomerulonephritis. This is followed by deposition of antibodies directed against glomerular tissues or antigen-antibody complexes in the nephron or invasion of the glomerulus by cellular elements of the immune system.

CLASSIFICATION AND MANAGEMENT

Minimal Change Disease

Patients with MCD, also called "nil disease" or "lipoid nephrosis," usually present with the nephrotic syndrome. Ninety percent of children between the ages of 1 and 6 years with the nephrotic syndrome will have MCD, whereas approximately 20% of adults with the nephrotic syndrome have MCD. The onset of the nephrotic syndrome may be acute and often follows an upper respiratory tract infection. Edema can be dramatic, while hypertension and hematuria occur in 20–30% of affected children. Creatinine clearance is usually near normal; however, renal failure can be seen that may be due, at least in part, to volume contraction secondary to severe hypoalbuminemia, i.e., "prerenal" azotemia.

MCD has normal glomeruli on light microscopy. Immunofluorescence microscopy is negative, but electron microscopy reveals fusion or effacement of the foot processes of the glomerular visceral epithelial cell.

Because MCD is by far the most common cause of childhood nephrotic syndrome, an empiric course of corticosteroids is usually administered and biopsy withheld unless a remission is not induced. More than 90% of children with MCD will experience a complete remission, but less than 25% will be cured with one course of corticosteroids. The rest will relapse at varying intervals but are generally responsive to another course of corticosteroids. Cyclophosphamide and chlorambucil can decrease the frequency of relapse, but this therapy must be weighed against the risk of using a cytotoxic agent for a benign disease in childhood, especially since relapses usually end by adulthood. Those who fail to respond to corticosteroids require a kidney biopsy to establish the diagnosis. Because more than two-thirds of adult patients with the nephrotic syndrome will have a lesion that does not respond to corticosteroids, most nephrologists obtain a kidney biopsy before initiating therapy. Prednisone is effective in inducing a remission in adults with MCD, albeit at a much lower rate than in children, and frequent relapses are the rule. Treatment failures will often respond to cyclophosphamide, but again the risk of using this agent in a benign disease must be considered carefully.

Focal Segmental Glomerulosclerosis

Typically, patients with focal segmental glomerulosclerosis (FSGS) will have the nephrotic syndrome or nephrotic-range proteinuria. However, patients may also present with a "nephritic" urinary sediment or with isolated proteinuria. FSGS is a common cause of the nephrotic syndrome in adults, comprising 20–30% of all cases in some series. A light microscopic picture similar to FSGS can also be seen in IgA nephropathy, Alport's syndrome, reflux nephropathy, or human immunodeficieny virus nephropathy or in association with intravenous drug abuse.

There is segmental or total sclerosis of glomerular tufts, and increased mesangial matrix and cellularity are common. Diseased and normal glomeruli are interspersed, and there is a predisposition for involvement of juxtamedullary glomeruli. IgM and C_3 deposits are present in the sclerotic segments.

Usually FSGS does not respond to treatment; however, a subset of patients with the nephrotic syndrome (approximately 25%) will improve their proteinuria with prednisone. Most nephrotic patients with FSGS progress to end-stage renal failure. Patients with FSGS and nonnephrotic proteinuria do not respond to therapy but have a slower progression to end-stage renal failure.

Membranous Glomerulonephritis

Patients with membranous glomerulonephritis usually present with the nephrotic syndrome, but many are asymptomatic and proteinuria is discovered on routine urinalysis. This disease accounts for approximately 30% of all adults with the nephrotic syndrome. The peak age of incidence is 35–50 years, and males predominate by a ratio of 2:1. Patients can lose 10–20 g protein/day and experience severe disability. No specific laboratory or clinical features are pathognomonic, and kidney biopsy is required to make the diagnosis. Pathologically, the subepithelial surface of the glomerular capillary loops is irregular or "spikelike" owing to extension of basement membrane material that is best seen on silver stain of kidney tissue. On immunofluorescence microscopy of capillary loops, granular subepithelial immune deposits that stain for IgG and C_3 are present. Electron microscopy delineates the deposits from the spike-like deformities.

Membranous glomerulonephritis is usually idiopathic, but up to 25% of patients can have an underlying disease such as systemic lupus erythematosus, hepatitis B and C, tumors, adverse drug reactions, or parasitic diseases. In addition to the laboratory tests mentioned earlier, antithyroid antibodies, serologic tests for syphilis, and anti-DNA antibodies should be obtained. Controversy exists regarding the likelihood of an underlying malignancy with idiopathic membranous glomerulonephritis; however, an evaluation for common malignancies should be undertaken, especially in older adults.

Approximately one-third of untreated patients require dialysis after 10 years, whereas another 20–30% have improvement in proteinuria or complete resolution of their disease. There are various therapies, but none has been proven superior. These include corticosteroids or cytotoxic agents or a combination of the two. Treatment should be tailored to the severity of symptoms, including proteinuria, as well as to the age and physical status of the patient.

Postinfectious Proliferative Glomerulonephritis

Postinfectious proliferative glomerulonephritis is usually described after a streptococcal infection of either the upper respiratory tract or the skin. However, similar clinical and pathologic features can occur after any infectious process including subacute bacterial endocarditis, visceral abscesses, osteomyelitis or bacterial sepsis. Poststreptococcal glomerulonephritis (PSGN) will be discussed as a representative of this class of diseases.

Typically PSGN presents with hematuria, hypertension, edema, proteinuria, and acute renal failure. In many patients, these signs may not be present or may be mild. Nephrotic-range proteinuria is uncommon in PSGN. Subclinical cases are common, especially in household contacts of the index case. PSGN is rare before the age of 2 years but is the most common glomerulonephritis in school-age children presenting with a nephritic urine sediment. It occurs at any age in adults and has a 2:1 male predominance. PSGN follows an infection with group A β-hemolytic streptococcus of the throat, upper respiratory tract, or skin. There is typically an 8- to 14-day latent period after infection before the onset of glomerulonephritis. This period may last as long as 21–28 days after skin infections. Cultures are usually negative when active glomerulonephritis is detected, but the antistreptolysin O titer is positive in 90% of patients after upper respiratory tract infections and in 50% after skin infections.

Because PSGN is the most common etiology of an acute nephritic urinalysis in children, an antistreptolysin O titer and a complement profile are indicated initially. Kidney biopsy should be reserved for patients who present atypically or in whom the disease does not resolve spontaneously. In adults, postinfectious glomerulonephritis may mimic other types of glomerulonephritis. A kidney biopsy is indicated to establish the diagnosis.

In mild cases there is glomerular mesangial cell proliferation with an increase in mesangial matrix. Severe cases will also have diffuse endothelial cell proliferation with loss of glomerular capillary lumens, and crescents may be present. Electron microscopy reveals irregular, subepithelial deposits or "humps" along the capillary loops.

Therapy is largely supportive, utilizing fluid and sodium restriction to control blood pressure and edema. Protein restriction is indicated in azotemic patients, and antihypertensive agents should be used to control blood pressure in those who fail to respond to conservative measures. Immunosuppressive agents are not indicated.

Family members of patients should have throat cultures, and those with streptococcal infection require antibiotic treatment. Children, even with severe disease, do well with supportive management; however, the presence of crescents on biopsy indicates a more guarded prognosis. Complete recovery is less certain in adults, particularly in those with a creatinine clearance of <40 mL/min/1.73 m^2, persistent proteinuria of >2 g/day, or increased age. Recurrence of PSGN is rare.

Rapidly Progressive Glomerulonephritis

Rapidly progressive glomerulonephritis presents clinically as acute renal failure and is associated with extensive glomerular crescent formation. It can be seen with an infectious etiology, vasculitis, or anti-GBM disease but is idiopathic in approximately 40% of patients. In half the patients it begins with a viral-like prodrome with myalgias, arthralgias, back pain, fever, and malaise. It may present with manifestations similar to a vasculitis. The urine often contains red blood cell casts.

The kidney reveals extensive cellular crescents with or without immune complex localization on immunofluorescence microscopy. Anti-GBM antibodies or antineutrophilic cytoplasmic antibodies may be present. When glomerulosclerosis, crescents, or interstitial fibrosis is extensive, the lesion is usually irreversible.

Treatment for rapidly progressive glomerulonephritis is usually intravenous corticosteroids and cyclophosphamide. Plasmapheresis is useful only if the underlying disease, such as anti-GBM disease, is known to be responsive. Early diagnosis and treatment are key to a successful therapeutic response. The prognosis is poor when treatment is initiated after the serum creatinine is greater than 6 mg/dL or when oliguria is present. Red blood cell casts on urinalysis warrant aggressive diagnosis and treatment. Rapid loss of renal function may require empiric therapy with corticosteroids and cyclophosphamide until a specific diagnosis is obtained.

Goodpasture's Syndrome (Anti-GBM Disease)

Patients with Goodpasture's syndrome classically present with pulmonary hemorrhage and nephritis. Pulmonary involvement can range from frank hemoptysis to simple pulmonary infiltrates on chest x-ray and may not be concurrent with the presentation of nephritis. Most patients, however, will give some history of recent pulmonary complaints. Occasionally, patients present with pulmonary involvement in the absence of renal lesions. The peak incidence is in the third decade with a second peak in patients older than 60 years. The disease has a 2:1 male predominance.

The disease results from the formation of antibodies directed against an antigen in the GBM that cross-reacts with pulmonary tissue antigens. Linear deposits of IgG are found along the GBM, and circulating anti-GBM antibodies can be measured in the serum.

Treatment involves a 14-day course of plasma exchange with albumin, accompanied by the administration of corticosteroids and a cytotoxic agent such as cyclophosphamide. Unless patients present near end-stage, they usually respond to therapy and eventually can be withdrawn from all agents. Recurrence is rare but is usually responsive to a second course of therapy. However, a significant number of patients eventually progress to end-stage renal failure.

Membranoproliferative Glomerulonephritis

Membranoproliferative glomerulonephritis (MPGN) frequently presents with a vague systemic illness (often described as similar to flu), accompanied by edema and gross hematuria. Edema and hematuria without systemic complaints are also commonly seen. Acute nephritis or rapidly progressive renal failure is less common. Complement levels are decreased in approximately 75% of patients. A serum IgG antiglobulin, C_3 nephritic factor, is present in some patients and may explain the decreased complement levels.

MPGN has been divided into three categories based on the histologic findings. Clinical differentiation of these subtypes is impossible. Type I is most common and is mediated by immune complexes with activation of the classical complement pathway. It is often associated with a chronic immunologic disease. Histologically there is an increase in mesangial cells with mesangial interposition in the capillary walls, which gives the appearance of reduplication of the GBM. Immune complex deposits are seen along peripheral capillary walls and in the mesangium. Type II MPGN, also known as dense-deposit disease, is characterized by activation of the alternate complement pathway. Most patients have C_3 nephritic factor in their serum. Histologically, there are intramembranous dense deposits in the basement membrane of the glomerulus, Bowman's capsule, and renal tubules as seen on electron microscopy. Type II MPGN is often associated with partial lipodystrophy but not with other immunologic diseases.

Type III MPGN has histologic lesions similar to type I, although less mesangial cell proliferation is seen. Electron microscopy usually reveals GBM spikes that are similar to those of membranous glomerulonephritis.

There is no definitive therapy for MPGN. The natural history is one of acute deterioration in renal function and proteinuria followed by spontaneous improvement. Progressive loss of renal function or worsening proteinuria for more than 6 months is associated with a poor prognosis, as is diffuse glomerulosclerosis or the presence of large numbers of crescents on kidney biopsy. Focal and segmental involvement is associated with a more benign prognosis.

IgA Nephropathy (Berger's Disease)

IgA nephropathy is the most common form of glomerulonephritis worldwide, comprising 20–40% of all biopsy-proven glomerulonephritis. It occurs most frequently in the second or third decade with a male predominance of 3:1. IgA nephropathy typically presents with an episode of macroscopic hematuria, often after an upper respiratory tract infection and without other renal manifestations. It is often suspected on routine urinalysis because of microscopic hematuria. Proteinuria is usually mild, but the nephrotic syndrome is occasionally present. A kidney biopsy is required for diagnosis.

IgA nephropathy is characterized by the deposition of IgA often accompanied by C_3 in the glomerular mesangium as seen on immunofluorescence microscopy. There is less prominent localization of IgG and IgM in various combinations. This is usually accompanied by widening of the mesangium and cellular proliferation.

IgA nephropathy typically progresses slowly to chronic renal failure; however, a significant number of patients do not have progressive disease. The 20-year kidney survival is about 75%. Aggressive therapy with corticosteroids or cytotoxic agents is indicated only for patients with acute renal failure or crescentic glomerulonephritis.

Fibrillary Glomerulonephritis

Fibrillary glomerulonephritis typically occurs in adults older than 50 who present with proteinuria in the nephrotic range, hematuria, elevations in serum creatinine, and hypertension. No specific laboratory finding or symptom is characteristic of this disease.

Histologically, there is mild hypercellularity of the mesangium with an increase in mesangial volume. There is infiltration of the mesangial matrix and capillary basement membrane with an amorphous material that is distinct from amyloid. This material is composed of nonbranching, randomly arranged fibrils approximately twice the diameter of amyloid. Immunofluorescence microscopy reveals immunoglobulins and C_3 in the mesangium and capillary walls in a granular pattern. No effective therapy has yet been described. In a small series, 50% progressed to end-stage renal failure.

Suggested Readings

Couser WG. Mediation of immune glomerular injury. J Am Soc Nephrol 1990;1:13–29.

Falk RJ. ANCA-associated renal disease. Nephrology forum. Kidney Int 1990;38:998–1010.

Falk RJ, Hogan SL, Maller KE, Jennette C, Glomerular Disease Collaborative Network. Treatment of progressive membranous glomerulopathy. Ann Intern Med 1992;116:438–445.

Tisher CC, Brenner BM, eds. Renal pathology with clinical and functional correlations, 2nd ed. Philadelphia: Lippincott, 1994.

Chapter 6

Renal Involvement in Systemic Diseases

Geraldine S. Shaw and C. Craig Tisher

SYSTEMIC LUPUS ERYTHEMATOSUS

Systemic lupus erythematosus is an autoimmune disease chiefly affecting the skin, kidneys, joints, serous membranes, and blood vessels.

Clinical Picture

Systemic lupus erythematosus is more common in women aged 20–40 years (female-to-male ratio 9:1) and affects approximately 1 in 500 adult women in the United States. Fever, arthralgia, and a malar or butterfly rash are among the most common presenting symptoms. Photosensitivity, alopecia, serositis, cerebritis, and peripheral neuritis can occur.

Several drugs are associated with a systemic lupus erythematosus-like syndrome including hydralazine, sulfonamides, procainamide, carbamazepine, and isoniazid, but renal involvement is rare.

Investigations may show a markedly elevated erythrocyte sedimentation rate, thrombocytopenia, anemia, and leukopenia. Antinuclear antibodies are positive in 90–95% of patients, but antibodies to double-stranded DNA are more specific. Hypocomplementemia is especially associated with certain types of lupus nephritis (LN).

Renal Involvement

Initial presentation may include mild proteinuria, microscopic hematuria, or hypertension or may be more severe with acute nephritis, nephrotic syndrome, rapidly progressive renal failure, chronic renal insufficiency, or even end-stage renal failure. Renal involvement is clinically apparent in 50% of patients at diagnosis, yet up to 95% have evidence of LN on kidney biopsy even in the absence of a clinical abnormality. Within 10 years of the diagnosis of LN, 20% of patients will have end-stage renal failure

LN is extremely diverse in its presentation and pathology. Hematoxylin bodies, consisting of a basophilic amorphous substance found in areas of necrosis, are thought to be pathognomonic. The World Health Organization (WHO) classification (Table 6.1) is useful in determining prognosis and management. Transformation between classes may occur. In addition to glomerular involvement, tubulointerstitial disease with immunoglobulin and complement deposits in association with cellular infiltration may be seen in up to 50% of patients. Usually this accompanies glomerular disease, especially class IV LN, but it is occasionally seen alone. Certain clinical patterns are more closely associated with a particular pathological class, but no clinical or laboratory parameters reliably predict findings on biopsy.

Management and Prognosis

Patients who present with WHO classes I (normal) and II (mesangial) disease, and those who present with slowly progressive renal insufficiency or advanced renal failure, are managed with blood pressure control and corticosteroids limited to the minimal dose that will control extrarenal disease. Class V (membranous) LN is also usually treated conservatively. Classes III (focal proliferative) and IV (diffuse proliferative) lesions, or patients presenting with a rapidly progressive renal failure, are treated aggressively with high-dose methylprednisolone followed by oral corticosteroids. Cytotoxic agents are often added, especially for the more active forms of class IV LN, which carry a worse prognosis. Pulse intravenous cyclophosphamide is often advocated for these patients.

WHO classes I, II, and III LN generally have a good prognosis. However, changes consistent with class IV disease may

Table 6.1
Lupus Nephritis According to WHO Classification

	Normal Class I	Mesangial Class II
Overall incidence (%)	0–4	10–20
Light microscopy	Normal	Normal or diffuse mesangial proliferation
Immunofluorescence microscopy	Negative	Granular deposits of IgG and C_3 in mesangium ± subendothelium and capillary wall
Electron microscopy	Normal	EDD in mesangium
Notes	Very rarely seen; complete absence of any structural abnormality or immune deposit	May have no detectable clinical abnormality or mild abnormality on urinalysis only; excellent prognosis

EDD, electron dense deposits.

develop, and for this reason many nephrologists advocate aggressive treatment for class III lesions with features of highly active disease or if rapidly progressive renal failure supervenes. Also, the differentiation between "focal" (class III) and "diffuse" (class IV) proliferative glomerulonephritis is arbitrary (<50% glomeruli involved = focal). Class IV is the most ominous form of LN. This commonly progresses to end-stage renal failure (50% within 2 years if untreated), and, because it is often associated with severe extrarenal disease, up to 35% of patients die within 5 years. Membranous (class V) is generally associated with a good renal prognosis with remissions occurring in one-third of pa-

Focal Segmental Proliferative Class III	Diffuse Proliferative Class IV	Membranous Class V
10–20	40–60	10–20
Focal segmental mesangial and endothelial proliferation ± segmental necrosis ± hyaline thrombi	Pronounced diffuse proliferation in mesangium and endothelium ± wire loops, crescents, and necrosis	Diffuse basement membrane thickening and mild mesangial proliferation
Diffuse deposits of IgG, C_3, and C_4 in mesangium ± subendothelium and capillary wall	Irregular diffuse granular deposits of IgG, IgM, IgA, C_3, C_4 throughout glomerulus	Diffuse granular deposits of IgG and C_3 in mesangium and along capillary walls
Diffuse EDD in mesangium ± subendothelium	EDD throughout glomerulus	EDD in subepithelium and mesangium
Hematuria or proteinuria on urinalysis occasionally nephrotic; hypertension, renal insufficiency (usually indicates transformation)	Renal insufficiency, nephrotic syndrome; hypertension common; if untreated, progresses to end-stage within 2–4 years	Proteinuria is universal; 50% nephrotic initially; 90% eventually develop nephrotic syndrome; may slowly progress to end-stage

tients. However, persistent nephrotic-range proteinuria or transformation to class IV LN is associated with a more rapid progression. Recurrence of LN in the transplanted kidney is rare.

SYSTEMIC VASCULITIS

Systemic necrotizing vasculitis is characterized by inflammation and necrosis of blood vessels. Virtually any size or type of blood vessel in any organ can be affected. Classification is difficult, and there is much overlap between each disease; however, certain general patterns can be recognized.

Wegener's Granulomatosis

Wegener's granulomatosis is a granulomatous systemic vasculitis affecting predominantly the small and medium-sized arteries of the respiratory tract and kidneys. It is uncommon.

Clinical Picture

Wegener's granulomatosis mostly affects middle-aged adults of either gender. The classic triad includes necrotizing granulomata of the upper and lower respiratory tract and a necrotizing glomerulonephritis. Clinical renal disease is almost always preceded by extrarenal manifestations, and patients commonly present with epistaxis or painful sinusitis and hemoptysis. Chest x-ray may show flitting pulmonary nodules that may cavitate. Fever, rashes, digital infarction and arthritis, coronary artery disease, serositis, and mononeuritis multiplex occur. Antineutrophilic cytoplasmic antibodies (ANCA) are seen in many forms of vasculitis. "C" ANCA with a coarse, granular cytoplasmic staining pattern are highly specific for Wegener's granulomatosis. Moreover, titers of ANCA appear to correlate with disease activity and may be important in pathogenesis.

Renal Involvement

Renal disease is evident at presentation in about 85% of patients, with urinalysis revealing hematuria, red cell casts, and proteinuria. Only 10% of patients will have renal impairment initially, but characteristically there is progressive deterioration in function. Kidney biopsy usually shows a focal segmental or diffuse necrotizing glomerulonephritis. Rapidly progressive renal failure can occur and is associated with a large number of crescents. The pathognomonic granulomas as seen in the respiratory tract are typically absent. Immunofluorescence microscopy is usually negative, but there may be irregular granular deposits of IgG, IgM, and C_3 along glomerular capillary walls.

Management and Prognosis

Untreated, 80% of patients with Wegener's granulomatosis die within 1 year. Early, aggressive treatment is indicated in the presence of major organ disease because tissue necrosis is irreversible. The necessity of dialysis for acute renal failure should not preclude the use of aggressive therapy, because significant recovery of function can occur. The mainstay of treatment remains methylprednisolone (usually 500–1000 mg depending on body weight on 3 successive days) followed by oral prednisone (1 mg/kg/day). This is tapered after 4 weeks and discontinued at 6 months. Cyclophosphamide is used in combination with corticosteroids either orally (starting at 2 mg/kg/day) or intravenously (0.5–1.0 mg/m^2/month). It is generally recommended that some form of immunosuppressive therapy be continued for at least 1 year, because relapses are common. Plasma exchange is effective in controlling rapidly progressive renal failure or massive pulmonary hemorrhage. It is used in combination with prednisone and cyclophosphamide. With care and correct management, more than 90% of patients can be brought into remission.

Polyarteritis Nodosa

This is a vasculitis of small and medium-sized muscular arteries involving many organs, notably the kidneys, nervous system, and heart. The necrosed blood vessels heal by fibrosis, and the weakened wall develops aneurysms, hence the term "nodosa."

Clinical Picture

Polyarteritis nodosa (PAN) is most common in men aged 30–50 years. It presents with nonspecific symptoms of fever, weight loss, and arthralgia. Hypertension, due to hypereninism secondary to glomerular ischemia, is present in 50% of patients at presentation and will eventually occur in almost all. About 70% will develop cardiac manifestations including angina, infarction, and pericarditis. Mononeuritis multiplex occurs, and PAN is the principal cause of polyneuropathy in the United States after diabetes mellitus. Involvement of the central nervous system may cause strokes, seizures, and cerebellar dysfunction. Hepatitis B infection, intravenous drug use, and hairy cell leukemia can be associated with PAN.

Diagnosis is based on histology of a clinically affected organ such as a peripheral nerve or the kidney. Alternatively, celiac and renal angiography may show characteristic aneurysms and segments of irregularly constricted larger vessels. ANCA are frequently detected, but the staining pattern is often perinuclear

("P" ANCA). Their significance is not as well established as that in Wegener's granulomatosis.

Renal Involvement

The kidneys are affected in 65–100% of patients who may be asymptomatic, have minimal findings on urinalysis, or present with gross hematuria or renal failure. Lesions primarily affect the arcuate and interlobular arteries. Glomerular ischemia leads to fibrinoid necrosis, sclerosis, patchy cortical infarction, but little cellular proliferation. The fall in glomerular filtration rate results from reduced glomerular perfusion rather than direct inflammation. Although circulating immune complexes are suspected in the pathogenesis of these lesions, they are rarely found on biopsy. This has lead to the term, "pauci-immune," which encompasses many ANCA-associated forms of vasculitis.

Necrotizing and crescentic glomerulonephritis are rare in classic PAN. Both are more common in the microscopic form of the disease. Resolving inflammation of the vessel walls leaves changes similar to those of chronic hypertensive vascular disease, but in the latter the elastic lamina is reduplicated, whereas it is destroyed in vasculitis.

Management and Prognosis

Rapid evaluation and initiation of treatment are important in PAN, because the lesions are irreversible and the disease is potentially fatal. Treatment consists of cyclophosphamide and corticosteroids and has resulted in a 5-year survival rate as high as 80%.

Microscopic Polyarteritis

This disease may be considered a variant of PAN, but it tends to involve smaller vessels.

Clinical Picture and Renal Involvement

Microscopic polyarteritis may present with all features of classic PAN including multisystem involvement. However, hypertension is unusual, and glomerulonephritis is more common. There is inflammation of the glomerular capillaries, distal interlobular arteries, and afferent arterioles. Glomerular capillaries surrounding areas of fibrinoid necrosis collapse; the glomerular basement membrane is thickened, and there is cellular proliferation of the mesangium and endothelium. Crescent formation and a clinical picture of rapidly progressive glomerulonephritis may occur. The typical picture is one of focal, segmental glomerulonephritis with no immune deposits, although involvement may be diffuse. There is usually proteinuria and an active urinary sediment.

Management and Prognosis

Treatment guidelines are the same as those for PAN. Microscopic polyarteritis tends to have a better prognosis than classic PAN.

Schönlein-Henoch Purpura

This is another vasculitis involving small vessels. Immune complexes containing IgA are deposited in vessels of the skin and kidneys.

Clinical Picture

Schönlein-Henoch purpura is a relatively common vasculitis that is most often seen in young children. Its incidence increases in winter and spring when upper respiratory tract infections are epidemic, suggesting the possibility of an infectious etiology in some patients.

The skin is involved in all patients, and any rash from urticaria to the classic "palpable purpura" may be seen over the buttocks and the dependent extensor surfaces of the arms and legs. Skin biopsy reveals a leukocytoclastic vasculitis. IgA deposits are seen if new lesions are biopsied. Abdominal pain, arthralgia, and dorsopedal edema also occur.

Renal Involvement

The kidneys are commonly involved in Schönlein-Henoch purpura, and findings range from microscopic or macroscopic hematuria with proteinuria to acute nephritis with oliguria, a fall in glomerular filtration rate, and hypertension. Proteinuria in the nephrotic range may also be present.

Histological changes are identical to those in IgA nephropathy with IgA deposits located in the glomerular mesangium.

Usually a mild glomerulonephritis with focal and segmental changes is present. In severe cases necrosis and crescents are seen. In addition to IgA, less intense IgG and C_3 deposition may be detected with immunofluorescence microscopy. Serum complement levels usually remain normal. The severity of glomerulonephritis does not correlate with the extent of extrarenal disease.

Management and Prognosis

Schönlein-Henoch purpura is usually self-limiting over weeks to months. However, relapses that are usually milder than the original presentation, with episodes of purpura and hematuria, may occur. Because the disease follows a benign course in most patients, specific treatment (corticosteroids) is limited to those with unusually debilitating or progressive disease. However, the value of corticosteroids is not proven.

Risk factors for developing progressive renal disease include the nephrotic syndrome, acute renal failure, and crescents on kidney biopsy. Methylprednisolone, cyclosphosphamide, and even plasma exchange have been used with varying success in patients with a picture of rapidly progressive glomerulonephritis.

The most important determinant of long-term prognosis is the extent of renal disease. For most patients the glomerulonephritis is self-limiting, and persistent hematuria does not necessarily indicate future renal insufficiency. Recurrence in the allograft after transplantation occurs in some 15% of patients.

THROMBOTIC MICROANGIOPATHY

This is a disease characterized by microangiopathic hemolytic anemia, thrombocytopenia, and variable renal and neurological manifestations. Adult and childhood hemolytic-uremic syndrome (HUS) and thrombotic thrombocytopenic purpura (TTP) are included. Thrombotic microangiopathy may also be associated with preeclampsia, various malignancies, and the use of oral contraceptives.

Clinical Picture

HUS and TTP occur with a female-to-male predominance of 10:1. Whether they should be regarded as separate diseases is still controversial. HUS tends to occur in childhood with an annual incidence of 2.65 per 100,000 children who are younger than 5 years in the United States, whereas most cases of TTP occur in the third to fourth decade with an incidence of 0.1 per 100,000 adults. However, a patient of any age can be affected by either disease.

HUS may be associated with infections, especially enteric. Neurological features including confusion, seizures, and paresis occur in both diseases but are much more common in TTP. These symptoms often wax and wane. More than 90% of patients in both groups present with purpura, variably associated with epistaxis, hematuria, and gastrointestinal hemorrhage. These problems are related to a thrombocytopenia that is present in virtually all patients, as is a Coomb's negative hemolytic anemia. One of the most helpful findings for diagnosis is evidence of erythrocyte fragmentation on a peripheral blood smear with schistocytes, burr cells, and helmet cells. Myalgia and arthralgia are also well described.

Renal Involvement

The kidneys are affected in both groups, but the process tends to be more common and more severe in HUS. About 90% of all patients will have proteinuria and microscopic or gross hematuria, and renal failure of varying severity occurs in 40–80%.

It is thought that the target organ damaged in TTP is the endothelium. In the acute stages, platelet and fibrin thrombi occlude the glomerular capillaries and arterioles, leading to ischemia and sometimes necrosis. Endothelial cell hypertrophy adds to the narrowing of the lumen. Immunofluorescence microscopy for immunoglobulins and complement is usually negative. The typical thrombotic angiopathy is also seen in the pancreas, adrenal glands, brain, and heart.

Management and Prognosis

Untreated TTP is almost invariably fatal within 3 months. HUS has a mortality of 50% if there is no intervention. Relapses are less common than in TTP and are usually mild.

Nearly all patients with TTP-HUS now receive corticosteroids, but this alone is usually inadequate to induce remission. The antiplatelet agents aspirin and Dextran 70 have been used in

TTP but do not appear to be beneficial in HUS. Splenectomy, prostacyclins, and immunosuppressive agents have also been used with variable success. The most consistently useful form of management is plasma therapy, and sometimes plasma infusion alone is effective. More commonly, however, plasma exchange with fresh frozen plasma as a replacement fluid is required. A typical schedule consists of daily plasma exchanges for 7 days, followed by alternate-day exchanges until hematological remission is achieved. Plasma therapy is successful in up to 90% of patients, although relapses occur.

Supportive therapy alone (including control of hypertension, blood transfusions, attention to fluid balance, and dialysis if indicated) is often sufficient for HUS, which may remit spontaneously.

Recurrence after renal transplantation occurs in up to 25% of patients and may be associated with the use of cyclosporine in some cases.

PROGRESSIVE SYSTEMIC SCLEROSIS

This is a systemic disease of collagen associated with obliterative vascular lesions. It mainly affects the skin, lungs, gastrointestinal tract, and kidneys.

Clinical Picture

Progressive systemic sclerosis (PSS) or scleroderma is a relatively rare disease that is most common in middle-aged women. Vessel walls are inflamed and thickened, with narrowed and eventually obliterated lumens. The skin is involved in 90% of patients: ischemic ulcers, subcutaneous calcinosis, Raynaud's phenomenon, telangiectasis, and sclerodactyly may occur. Esophageal dysmotility, pulmonary interstitial fibrosis, cardiomyopathy, polymyositis, and arthralgia are also seen.

Various immunological abnormalities may be present. More than 90% of patients are antinuclear antibody positive (usually a speckled pattern on immunofluorescence microscopy). Highly specific for PSS and its variants are anticentromere antibodies and antibody to topoisomerase. These antibodies are found in 20% of the patients and correlate with the more severe, diffuse form of PSS.

Renal Involvement

The kidneys are involved in up to 50% of patients with PSS, and renal failure accounts for about 40% of deaths. Kidney biopsy characteristically reveals obliterative arterial lesions predominantly of the interlobular arteries. There is concentric proliferation of smooth muscle cells in the media that migrate into the intima to produce "onion-skin" thickening. The glomerulus and tubulointerstium may be affected by basement membrane thickening and areas of fibrinoid necrosis. There is interstitial edema and tubular atrophy. Immunofluorescence microscopy may show IgM or C_3 deposits, but they are rarely present in the glomerulus.

Because the disease is basically noninflammatory, the urinary sediment is often inactive. Ischemia-induced glomerulonecrosis may cause hematuria. Glomerular ischemia commonly leads to elevated renin levels and hypertension.

An important complication is the scleroderma renal crisis. This usually develops within 4 years after the onset of extrarenal disease, and hypertension is a prominent, but not absolute, feature. Scleroderma renal crisis is of abrupt onset and involves a rapid progression to renal failure over 1–2 months. Throughout this time the urinary sediment may remain inactive. Scleroderma renal crisis occurs in up to 25% of patients with PSS and is more common in the colder months. It is postulated that renal vasoconstriction caused by hypovolemia, cold-induced vasospasm, or heart failure superimposed on an already compromised circulation is the cause of this rapid deterioration. Renin levels are elevated.

Management and Prognosis

The general course of PSS depends on the distribution and severity of organ involvement. The overall mortality from renal, cardiac, or respiratory failure is about 65% at 7 years. Before the advent of angiotensin-converting enzyme inhibitor therapy, scleroderma renal crisis was almost invariably fatal.

The most important therapeutic step in the management of PSS is adequate control of blood pressure. Corticosteroids and cytotoxic agents do not affect the course of the disease. In scleroderma renal crisis, angiotensin-converting enzyme inhibitors successfully control hypertension in up to 90% of patients and, if instituted early, can stabilize or even improve deteriorating renal function. This improvement is often associated with a remission in extrarenal disease. Supportive therapy is also important and includes adequate nutrition, avoidance of cold, calcium antagonists for digital vasospasm, skin emollients, and dialysis. The 1-year survival has now increased to 75% with the use of angiotensin-converting enzyme inhibitors. Hemodialysis is often problematic because of the lack of good vascular access. Continuous ambulatory peritoneal dialysis is usually more successful, but impaired peritoneal blood flow sometimes reduces the efficiency of dialysis. After transplantation, the allograft may be involved in disease recurrence, but the incidence may be overestimated since the histological features of chronic rejection are very similar to those seen in PSS.

MULTIPLE MYELOMA

This is a tumor of plasma cells in the bone marrow that produces excessive immunoglobulin (M protein). The light chains of this immunoglobulin are detected in the urine as Bence Jones protein.

Clinical Picture

Multiple myeloma usually affects adults older than 50 years. Many symptoms at presentation are due to the abnormal protein, which may elevate the erythrocyte sedimentation rate, lead to renal failure, and cause the hyperviscosity syndrome. Bone involvement with pain, fractures, and hypercalcemia is common. Marrow infiltration causes anemia, thrombocytopenia, leukopenia, and immunoparesis, permitting opportunistic infections such as herpes zoster.

Renal Involvement

Renal dysfunction occurs in more than 50% of patients but does not dramatically alter prognosis. Proteinuria in the nephrotic range is quite common. The main pathology occurs in the tubules where filtered proteins such as albumin and fibrinogen, along with Tamm-Horsfall mucoprotein, obstruct the lumen and form large glassy eosinophilic casts, which are accompanied by inflammation, interstitial fibrosis, and tubular atrophy. Free light chains spill into the urine and are in themselves nephrotoxic, causing tubular dysfunction. Amyloid deposition in the kidney can complicate the picture. Renal failure in multiple myeloma may be precipitated by hypercalcemia and dehydration, chemotherapy and hyperuricemia, and nephrotoxins such as nonsteroidal antiinflammatory drugs prescribed for bone pain.

Management

One aim of treatment is to reduce production of the nephrotoxic light chains. Corticosteroids and melphalan are both effective. Advanced disease may be treated more aggressively with doxorubicin and vincristine and dialysis as indicated. Recently, plasma exchange has been recognized as an important part of treatment, although a small group of patients remain resistant. General measures such as avoiding dehydration, treating infections and hypercalcemia, and minimizing nephrotoxic drugs are important.

AMYLOID

Amyloid is a fibrous protein that produces a bright green birefringence with polarization of tissue sections stained with Congo red. Its deposition gradually destroys normal tissue and is seen in two basic patterns: primary amyloid and secondary amyloid (AA).

Clinical Picture

Primary amyloid mainly involves the kidneys, heart, gastrointestinal tract, nerves, and blood vessels. It is often associated with myeloma. In secondary amyloid, deposits are seen principally in the kidneys, spleen, and liver. Secondary amyloid is associated with chronic diseases such as rheumatoid arthritis, seronegative arthritis, tuberculosis, osteomyelitis, systemic lupus erythematosus, paraplegia, and Crohn's disease.

Renal Involvement

The kidneys are affected in more than 90% of patients both in primary and secondary amyloid, and up to 50% of patients have an elevated serum creatinine at presentation. Renal involvement may be the only clinically significant abnormality in secondary amyloid and usually manifests as proteinuria. Renal secondary amyloid tends to be a more slowly progressive entity than renal primary amyloid. Nephrotic syndrome caused by glomerular deposition of the abnormal protein is a common finding in both. If amyloid deposition is primarily tubular, nephrogenic diabetes insipidus, renal tubular acidosis, or hyperkalemia caused by diminished distal potassium secretion may be the predominant clinical picture. In primary amyloid, M protein is often detectable in the serum or urine, and malignant transformation to myeloma may occur.

Amyloid should be considered in any patient with nephrotic syndrome or renal insufficiency who has an associated chronic inflammatory disease or has evidence of multisystem involvement such as malabsorption, congestive heart failure, hepatomegaly, or neuropathy.

Management and Prognosis

Once suspected, amyloid may be confirmed by abdominal fat pad or bone marrow aspiration or by biopsy of the kidney, tongue, or rectum. Proteinuria may be relatively small in amount for many years, especially in secondary amyloid. Once azotemia or the nephrotic syndrome appears, the prognosis is poor. Approximately 20% of the patients will die within 3 years.

Treatment of amyloidosis is difficult and usually centers on standard nephrotic syndrome therapy such as salt restriction and diuretics and dialysis when needed. Associated autonomic dysfunction or cardiac involvement may adversely affect hemodialysis. In secondary amyloid, treatment is directed toward control of the underlying disease, which also dictates the ultimate prognosis. In primary amyloid, melphalan and prednisone have been used with some success. Recurrence of disease can occur in up to 30% of renal allografts after transplantation, but the associated decline in function is often less severe than with native kidneys.

Suggested Readings

Croker BP, Ramos EL. Pathology of the renal allograft. In: Tisher CC, Brenner BM, eds. Renal pathology with clinical and functional correlations, 2nd ed. Philadelphia: Lippincott, 1994:1591–1640.

D'Agati VD, Cannon PJ. Scleroderma (systemic sclerosis). In: Tisher CC, Brenner BM, eds. Renal pathology with clinical and functional correlations, 2nd ed. Philadelphia: Lippincott, 1994:1059–1086.

Falk RJ, Jennette JC. Systemic vasculitis. In: Glassock RJ, ed. Current therapy in nephrology and hypertension, 3rd ed. St. Louis: Decker, 1992:168–173.

Habib R, Niaudet P, Levy M. Schönlein-Henoch purpura nephritis and IgA nephropathy. In: Tisher CC, Brenner BM, eds. Renal pathology with clinical and functional correlations, 2nd ed. Philadelphia: Lippincott, 1994:472–523.

Hayslett JP, Kashgarian M. Nephropathy of systemic lupus erythematosus. In: Schrier RN, Gottschalk CW, eds. Diseases of the kidney, 5th ed. Boston: Little, Brown, 1993:2019–2039.

Kyle RA, Gertz MA. Renal complications of amyloidosis. In: Glassock RJ, ed. Current therapy in nephrology and hypertension. 3rd ed. Philadelphia: Decker, 1992:188–195.

Chapter 7

Diabetic Nephropathy

C. Craig Tisher

Nephropathy is a complication of diabetes mellitus that often leads to end-stage renal failure. In type I or insulin-dependent diabetes mellitus, 30–50% of the patients will develop nephropathy and renal failure, whereas in type II or noninsulin-dependent diabetes mellitus, the number is approximately 20%.

INCIDENCE

Currently 2–4% of the United States population or 5–10 million individuals have diabetes mellitus. The yearly incidence is approximately 750,000 individuals, and the yearly incidence rate is about 0.3%. In 1989, diabetes mellitus ranked sixth in causes of death by disease in the United States of which approximately 3850 deaths could be attributed to renal failure. At present, approximately 35% of all patients hospitalized for the treatment of end-stage renal failure have diabetes as the underlying cause. The prevalence of diabetic nephropathy increases with the duration of the disease. Poor glycemic control and hypertension are associated with a greater prevalence of renal disease.

CLINICAL PRESENTATION AND PATHOPHYSIOLOGY

Insulin-Dependent Diabetes Mellitus

The progression of renal disease in insulin-dependent diabetes mellitus can be divided into five stages as described by Mogensen and Christensen (listed under "Suggested Readings").

Stage I (Hyperfiltration-Hypertrophy Stage)

Characteristic clinical features relative to the kidney at initial presentation include the following:

- Hyperfiltration (increase in glomerular filtration rate (GFR) that is 20–50% above age-matched control subjects);
- Hypertrophy of kidneys (visible by x-ray);
- Glucosuria with polyuria;
- Microalbuminuria (>20 but <200 µg/min).

With insulin treatment of several weeks duration, the hyperfiltration and hypertrophy correct in most patients, and the microalbuminuria falls below 20 µg/min.

Stage II (Silent Stage)

- Normal or near normal microalbuminuria (<20 µg/min);
- Normalization of elevated GFR in most patients;
- Development of structural damage in the kidney (see explanation below).

Those patients destined to develop diabetic nephropathy often manifest a persistently elevated GFR (>150 mL/min), early hypertension, and poor metabolic control. From 30 to 50% of diabetic patients will proceed into stage III and beyond and develop structural damage in the kidney.

Stage III (Incipient Nephropathy Stage)

- Persistent hyperfiltration early, but GFR starts to decrease later;
- Microalbuminuria (20–200 µg/min, which correlates with an excretion rate of 30–300 mg/24 hr);
- Early hypertension.

This stage can last for several years. The level of protein excretion can be decreased, and the decline in GFR can be slowed with improved control of hyperglycemia and aggressive control of hypertension.

Stage IV (Overt Nephropathy Stage)

- Fixed and reproducible proteinuria (>0.5 g/24 hr, detectable with dipstick);

- Hypertension;
- Declining GFR.

Stage V (End-Stage Renal Failure)

In those patients who progress to end-stage, the time required to develop overt diabetic nephropathy (stage IV) is highly variable but averages 15–17 years. However, subsequent progression to end-stage (stage V) is relatively predictable and averages 5–7 years.

Noninsulin-Dependent Diabetes Mellitus

Far less is known regarding the development of diabetic nephropathyn noninsulin-dependent or type II diabetes mellitus. At diagnosis, microalbuminuria is frequently present and is often reversible with proper metabolic control. In contrast to insulin-dependent or type I disease, hyperfiltration is detected only rarely, and there is no evidence of glomerular hypertrophy. It is clear, however, that in comparison with an age-matched population, the presence of microalbuminuria in noninsulin-dependent diabetes mellitus carries a worse prognosis.

Other manifestations of renal disease in any diabetic patient include the following:

- Bacteriuria;
- Cystitis;
- Acute pyelonephritis;
- Papillary necrosis;
- Perinephric abscess;
- Atonic bladder with hydronephrosis.

PATHOLOGY

The histopathologic alterations observed in diabetic nephropathy typically affect the glomeruli, vasculature, and tubulointerstitial compartment (Table 7.1).

Nodular intercapillary glomerulosclerosis, although not pathognomonic of diabetic nephropathy, is the most characteristic of the renal lesions observed in this disease. However, a very similar lesion can be observed in light chain deposition disease. Therefore, caution must be exercised when this lesion is found in patients with proteinuria in the absence of hyperglycemia or other signs and symptoms of diabetes mellitus.

Table 7.1
Histopathologic Alterations in Diabetic Nephropathy

Glomerular lesions
   Diffuse intercapillary glomerulosclerosis
   Nodular intercapillary glomerulosclerosis
   Capsular drop lesion
   Fibrin-cap lesion
   Glomerular basement membrane thickening
Vascular lesions
   Subintimal hyalin arteriolosclerosis
   Benign arteriosclerosis
Tubular and interstitial lesions
   Hyaline droplets in proximal tubules (representing reabsorbed protein in lysosomes)
   Glycogen deposits in the pars recta of the proximal tubule (so-called Armanni-Ebstein change)
   Tubular atrophy
   Interstitial fibrosis

PATHOGENESIS

The pathogenesis of diabetic nephropathy is undoubtedly multifactorial and remains to be clearly elucidated. However, one important factor is the presence of glomerular hyperfiltration early in the disease, which, if persistent, is more likely to be associated with renal failure later. An abnormal metabolic milieu must also be present for development of the characteristic renal lesions. These hemodynamic and metabolic abnormalities are associated with a complex set of events that eventually results in renal destruction and includes abnormal glycosylation of proteins that form the glomerular basement membrane and mesangial matrix, hyperperfusion of the glomerular capillaries with an associated increase in the transcapillary pressure gradient, and growth of the glomerular capillaries. The combination of these events, if left unchecked, leads to progressive glomerulosclerosis and hypertrophy of residual nephrons, which, in turn, undergo eventual destruction as the kidney reaches end-stage. Improved control of hyperglycemia and reduction in intraglomerular and systemic hypertension can delay progression of these functional and histologic changes.

EVALUATION

The presence of proteinuria, with or without hypertension and renal insufficiency, in a patient with diabetes mellitus of several years duration is diabetic nephropathy until proved otherwise. The presence of diabetic retinopathy, which is observed in more than 90% of those patients with diabetic nephropathy, strengthens the diagnosis. In the absence of diabetic retinopathy, other causes should be entertained to explain the presence of proteinuria. However, only one-fourth to one-third of those patients with diabetic retinopathy have clinically detectable renal disease.

There are situations in which renal disease other than diabetic nephropathy should be considered in the diabetic patient. For instance, sudden onset of the nephrotic syndrome, especially early in the course of diabetes mellitus, or renal insufficiency in association with an active urinary sediment (red blood cells, white blood cells, red cell casts, granular casts) may indicate the presence of a primary glomerular disease (e.g., minimal change disease, membranous glomerulonephritis, or proliferative glomerulonephritis). In these situations a percutaneous renal biopsy is often indicated to establish the diagnosis, determine the prognosis, and aid in management.

Occasionally, a patient may present with proteinuria and on kidney biopsy will have pronounced subintimal hyalin arteriolosclerosis in the absence of other renal lesions. Diabetes mellitus should be excluded in this situation.

MANAGEMENT

Management of the renal disease associated with insulin-dependent diabetes mellitus depends on the point in the disease at which the patient is encountered.

Hypertension

Today most physicians would agree that one of the most important factors in the management of diabetic renal disease is control of hypertension. Intraglomerular hypertension is thought by many to cause progressive glomerular destruction. Although lowering systemic blood pressure can lower intraglomerular pressures, angiotensin-converting enzyme inhibitors lower intraglomerular hypertension more predictably by reducing postglomerular vascular resistance. Lowering the blood pressure in the hypertensive diabetic patient can slow the rate of decline in GFR by 5–6 mL/min/year.

Cardioselective β-blockers are preferable to nonselective agents, such as propranolol, to avoid masking symptoms of hypoglycemia. α-Receptor antagonists, such as prazosin and calcium channel blockers, are also useful in the control of hypertension in the diabetic patient.

Hyperglycemia

At the onset of diabetes mellitus, before insulin therapy is initiated (hyperfiltration-hypertrophy stage), the GFR is elevated and the kidneys are enlarged. With insulin therapy and proper diet, both the GFR and the size of the kidneys usually decrease. Because studies in animals and long-term clinical observations provide evidence that failure to correct the elevated GFR increases the likelihood of the development of progressive renal disease later, proper control of blood glucose levels early in the disease is important. Clinical studies have also demonstrated that normalization of blood glucose levels will reduce microalbuminuria, especially in patients in the so-called incipient nephropathy stage (stage III). Thus, proper control of blood glucose levels in any diabetic patient is an important treatment goal.

Urinary Tract Infection

In general, asymptomatic bacteriuria (>100,000 organisms/mL) should be treated in the diabetic patient. The development of acute pyelonephritis, especially if associated with obstruction, can result in papillary necrosis that can be life threatening (see Chapter 15 for management of urinary tract infections).

Renal Insufficiency

Once it is established that renal insufficiency in a diabetic patient is due to the underlying disease and not to a superimposed or secondary problem that may be reversible, management is essentially the same as in any patient with renal insufficiency (see Chapter 9). Blood pressure control is essential.

Transplantation and Dialysis

Hemodialysis and continuous ambulatory peritoneal dialysis offer a 3-year survival rate of approximately 50%. In the younger diabetic patient, and especially in the absence of severe peripheral vascular disease, renal transplantation offers the best chance for survival. The 3-year patient survival with a living related donor allograft is close to 85%. The disease does recur in the transplanted kidney and can cause destruction of the graft in 5–10 years or less. Unfortunately, the successful rehabilitation of the transplant patient often depends largely on the rate of progression of the disease in other organs.

Suggested Readings

Diabetes Control and Complications Trial Research Group. The effect of intensive treatment of diabetes on the development and progression of long-term complications in insulin-dependent diabetes mellitus. N Engl J Med 1993;329:977–986.

Friedman EA. Management of diabetes and diabetic complications in the patient with diabetic renal disease. In: Jacobson HR, Striker GE, Klahr S, eds. The principles and practice of nephrology, 1st ed. Philadelphia: Decker, 1991:483–490.

Kimmelstiel P, Wilson C. Intercapillary lesions in glomeruli of kidney. Am J Pathol 1936;12:83–97.

Lewis EJ, Hunsicker LG, Bain RP, Rohde RD. The effect of angiotensin-converting-enzyme inhibition on diabetic nephropathy. N Engl J Med 1993;329:1456–1462.

Mogensen CE, Christensen CK. Predicting diabetic nephropathy in insulin-dependent patients. N Engl J Med 1984;311:89–93.

Parving H, Smidt UM, Andersen AR, Svendsen PA. Early aggressive hypertensive treatment reduces rate of decline in kidney function in diabetic nephropathy. Lancet 1983;1:1175–1179.

Tisher CC, Hostetter TH. Diabetic nephropathy. In: Tisher CC, Brenner BM, eds. Renal pathology with clinical and functional correlations, 2nd ed. Philadelphia: Lippincott, 1994:1387–1412.

Chapter 8

Acute Renal Failure

Nicolas J. Guzman and John C. Peterson

Acute renal failure (ARF) represents an abrupt decrease in the ability of the kidney to excrete nitrogenous wastes, resulting in azotemia. ARF may be prerenal, parenchymal, or postrenal in origin.

PRERENAL ARF

ARF that is prerenal in nature represents a rapidly reversible decrease in glomerular filtration rate caused by renal hypoperfusion. It is responsible for 50% of the cases of ARF observed in hospitalized patients.

Pathophysiology

Renal autoregulation maintains normal glomerular filtration rate and capillary hydrostatic pressure over a wide range of perfusion pressures (mean arterial pressure 60–120 mmHg). However, systemic hypotension also stimulates the renin-angiotensin-aldosterone axis, antidiuretic hormone release, and the sympathetic nervous system, which results in redistribution of blood flow away from the renal cortex and avid tubular reabsorption of sodium, water, and urea. Consequently, urine and sodium output decline, and osmolality increases. Blood urea nitrogen increases before changes in serum creatinine concentration become apparent. Further reductions in renal blood flow decrease glomerular filtration rate. If renal hypoperfusion is sustained or severe, acute tubular necrosis (ATN) may ensue.

Etiology

Intravascular Volume Depletion

Hemorrhage;
Gastrointestinal fluid losses;
Renal fluid losses;
Skin loss of sweat;
Sequestration of fluid in third spaces;
Inadequate fluid replacement.

Reduced Cardiac Output

Cardiogenic shock;
Congestive heart failure;
Pericardial tamponade;
Massive pulmonary embolism.

Systemic Vasodilatation

Anaphylaxis;
Antihypertensive drugs;
Sepsis;
Drug overdose.

Systemic or Renal Vasoconstriction

Anesthesia;
Surgery;
α-Adrenergic agonists or high-dose dopamine;
Hepatorenal syndrome.

Hyperviscosity Syndromes

Multiple myeloma or macroglobulinemia.

Clinical Presentation

History and Symptoms

History of fluid losses (vomiting, diarrhea, polyuria, burns);
Use of nonsteroidal antiinflammatory drugs or angiotensin-converting enzyme inhibitors;
Fluid deficit by intake-output balance (output greater than intake);
Thirst.

Signs

Weight loss (catabolic patients may lose >1 lb/day);
Oliguria;
Orthostatic hypotension;
Tachycardia;
Flat neck veins in supine position;
Dry skin and mucosae with loss of skin turgor.

Laboratory Tests

Hemoconcentration (increased albumin and hematocrit);
Serum blood urea nitrogen/creatinine > 20 (however, this can also occur with increased protein catabolism seen with corticosteroid therapy, sepsis, burns, surgery, high fever, and gastrointestinal bleeding);
Urine specific gravity > 1.030;
Urine osmolality > 500 mOsm/kg H_2O;
Urinary sodium < 20 mEq/L;
Fractional excretion of sodium (FE_{Na}) < 1%

$$FE_{Na} = \frac{U_{Na} \times P_{cr}}{P_{Na} \times U_{cr}} \times 100$$

Special Monitoring

Low central venous pressure, pulmonary capillary wedge pressure, or cardiac output;
Congestive heart failure, tamponade, sepsis, cardiogenic shock.

Prerenal azotemia often results from failure to fully replace fluid and electrolyte losses. Body weight is a useful indicator of volume status.

Management

Rapid and aggressive volume replacement is essential to prevent ATN. A useful protocol consists of administering a fluid challenge of 300–500 mL *isotonic saline* iv over 30–60 min. A more gradual infusion of 100–150 mL/hr is required in the elderly or when the cardiovascular status is tenuous. The fluid challenge may be repeated once or twice at hourly intervals while the urine output and cardiovascular status are monitored closely. Thereafter, fluid replacement should maintain the urine output between 1 and 2 mL/min. If there are doubts regarding the patient's cardiovascular status, a Swan-Ganz catheter should be inserted to monitor central venous pressure, pulmonary capillary wedge pressure, and cardiac output. In patients with prerenal azotemia from causes other than volume depletion (e.g., congestive heart failure, pericardial tamponade, drug overdose), the underlying disorder should be corrected.

ACUTE PARENCHYMAL RENAL FAILURE: ACUTE TUBULAR NECROSIS

ATN is an abrupt decrease in glomerular filtration rate caused by tubular cell damage as a consequence of renal hypoperfusion, nephrotoxic injury, or severe tubulointerstitial nephritis. The incidence of ATN in a general hospital is approximately 5%, but it can be as high as 50% in patients undergoing emergency abdominal aortic surgery. Although ATN is usually accompanied by oliguria (urine output < 500 mL/24 hr), some patients will continue to excrete 1–2 L of urine/day. The hallmark of ATN is the acute onset or worsening of azotemia, which is not immediately reversible after withdrawal of the causative agent or fluid replacement.

Etiology

Renal hypoperfusion leading to ischemia accounts for 50% of all cases of ATN. Ischemic damage also may occur without overt hypotension. Another major cause of ATN is nephrotoxicity from either exogenous (25%) or endogenous (20%) toxins (Table 8.1). Approximately 70% of patients with ATN will have more than one etiology.

Aminoglycosides

ATN occurs in 10–26% of patients receiving gentamicin, tobramycin, or amikacin, even when plasma levels are maintained within the therapeutic range. Nephrotoxicity correlates better with the total cumulative aminoglycoside dose than with the plasma levels. ATN, which is usually nonoliguric, becomes clinically apparent after 5–10 days therapy. The following predispose to ATN during aminoglycoside therapy: advanced age, preexisting renal disease, volume depletion, and recent exposure to

Table 8.1
Some Toxic Causes of ATN

Exogenous
  Antibiotics (e.g., aminoglycosides, cephalosporins, tetracyclines, amphotericin B, pentamidine)
  Radiographic contrast media
  Heavy metals (e.g., mercury, lead, arsenic, bismuth)
  Chemotherapeutic agents (e.g., cisplatin, methotrexate, mitomycin)
  Immunosuppressive agents (e.g., cyclosporine)
  Organic solvents (e.g., ethylene glycol)
Endogenous
  Myoglobin
  Hemoglobin
  Calcium phosphate precipitation

other nephrotoxins. Early findings include isosthenuria caused by nephrogenic diabetes insipidus, tubular proteinuria, and Fanconi's syndrome with proximal renal tubular acidosis, glycosuria, and aminoaciduria. Magnesium and potassium wasting may lead to hypomagnesemia and hypokalemia. With more severe nephrotoxicity, azotemia ensues. Recovery may be slow (months) or incomplete. Tobramycin appears to be as nephrotoxic as gentamicin.

Amphotericin B

Nephrotoxicity is rare with cumulative doses of <600 mg. Distal nephron damage is manifested as polyuria with isosthenuria (nephrogenic diabetes insipidus), hypokalemia, hypomagnesemia, and distal renal tubular acidosis. Salt repletion and mannitol may be protective.

Radiographic Contrast Agents

The incidence of ATN with contrast agents is as high as 50%. Renal failure usually occurs 1–2 days after exposure and is characterized by a persistent nephrogram, a low FE_{Na}, and a high urine specific gravity. ATN can be prevented by adequate hydration with saline and/or mannitol given immediately before the contrast load. New nonionic agents do not appear to be less nephrotoxic. Risk factors for contrast-induced ATN include advanced age, preexisting renal disease, volume depletion or any other prerenal state, diabetes mellitus, multiple myeloma, large or repeated doses of a radiographic contrast agent, and recent exposure to other nephrotoxic agents. Calcium channel blockers and adenosine antagonists (theophylline) may protect against contrast-induced ATN.

Cisplatin

Cisplatin nephrotoxicity usually causes severe magnesium wasting, and ATN and chronic renal insufficiency have also been described. Toxicity can be reduced by hydration, mannitol, and a slow infusion of cisplatin in chloride-containing solutions. The newer compounds, carboplatin and iproplatin, appear to be less nephrotoxic.

Organic Compounds

Renal failure from ethylene glycol is due to tubular deposition of calcium oxalate crystals and can be diagnosed by identifying these crystals in the urine. Treatment includes hemodialysis together with ethanol infusion to block ethylene glycol metabolism.

Endogenous Nephrotoxins

Pigments

Rhabdomyolysis sufficient to cause ATN can be caused by the following mechanisms:

- Direct muscle damage (e.g., trauma, crush injury, burns);
- Ischemia and/or increased muscle metabolism (e.g., seizures, exercise, heat stroke, hyperthermia, shock, vascular occlusion);
- Metabolic disorders (e.g., ketoacidosis, hypokalemia, hypophosphatemia);
- Toxins (e.g., alcohol, heroin, CO poisoning, snake bite);
- Severe infections.

The clinical features of rhabdomyolytic ATN include muscle pain, dark brown urine, a positive orthotoluidine test for blood in the urine by dipstick, hyperkalemia, hyperphosphatemia, hyperuricemia, early hypocalcemia, and late hypercalcemia.

Rising serum creatine phosphokinase and myoglobin levels indicate ongoing rhabdomyolysis.

ATN can be prevented by vigorous volume replacement with isotonic saline (200–300 mL/hr) to achieve euvolemia, followed by intravenous mannitol (12.5–25 g in 30 min) or furosemide (40–300 mg every 4–6 hr) to maintain a urine output of 100–200 mL/hr and urine alkalinization to a pH above 6 with intravenous sodium bicarbonate (1 mEq/kg/dose). This last goal is often difficult to achieve, and the use of large amounts of alkali may induce tetany in hypocalcemic patients. When ATN develops, the patient is usually so severely hypercatabolic that early and frequent hemodialysis is almost always required. The prognosis for recovery of renal function is good. Mortality, however, varies from 5 to 10%.

Crystals

ATN may result from intratubular deposition of uric acid crystals during chemotherapy for malignancies with high cell turnover (e.g., leukemia, lymphoproliferative and germ cell neoplasms). Hemodialysis is the treatment of choice. Preventive measures include vigorous hydration, alkaline diuresis, and allopurinol. These measures should be initiated several days before chemotherapy and maintained during induction. Hyperkalemia and hyperphosphatemia commonly complicate hyperuricemic ATN.

Multiple Myeloma

ATN occurs in patients with multiple myeloma from tubular damage by light chains, from intratubular casts, or from complications, such as hypercalcemia, hyperviscosity, and volume depletion. These patients are also very susceptible to contrast-induced ATN.

Pregnancy

ATN can occur early after septic abortion or during late pregnancy associated with eclampsia, abruptio placentae, peripartum hemorrhage, amniotic fluid embolism, or prolonged intrauterine fetal death. The pathogenesis includes a combination of renal hypoperfusion from vasospasm and formation of fibrin thrombi inside the glomerular capillaries. Disseminated intravascular coagulation is seen frequently. Cortical necrosis leading to end-stage renal failure can also occur.

Rare forms of pregnancy-associated ARF include acute fatty liver with ATN and postpartum ARF. In the former, the only effective treatment is termination of the pregnancy. Postpartum ARF is a form of thrombotic microangiopathy. There is no effective therapy.

Hepatorenal Syndrome

This is a progressive decline in renal function in patients with advanced liver disease (usually cirrhosis) in the absence of other identifiable causes. There is marked renal vasoconstriction with oliguria. Urine sodium concentration is usually <10 mEq/L (and remains low after a volume challenge), and the FE_{Na} is <1%. The syndrome usually develops in the hospital after aggressive diuretic therapy, paracentesis without intravascular volume replacement, infection, surgery, or gastrointestinal bleeding. Mortality is very high (>95%) and is usually due to liver failure, infection, or hemorrhage. There is no effective therapy.

Pathophysiology

Back-leak of filtered tubular fluid across a disrupted tubular epithelial barrier is an important mechanism in nephrotoxic ATN. *Deposition of tubular debris with tubular obstruction* is important in early ischemic ATN. *Reduction in total renal blood flow and redistribution of renal blood flow away from the outer cortex* may be involved in both types of ATN. Regardless of the pathogenetic mechanism, the final result is always impaired renal function with progressive azotemia and, in most cases, impaired water and electrolyte handling.

Clinical Presentation and Laboratory Findings

Most patients with ATN present with an acute rise in serum creatinine and oliguria. Some, particularly those with nephrotoxic injury, are nonoliguric initially. Complete anuria rarely occurs in ATN, and its presence should suggest urinary obstruction, bilateral cortical necrosis, vascular occlusion, or rapidly progressive glomerulonephritis. A smaller number of patients will present with volume overload leading to congestive heart failure and pulmonary edema, peripheral edema, dyspnea, hypertension, or hyperventilation from metabolic acidosis. Occasionally uremia, which is characterized by lethargy, anorexia, nausea, vomiting, and abdominal pain, is the presenting feature. Frequently, patients will have marked electrolyte disturbances consisting of severe azotemia, hyperkalemia, high anion gap, metabolic acidosis, and hyponatremia. The daily rate of rise in serum creatinine with total renal failure ranges between 0.5 and 1.0 mg/dL. A more rapid increase should suggest a hypercatabolic state or massive muscle destruction. Other metabolic abnormalities include hyperphosphatemia, hypermagnesemia, hypocalcemia, and hyperuricemia.

Examination of the urine sediment reveals renal tubular epithelial cells, cellular debris, and cellular and coarse granular casts. Hematuria and red blood cell casts are rare. White blood cells or white blood cell casts suggest acute interstitial nephritis.

In the setting of oliguria and acute azotemia, and in the absence of recent diuretic therapy, a FE_{Na} of >1%, a urine osmolality of <350 mOsm/kg H_2O, and a urine sodium concentration of >40 mEq/L are characteristic of ATN. However, a FE_{Na} of <1% can occur in ATN (particularly the nonoliguric types) when associated with radiocontrast agents, sepsis, burns, liver failure, and edematous states, in interstitial nephritis, in acute obstruction, and in acute poststreptococcal glomerulonephritis.

DIAGNOSTIC APPROACH TO THE PATIENT WITH ACUTE RENAL FAILURE AND THE DIFFERENTIAL DIAGNOSIS OF ATN

After excluding a spurious elevation in the serum creatinine concentration, the next step is to determine whether the ARF is acute or chronic. The presence of one or more of the features shown in Table 8.2 suggests chronic renal disease.

Table 8.2
Features Suggestive of Chronic Renal Disease

Family history of renal disease (e.g., polycystic kidney disease) or history of chronic disease causing renal insufficiency (e.g., diabetes mellitus)
Polyuria, nocturia, or symptoms of chronic urinary obstruction or infections
Normocytic, normochromic anemia
Radiologic evidence of renal osteodystrophy
Bilateral small (<10 cm) or scarred kidneys on ultrasound

Table 8.3
Features Suggestive of Obstructive Uropathy

Elderly male with acute or progressive renal failure
History of previous urinary tract obstruction or infections
Findings suggestive of bladder outflow obstruction (e.g., dysuria, nocturia, frequency, hesitation)
History of diseases known to predispose to papillary necrosis (e.g., diabetes mellitus, sickle cell disease, or analgesic abuse)
Pelvic or retroperitoneal disease or surgery
Complete anuria or wide variations in urine output
Normal urinalysis with progressive renal failure

Once chronic renal failure has been excluded, the next step is to identify patients with ARF that is prerenal in origin or with urinary tract obstruction, the major cause of postrenal ARF (Table 8.3). Oliguric patients should have a single bladder catheterization. All patients should have a complete urinalysis and renal ultrasound to search for obstruction. Renal ultrasound may be nondiagnostic for obstruction early in its course. If suspicion of obstruction is high, ultrasound should be repeated and further diagnostic tests (e.g., retrograde pyelogram, computed tomography, furosemide renogram) undertaken.

Acute Renovascular Disease

Acute renovascular disease can present with various clinical manifestations (Table 8.4). Its etiology follows:

- Aortic aneurysm (dissection, thrombosis);
- Renal artery dissection or thrombosis (trauma, postangioplasty);
- Embolism (thrombus, cholesterol);
- Thrombotic microangiopathy;
- Renal vein thrombosis.

Acute Interstitial Nephritis (see Chapter 16)

Acute Glomerulonephritis and Vasculitis

Features suggestive of glomerulonephritis or vasculitis include fever, skin rash, arthralgias, or evidence of systemic disease or pulmonary involvement. Helpful laboratory findings include an

Table 8.4
Features Suggestive of Acute Renovascular Disease

Hypertension (new onset or accelerated)
Evidence of aortic or renal arterial disease (aortic aneurysm, abdominal bruits, reduced or absent femoral pulses)
Vascular disease elsewhere (peripheral, cerebral)
Source for arterial embolization (infective endocarditis, atrial fibrillation, recent myocardial infarction)
Evidence of cholesterol embolization (recent aortic catheterization, livedo reticularis, elevated erythrocyte sedimentation rate, peripheral eosinophilia, low complement levels, thrombocytopenia)
Evidence of thrombotic microangiopathy (thrombocytopenia, microangiopathic anemia, fever, neurologic abnormalities)
Nephrotic syndrome associated with proximal tubular dysfunction (suggests renal vein thrombosis)

---

elevated erythrocyte sedimentation rate, low complement levels, positive tests for collagen vascular disease, and hematuria or red blood cell casts.

Acute Tubular Necrosis

The diagnosis of ATN is made only after exclusion of all other conditions mentioned. In most patients the etiology of ARF will be identified on clinical grounds alone. Patients will remain, however, in whom the diagnosis is unclear and a kidney biopsy is needed. Also, biopsy should normally be performed in patients with suspected ATN in whom ARF persists beyond 4 weeks in the absence of a known etiology.

Clinical Course

The clinical course of ATN can be divided into three phases.

Initiating Phase. This period between the onset of decreased renal function and established renal failure is usually reversible by treating the underlying disorder or removing the offending agent.

Maintenance Phase. Renal failure is not immediately reversible. Duration may vary from a few hours to several weeks. Renal function usually improves spontaneously after 10–16 days in oliguric patients and 5–8 days in nonoliguric patients.

Recovery Phase. Renal function begins to improve, and blood urea nitrogen and serum creatinine return toward normal. Oliguric patients increase their urine output and may sometimes enter a polyuric phase that can result in fluid and electrolyte imbalance. Recovery of renal function usually occurs within 4 weeks. In a few patients, particularly those with previous renal disease, renal function may never return to baseline.

Management

First, reversible factors must be rapidly and exhaustively sought and treated. Conversion of oliguric to nonoliguric ATN may facilitate management but does not clearly reduce morbidity or mortality. This may be achieved with a loop diuretic such as furosemide (80–400 mg iv). The dose can be repeated once if no response is seen after 1 hr. However, high doses of loop diuretics may impair hearing and should not be administered indiscriminately. Complications can be prevented by close monitoring of fluid and electrolyte balance and by serial assessment of clinical and biochemical parameters as indicated below.

Fluid Intake. Restrict fluids (<1 L/day in oliguric patients) to match measurable plus insensible losses.

Electrolytes. Restrict to match measured losses. This is usually <2 g or 86 mEq/day for sodium and <1.5 g or 40 mEq/day for potassium.

Diet. Restrict *protein* to 0.6 g/kg/day (high biologic value). Provide at least 35 kCal/kg nonprotein *calories*. Allow for *weight loss* of 0.5 lb/day owing to catabolism. Consider *hyperalimentation* early, especially in catabolic patients.

Biochemical Monitoring.

Serum Sodium. Avoid hyponatremia by restricting free water.

Serum Potassium. Treat hyperkalemia with sodium bicarbonate, glucose plus insulin, Kayexalate, or dialysis. Use calcium gluconate to antagonize the cardiac effects of potassium (see Chapter 11).

Serum Bicarbonate. Maintain serum pH at >7.20 or serum bicarbonate at 20 mEq/L or above.

Serum Phosphate. Control hyperphosphatemia with calcium-containing phosphate binders.

Table 8.5
Indications for Dialysis in Oliguric Patients

Uremic pericarditis
Severe hyperkalemia, particularly in catabolic patients
Volume overload resulting in pulmonary edema or severe hypertension
Severe refractory metabolic acidosis (pH < 7.20)
Symptomatic uremia

Serum Calcium. Hypocalcemia rarely requires therapy; treat only if symptomatic.

Drugs. *Avoid* magnesium-containing medications. *Adjust* drug dosages for level of renal function (see Chapter 26).

Dialysis. Early dialysis simplifies management and nutritional support. Hemodialysis, continuous arteriovenous hemofiltration, and peritoneal dialysis are all effective (see Chapters 22 and 23). Indications for dialysis are listed in Table 8.5. The predialysis blood urea nitrogen and serum creatinine should be maintained below 100 and 8 mg/dL, respectively.

Prognosis

Mortality from ATN is 20–50% in a medical setting and 60–70% when surgically related. Factors associated with an increased mortality include advanced age, severe underlying disease, and multiple organ failure. Leading causes of death are infections, progression of the underlying disease, gastrointestinal hemorrhage, and fluid and electrolyte disturbances. Patients who survive usually regain enough renal function to avoid chronic dialysis. Despite advances in critical care, mortality has not changed significantly during the past 20 years. Therefore, the importance of prevention of ATN cannot be overemphasized.

Suggested Readings

Agmon Y, Brezis M. Acute renal failure: a multifactorial syndrome. Pathogenesis and prevention strategies. Contrib Nephrol 1993;102:23–36.

Anderson RJ. Prevention and management of acute renal failure. Hosp Pract 1993;28:61–75.

Epstein M. Calcium antagonists and the kidney: future therapeutic perspectives. Am J Kidney Dis 1993;21(suppl 3):16–25.

Hays SR. Ischemic renal failure. Am J Med Sci 1992;304:93–108.

Lieberthal W, Levinsky NG. Treatment of acute tubular necrosis. Semin Nephrol 1990;10:571–583.

Mehra MJ, Sharif K, Bode FR. Radiocontrast-induced nephropathy. Prevention is better than cure. Postgrad Med J 1992;92:215–223.

Chapter 9

Chronic Renal Failure

John C. Peterson

Chronic renal failure (CRF) exists when renal function has been diminished by parenchymal renal damage. End-stage renal failure is present when there is so little remaining function that patients require replacement therapy in the form of dialysis or transplantation (see Chapters 22–24).

INCIDENCE

More than 200,000 patients are being treated for end-stage renal failure in the United States. Similar data are not available for patients with CRF.

ETIOLOGY

- Diabetic nephropathy;
- Hypertension (nephrosclerosis);
- Glomerulonephritis;
- Hereditary renal disease;
- Polycystic kidney disease;
- Alport's syndrome;
- Obstructive uropathy;
- Interstitial nephritis.

PATHOPHYSIOLOGY

Irrespective of the nature of the initial injury, when the plasma creatinine exceeds 2.0 mg/dL (177 mmol/L), progression to end-stage is common. The reason is unknown, but suggested causes include systemic and glomerular hypertension, secondary hyperparathyroidism, and unknown "toxic factors" related to the uremic state.

Glomerular hypertension leading to hyperfiltration injury in remnant nephrons has been proposed as a factor in the progression of chronic renal disease. Human studies suggest a delay in progression of the hyperfiltration injury by the use of angiotensin-converting enzyme inhibitors to control systemic hypertension and "normalize" the glomerular transcapillary hydraulic pressure. Secondary hyperparathyroidism may be significant in the progressive loss of renal function. Human studies have shown a decline in the rate of progression of renal failure when phosphorus intake is restricted. Thus, an early and vigorous attempt to control serum calcium and phosphorus levels may be helpful in slowing the progression of renal failure.

UREMIA

Although initial injury to the kidney may arise from a wide spectrum of diseases, the ensuing renal failure produces clinical abnormalities that are similar in all such patients—the so-called "uremic syndrome." Uremia is a symptom complex characterized by the retention of waste products of protein metabolism and is also marked by abnormalities of fluid and electrolyte homeostasis with endocrine and metabolic derangements.

Fluid and Electrolyte Changes

As creatinine clearance (C_{cr}) decreases, the ability to concentrate or dilute the urine is impaired. Restriction of water intake may result in hypernatremia and volume contraction, whereas if water or salt intake is excessive, hyponatremia, edema, or both may occur.

In general, serum potassium is well regulated until the C_{cr} is <5 mL/min. Thus hyperkalemia with CRF usually implies excessive intake, use of potassium-sparing diuretics and other drugs, or hyperkalemic distal tubular acidosis (see Chapter 11). Finally, if metabolic acidosis develops acutely, the transcellular shift of potassium may result in hyperkalemia.

The fractional excretion of calcium, magnesium, and phosphorus increases as glomerular filtration rate (GFR) declines. Serum levels of parathyroid hormone are increased when the GFR is 70–80% of normal, and 1,25-dihydroxyvitamin D_3 levels

Table 9.1
Hormonal Changes

Decreased production: testosterone, erythropoietin, and 1,25-dihydroxyvitamin D_3
Decreased degradation: elevated levels of prolactin, luteinizing hormone, gastrin, insulin, glucagon, and parathyroid hormone
Renal ischemia: elevated levels of renin, angiotensin II, and aldosterone
Adaptive response to regulate fluid or electrolyte balance: elevated parathyroid hormone

are depressed when C_{cr} reaches 40–50% of normal. Hypocalcemia is very common in CRF owing to decreased gastrointestinal absorption and bone resistance to the action of parathyroid hormone. These findings led to the concept of the "trade-off hypothesis," which states that maintenance of normal serum phosphorus and calcium levels is obtained through elevation of parathyroid hormone levels and resultant bone dissolution (renal osteodystrophy). In this process, the accumulated acid is buffered by bone salts to defend blood pH. Because of this "bone buffering" and the maintenance of tubular acid secretion until extremely low levels of C_{cr} are reached, the acidosis of renal failure is rarely severe (blood pH usually >7.31). Hormonal changes seen in uremia are listed in Table 9.1.

Retained Waste Products

Although blood urea nitrogen (BUN) represents the largest quantity of retained nitrogen in CRF, its role as a toxin remains unclear. Patients in whom urea was added to the dialysate during hemodialysis became symptomatic (fatigue, nausea, and vomiting) only when the BUN was >150 mg/dL for longer than 1 week. In CRF, an increase in BUN is invariably associated with elevations of other nitrogenous waste products (ammonia, guanidine, guanidinosuccinic acid, and methylguanidine), but definitive demonstration that any of the above can account for uremic symptomatology is lacking.

CLINICAL FEATURES

The initial symptoms of CRF are subtle and often ignored. A generalized symptom complex of lethargy, malaise, and weakness is common. Major symptoms are listed below.

- Dermal: pruritus, easy bruisability, edema;
- Cardiovascular: dyspnea on exertion, retrosternal pain on inspiration (pericarditis);
- Gastrointestinal: anorexia, nausea, vomiting, singultus;
- Genitourinary: nocturia, impotence;
- Neuromuscular: restless legs, numbness and cramps in legs;
- Neurologic: generalized irritability and inability to concentrate, decreased libido.

Physical examination often reveals only nonspecific findings that may include the following.

- General: sallow, debilitated appearance;
- Dermal: pallor, ecchymoses, excoriations, edema, xerosis;
- HEENT: uriniferous breath;
- Pulmonary: rales, pleural effusion;
- Cardiovascular: hypertension, flow murmur or pericardial friction rub, cardiomegaly;
- Neurologic: stupor, asterixis, myoclonus, neuropathy.

EVALUATION

It is important not only to document the degree of renal impairment (and its cause, if possible) but also to determine whether potentially reversible factors exist (see Table 9.2).

Urine culture and ultrasound yield valuable information. Infection rarely causes CRF in the absence of obstruction. Ultrasonography will reveal kidney size (usually <10 cm in CRF, although diabetes, multiple myeloma, and amyloid may produce normal to large kidneys in the presence of CRF) and contour (polycystic kidney disease). A 24-hr urine collection for C_{cr} and total protein excretion should be obtained. Once the C_{cr} is below 25 mL/min, this measurement exceeds the true GFR (measured by inulin clearance) by as much as 20–30% owing to secretion of creatinine. Once C_{cr} falls below 5 mL/min, the values again approximate inulin clearance.

MONITORING

After the initial evaluation has been performed and reversible factors have been excluded, the physician must focus on serial measurements of parameters reflecting the patient's clinical

Table 9.2
Potentially Reversible Factors in CRF

Reversible Factor	Evaluation Required
Infection	Urinalysis, culture, and sensitivity
Obstruction	Bladder catheterization, then ultrasonography
Nephrotoxic agents	Drug history (nonsteroidal antiinflammatory agents, analgesics, antibiotics, radiocontrast agents)
Extracellular fluid volume depletion	Evaluate diuretic use or severe sodium restriction; supine and upright blood pressure and pulse
Hypertension	Measure blood pressure, obtain chest x-ray
Congestive heart failure	Physical exam, chest x-ray
Pericarditis	Echocardiography, ECG
Metabolic abnormalities Hypokalemia Hypercalcemia Hyperuricemia (>15 mg/dL)	Serum electrolytes, calcium, phosphate, uric acid

course. C_{cr} and serum creatinine are useful in monitoring renal function. If precipitous deterioration occurs, reversible factors should be sought.

The parameters listed below are suggested at routine follow-up visits (usually monthly) until a definite pattern of decline of function is established:

- History: uremic symptoms (check for worsening);
- Physical examination: weight, supine and upright blood pressure and pulse, skin turgor, pericardial friction rub, edema, reflexes and sensation in extremities;
- Laboratory tests: BUN, creatinine, electrolytes, calcium, phosphorus, albumin, complete blood count, parathyroid hormone (6-month intervals).

TREATMENT

The goals of conservative therapy for CRF are listed in Table 9.3.

Correction of Reversible Factors

As previously discussed (under "Evaluation"), reversible factors, such as urinary tract infections, obstruction, extracellularlar

Table 9.3
Goals of Therapy

Correction of reversible factors hastening loss of renal function
Correction of fluid and electrolyte abnormalities
Prevention of further loss of renal function
Prevention or reduction of uremic symptoms by lowering quantity of retained nitrogenous waste products while maintaining adequate protein nutrition

fluid volume contraction, or congestive heart failure, should be assiduously sought and treated.

Drugs

The use of drugs in patients with CRF is a double-edged sword in that the effectiveness of an agent may be outweighed by toxicity, because many agents depend on renal degradation or excretion for elimination. A detailed analysis of the use of drugs in CRF is provided in Chapter 26. Certain drugs should not be used in the presence of CRF.

- Nitrofurantoin: causes peripheral neuropathy;
- Amiloride, triamterene, spironolactone: may cause hyperkalemia;
- Sulfonylureas: cause prolonged hypoglycemia;
- Nonsteroidal antiinflammatory agents: decrease renal function;
- Tetracyclines: increase protein catabolism.

Avoid the use of intravenous contrast agents. In the presence of renal dysfunction, they may cause irreversible renal failure (especially in patients with multiple myeloma or diabetic nephropathy).

Pregnancy may accelerate progression of CRF. Risks are greatest in patients with hypertension, with a serum creatinine of >1.5 mg/dL, and with active renal disease.

Correction of Fluid and Electrolyte Abnormalities

Sodium

The limits of salt excretion are narrowed in CRF. A fixed daily salt excretion predisposes patients to volume contraction during severe salt restriction. The 24-hr urinary sodium excretion can be measured during a period of stable weight and the dietary sodium intake adjusted accordingly to allow a trace of ankle edema in the early evening. In general, a 6-g NaCl diet ("no added salt") is a good starting point. Patients should be encouraged to keep a record of daily weights and notify their physician of any change in excess of 5 lb over a 48-hr period. At each routine clinic visit, the weight chart, as well as supine and upright blood pressure measurements, will allow assessment of volume status.

Because dietary sodium intake will frequently be a mixture of NaCl and $NaHCO_3$, the following equivalent measures are useful:

1 g $NaHCO_3$ contains 12 mEq Na;
1 g NaCl contains 17 mEq Na;
1 g Na = 43 mEq Na.

Patients should be warned to avoid "salt substitutes" because these compounds contain up to 45 mEq KCl/teaspoon and are potentially lethal.

Water

Because osmolality is well regulated until the C_{cr} is below 10 mL/min, hyponatremia in the CRF patient requires water restriction only with evidence of total body salt and water overload (edema). In the euvolemic or hypovolemic patient with hyponatremia, the most common etiology is diuretic therapy. Water restriction would only worsen extracellular fluid contraction. These patients frequently have an increased BUN-to-creatinine ratio and are best managed by withdrawal of diuretics or judicious replacement of salt.

Diuretics

Thiazide diuretics are ineffective when the GFR is below 30 mL/min. Loop diuretics (furosemide, ethacrynic acid, or bumetanide) are preferred. Because retained organic anions compete for tubular secretion, the patient with CRF requires higher doses of these diuretics. It is reasonable to start with 40 mg furosemide or 1 mg bumetanide and double the dose until the desired effect is achieved. If diuresis is not achieved with 240–300 mg furosemide as a single daily dose, addition of metolazone (2.5 or 5 mg every day) is a useful adjunct. The effectiveness of metolazone in this setting is due to its more distal tubular site of action, preventing the compensatory response to furosemide.

Acidosis

Patients with CRF are acidotic because their kidneys cannot excrete the 1 mEq/kg/day of acid generated by metabolism of dietary protein. In general, maintenance of serum total CO_2 levels above 18–20 mEq/L will provide symptomatic relief as well as prevent catabolism of skeletal muscle. $NaHCO_3$ can be given as 650-mg tablets three times a day and titrated to obtain a total CO_2 of 20 mEq/L. Alternatively, $CaCO_3$ has been suggested. However, it is not an effective buffer.

Potassium

Treatment of acute hyperkalemia is addressed in Chapter 11. Chronic hyperkalemia is treated by dietary potassium restriction or with sodium polystyrene sulfonate (Kayexalate). The usual dose is 15–30 g in either juice or sorbitol (acts as a cathartic) once per day. Potassium removal is estimated at 1 mEq/1 g polystyrene excreted in the stool.

Calcium and Phosphorus

The maintenance of normal serum phosphorus levels can prevent renal osteodystrophy and progression of CRF. The serum phosphorus should be maintained between 3.5 and 4.0 mg/dL (1.1–1.3 mmol/L). Dietary sources rich in phosphorus (e.g., meats, eggs, and dairy products) should be restricted. Most patients also require oral "phosphate binding" compounds. Because of the long-term risks of aluminum-induced bone disease, the standard regimen is now calcium acetate or $CaCO_3$ tablets. These tablets should be ingested with meals.

Until serum phosphorus is controlled, vitamin D should not be given. Patients with CRF require 1000–1500 mg calcium/day to maintain calcium balance. If supplements of $CaCO_3$ and/or calcium gluconate do not normalize serum calcium (and if serum phosphorus remains controlled), therapy with 1,25-dihydroxyvitamin D_3 may be initiated with 0.25 μg, which can be increased at 2- to 4-week intervals to normalize serum calcium.

Prevention of Further Loss of Renal Function

As discussed under pathophysiology, it may be possible to ameliorate the hyperfiltration injury by reduction of transcapillary hydraulic pressure through the use of converting enzyme inhibitors and a low protein diet.

Hypertension

Treatment with angiotensin-converting enzyme inhibitors is preferable, but serial checks of serum creatinine are important to detect an abrupt worsening of GFR, which can occur in cases of bilateral renal artery stenosis (GFR is angiotensin dependent), nephrotic syndrome, and volume depletion caused by diuretics. Recent evidence suggests that maintaining blood pressure at 125/75 mmHg will slow progression of CRF more effectively than usual levels of blood pressure control (140/90 mmHg).

Dietary Protein Restriction

Dietary protein increases renal plasma flow and GFR in humans and animals. It has been proposed that over long periods this can cause progressive injury in kidneys that are already damaged, resulting in glomerulosclerosis. Studies of the protective effect of low protein diets in patients with CRF suggest that protein restriction (with appropriate attention to increasing the biologic value of remaining dietary protein) may delay progression of CRF. The recommendation is 0.6 g/kg/day of protein of high biologic value supplemented by an amount equal to urinary protein loss. If attempted, it requires collaboration with a trained dietitian and regular assessments of dietary compliance with measurements of urea excretion (see Chapter 25).

Therapy of Specific Uremic Symptoms

Pruritus

If unresponsive to dietary protein restriction, normalization of serum phosphorus, or both, use of diphenhydramine at bedtime is frequently effective.

Gastrointestinal Symptoms

Anorexia, musty or metallic tastes, and early morning nausea and vomiting usually respond well to dietary protein restriction, but they may resurface as the patient approaches end stage. At this time, the abnormal taste may be treated with half-strength hydrogen peroxide gargles to decrease oral bacteria that contain urease, which can convert urea to ammonia.

Anemia

If the anemia is not normocytic and normochromic, a search should be instituted for iron, folic acid, or vitamin B_{12} deficiencies. Reversal of anemia by recombinant human erythropoietin is effective in relieving many symptoms previously ascribed to uremia.

When conservative management fails to control uremic signs and symptoms, dialysis (see Chapters 22 and 23) or transplantation (Chapter 24) should be undertaken. Indications for initiation of dialysis or transplantation include

- Volume overload unresponsive to diuretic therapy;
- Pericarditis;
- Progressive renal osteodystrophy;
- Progressive neuropathy;
- Bleeding diathesis;
- Noncompliant or irresponsible patient with hyperkalemia.

Suggested Readings

Baker LRI, Abrams SML, Roe CJ, et al. 1,25 $(OH)_2D_3$ administration in moderate renal failure: a prospective double blind trial. Kidney Int 1989;35:661–669.

Klahr S, MDRD Study Group. The effects of dietary protein restriction and blood pressure control on the progression of chronic renal disease. N Engl J Med 1994;330:877–884.

Lim VS, DeGowin RL, Zavala D, et al. Recombinant human erythropoietin treatment in pre-dialysis patients. Ann Intern Med 1989;110: 108–114.

Lopes-Hilker S, Dusso AS, Rapp NS, et al. Phosphorus restriction reverses hyperparathyroidism in uremia independent of changes in calcium and calcitriol. Am J Physiol 1990;259:F432–F437.

May RC, Kelly RA, Mitch WE. Pathophysiology of uremia. In: Brenner BM, Rector FC, eds. The kidney, 4th ed. Philadelphia: Saunders, 1991:1997–2018.

Ter Wee PM, Donker AJM. Clinical strategies for arresting progression of renal disease. Kidney Int 1992;42:S114–S120.

Chapter 10

Disorders of Water Balance

Bruce C. Kone and Charles S. Wingo

Under physiologic conditions, the osmolality of all body fluids is maintained within narrow limits (285–295 mOsm/kg H$_2$O) by appropriate changes in water intake and excretion. Water balance is dependent on (*a*) access to water and an intact thirst mechanism, (*b*) extrarenal water losses, (*c*) appropriate renal excretion of solutes and water, and (*d*) intact antidiuretic hormone (ADH) biosynthesis, release, and response. Derangements in serum osmolality (S$_{osm}$), which are generally reflected by abnormalities in serum sodium concentration (S$_{Na}$), can cause serious neurologic dysfunction and death.

NORMAL WATER BALANCE

Total body water (TBW) constitutes 50% of lean body mass in women and 60% in men. It is distributed between intracellular (two-thirds of TBW) and extracellular (one-third of TBW) fluid compartments. Roughly one-fourth of the extracellular fluid (ECF) volume is intravascular (plasma), and the remaining three-fourths is primarily interstitial lymph fluid. Because most cell membranes are freely permeable to water, osmotic equilibrium between the intracellular fluid and the ECF is strictly maintained by appropriate fluid shifts between these compartments.

The principal intracellular osmoles are potassium salts, whereas sodium salts are the major ECF osmoles. Because ECF osmolality is equivalent to S$_{osm}$, the S$_{Na}$ directly correlates with the S_{osm}. Because elevated concentrations of blood urea nitrogen (BUN) or glucose can also increase S_{osm}, they should be included in the formal calculation of S_{osm}:

Sosm (mOsm/kg H2O) =

$$2 S_{Na} (mEq/L) + \frac{glucose\ (mg/dL)}{2.8} + \frac{BUN\ (mg/dL)}{18}$$

This calculated result should agree to within 10 mOsm/kg H_2O with the measured value of S_{osm}. A greater disparity between these values, an "osmolar gap," suggests either an error in measurement, pseudohyponatremia, or the presence of another osmotically active solute (e.g., mannitol, ethylene glycol) in the serum. Notably, S_{osm} can be increased by membrane-permeant solutes, termed "ineffective osmoles" (e.g., ethanol and urea), without affecting water distribution between the intracellular fluid and ECF. In contrast, "effective osmoles" (e.g., sodium, glucose, mannitol) are distributed mainly in the ECF and cause water to leave cells.

Discrete osmoregulatory systems in the hypothalamus for thirst and for ADH secretion respond in an integrated manner to small changes in S_{osm}. In addition, significant hypovolemia (>10% reduction in plasma volume) or hypotension can stimulate both thirst and ADH release through nonosmotic mechanisms. Thirst is the principal defense against hyperosmolality, whereas renal water excretion is the ultimate defense against hypoosmolality. ADH binds to specific receptors in the collecting duct to effect an increase in water permeability that promotes net water reabsorption into the interstitium. Maximal ADH action reduces urine output to 500 mL/day and increases urine osmolality (U_{osm}) to 800–1400 mOsm/kg H_2O. Complete absence of ADH results in a large diuresis (15–20 L/day) with a U_{osm} of 40–80 mOsm/kg H_2O. Any factor that impairs ADH release, tubular responsiveness to ADH, or medullary hypertonicity will also limit urinary concentrating ability.

Finally, it is important to recall that the S_{Na} is a measurement of *concentration*. It reflects the balance of body sodium and water. Changes in total body sodium alter effective circulating volume, whereas changes in S_{Na} generally reflect alterations in water balance. Thus, S_{Na} does not necessarily correlate with either effective circulating volume or with renal sodium excretion.

HYPONATREMIA (S_{Na} < 135 mEq/L)

This is the most frequent serum electrolyte abnormality in hospitalized patients, with an incidence of 1–2%.

Pathophysiology

Hyponatremia occurs when water intake exceeds water excretion. This can occur by (*a*) excess water intake (water intoxication) with normal renal function or (*b*) a continued solute-free water intake with decreased renal diluting capacity. Appropriate excretion of a water load requires the following:

- Adequate glomerular filtration without excessive proximal reabsorption to deliver tubular fluid to the diluting segments of the nephron (ascending limb of Henle and early distal convoluted tubule);
- Normal function of diluting segments of the nephron;
- Suppression of ADH to prevent reabsorption of solute-free water in collecting ducts.

Classification

A diagnostic and therapeutic tree is presented in Figure 10.1. Initial evaluation includes measurement of S_{osm} and an assessment of the effective circulating volume (as an index of total body sodium). Accurate serial recordings of body weight and intake-output may be especially valuable. Signs of *hypovolemia* include poor skin turgor, dry mucous membranes, dry axillae, flat neck veins, tachycardia, and postural hypotension. Hemoconcentration (increased hematocrit and serum protein), an increased BUN-to-creatinine ratio, and U_{Na} of <20 mEq/L are often present. *Hypervolemia* is usually manifested by an elevated jugular venous pressure and peripheral or presacral edema. Hemodilution (decreased hematocrit and serum protein) and a decreased BUN-to-creatinine ratio are often observed, whereas the U_{Na} is diagnostically less helpful.

ISOOSMOLAR HYPONATREMIA

Artifactual depression of the S_{Na}, termed "pseudohyponatremia," can occur when the fraction of plasma that is water (normally 92–94%) is decreased by excessive amounts of lipids or proteins. This may occur with severe hyperlipidemias (usually

Measure Serum Osmolality

- **Isoosmolar** (280–295 mOsm/kg H$_2$O)
  - Pseudohyponatremia
  - Isotonic infusion of glucose, mannitol, glycine

- **Hypoosmolar** (<280 mOsm/kg H$_2$O)

  Assess effective circulating volume status

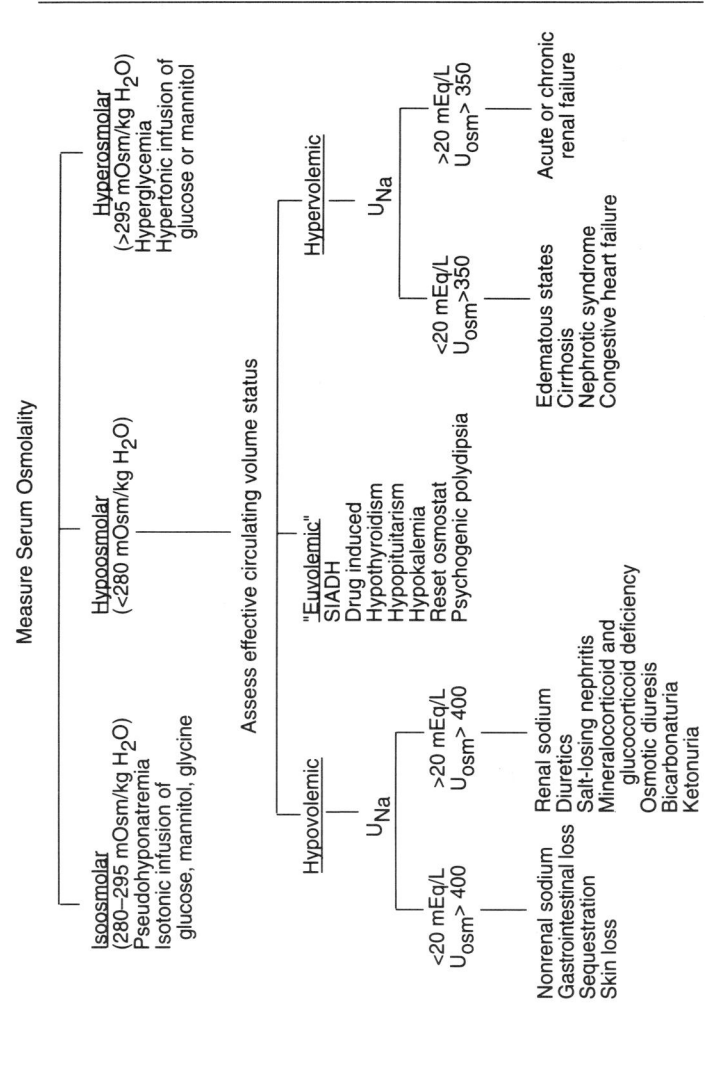

  - **Hypovolemic**
    - U_{Na}
      - <20 mEq/L, U_{osm} > 400
        - Nonrenal sodium
        - Gastrointestinal loss
        - Sequestration
        - Skin loss
      - >20 mEq/L, U_{osm} > 400
        - Renal sodium
        - Diuretics
        - Salt-losing nephritis
        - Mineralocorticoid and glucocorticoid deficiency
        - Osmotic diuresis
        - Bicarbonaturia
        - Ketonuria

  - **"Euvolemic"**
    - SIADH
    - Drug induced
    - Hypothyroidism
    - Hypopituitarism
    - Hypokalemia
    - Reset osmostat
    - Psychogenic polydipsia

  - **Hypervolemic**
    - U_{Na}
      - <20 mEq/L, U_{osm} > 350
        - Edematous states
        - Cirrhosis
        - Nephrotic syndrome
        - Congestive heart failure
      - >20 mEq/L, U_{osm} > 350
        - Acute or chronic renal failure

- **Hyperosmolar** (>295 mOsm/kg H$_2$O)
  - Hyperglycemia
  - Hypertonic infusion of glucose or mannitol

Figure 10.1. Hyponatremia.

serum triglycerides > 1500 mg/dL) or hyperproteinemias (serum protein > 10 g/dL). In these instances, the measured S_{osm} will be normal, but the serum osmolar gap will be increased. Pseudohyponatremia must be distinguished from the true, potentially serious hyponatremia with normal S_{osm} that can occur with infusions of isosmotic, sodium-free solutions (e.g., glycine in certain urologic procedures).

HYPOOSMOLAR HYPONATREMIA

Hypovolemic Hyponatremia

This condition implies a total body sodium deficit in excess of water losses and results primarily from renal or nonrenal sodium loss. The contracted effective circulating volume enhances isosmotic reabsorption of fluid in the proximal tubule and thereby limits fluid delivery to the distal diluting segments. With significant hypovolemia, nonosmotic stimulation of thirst and ADH also occur.

Nonrenal Sodium Loss

This usually results from the loss (e.g., vomiting, diarrhea) or sequestration (e.g., pancreatitis, peritonitis) of gastrointestinal fluids.

Renal Sodium Loss

Diuretic Administration. This is most frequently seen in elderly women receiving thiazides, which can impair fluid delivery to the diluting segments (owing to hypovolemia), inhibit NaCl reabsorption in the diluting segment, and potentiate ADH action and release.

Salt-Losing Nephritis. This can occur in patients with chronic renal failure given a sodium-deficient diet or in patients with relatively preserved glomerular filtration rate but significant interstitial disease (e.g., polycystic kidney disease, medullary cystic disease, chronic pyelonephritis).

Mineralocorticoid and Glucocorticoid Deficiency. A combination of volume depletion with enhanced proximal tubular reabsorption and nonosmotic stimulation of ADH may be implicated.

Osmotic Diuresis, Bicarbonaturia, Ketonuria. Excessive amounts of osmotically active solutes (e.g., glucose, bicarbonate, or ketones) in the urine can obligate excessive renal sodium and water excretion.

"Euvolemic" Hyponatremia

These patients generally have an increased TBW (by 3–5 L) but normal total body sodium content and no edema. This class of disorders results from nonphysiologic secretion, potentiation, or inappropriate action of ADH.

Syndrome of Inappropriate ADH Secretion (SIADH)

This is generally associated with (*a*) malignancies (e.g., bronchogenic carcinoma), (*b*) pulmonary disorders (e.g., pneumonia), (*c*) neuropsychiatric disorders, or (*d*) the postoperative period. SIADH is a diagnosis of exclusion and requires that the patient has no causes for nonosmotic ADH release (e.g., hypovolemia, nausea) and no other cause of decreased diluting capacity (e.g., thyroid, renal, adrenal, cardiac, or liver disease). The urine is less than maximally dilute (>100 mOsm/kg H_2O) despite serum hypoosmolality, and U_{Na} is usually >20 mEq/L. Hypouricemia (<4 mg/dL) is a useful diagnostic clue. Because hyponatremia itself implies impaired urinary dilution, the diagnosis is confirmed by an elevated ADH level and does not require a formal urine dilution test.

Reset Osmostat

This is most commonly seen in pregnant women and results from down-regulation of the central osmoreceptors. ADH release varies appropriately with changes in S_{osm}, but the S_{osm} threshold for ADH release is below normal. S_{Na}, although reduced, remains stable, because water excretion is normal.

Psychogenic Polydipsia

Psychotic patients can drink sufficient volumes of fluid to exceed their capacity to excrete free water. In addition, these patients often have a subtle impairment of urinary dilution.

Drugs

Drugs that potentiate ADH action:

Clofibrate;
Cyclophosphamide;
Nonsteroidal antiinflammatory agents;
ADH analogues.

Drugs that stimulate ADH release:

Vincristine;
Carbamazepine;
Narcotics;
Barbiturates.

Drugs that potentiate ADH action and stimulate its release:

Thiazide diuretics;
Chlorpropamide;
ADH analogues.

Hypervolemic Hyponatremia

Patients with edema (e.g., congestive heart failure, nephrotic syndrome, and cirrhosis with ascites) can have an increased TBW that exceeds the increase in total body sodium. In these patients, a reduced effective circulating volume (from reduced cardiac output or peripheral arterial vasodilation) decreases filtrate delivery to the diluting segment and stimulates ADH release. In the absence of concomitant diuretic use, U_{Na} is usually <15 mEq/L, and U_{osm} is >350 mOsm/kg H_2O. In addition, acute or chronic renal failure can cause hyponatremia because renal diluting capacity is reduced.

Clinical Presentation

Most patients with hyponatremia are asymptomatic. Symptoms generally occur only when significant hyponatremia (S_{Na} < 125 mEq) has evolved in <24 hr *(acute hyponatremia)*. Nausea, vomiting, and headache are common presenting symptoms, but the clinical course can rapidly deteriorate to seizures, coma, and respiratory arrest. Severe, acute hyponatremia (S_{Na} < 120 mEq/L, developing over <24 hr) has a mortality of up to 50% owing to complications of cerebral edema.

In *chronic hyponatremia* (hyponatremia developing over >48 hr), symptoms may be less specific (e.g., lethargy, confusion, muscle cramps) but can progress to serious neurologic dysfunction. Chronic hyponatremia has a lower mortality (<10%), with death generally attributable to the underlying disease. The slower onset of hyponatremia allows for compensatory loss of intracellular potassium and amino acids to normalize cellular water content in the brain.

Treatment

Acute Versus Chronic Hyponatremia

Correction of hyponatremia in patients who are asymptomatic or who have only subtle neurologic dysfunction (and thus likely have chronic hyponatremia) should be gradual. Administration of isotonic saline or water restriction, as appropriate (described below), and frequent measurements of S_{Na} should be employed. Overzealous correction of S_{Na} in patients with chronic hyponatremia has been associated with the cerebral demyelination syndrome (e.g., central pontine myelinolysis), which can result in flaccid paralysis and death.

In contrast, in patients with *acute symptomatic hyponatremia* (duration < 24 hr), more rapid correction of hyponatremia is indicated, because the risks of complications from cerebral edema outweigh any risk of treatment. The choice of 3% saline versus isotonic saline in the treatment of these patients remains somewhat controversial and should be guided by the severity of the clinical condition and the availability of intensive clinical monitoring. These patients should be admitted to an intensive care unit for monitoring of electrolytes, blood pressure, neurologic status, and renal function. S_{Na} must be measured frequently during its correction. A loop diuretic (e.g., furosemide, 1 mg/kg body weight) should be given to initiate and maintain a salt and water diuresis. Hourly urinary sodium and potassium losses should be measured and replaced with 3% NaCl (513 mEq sodium/L) and KCl until S_{Na} has increased by 10% or symptoms have resolved. Thereafter, slower correction of S_{Na} by water restriction should be prescribed. The rate of S_{Na} correction should never exceed 1.5–2.0 mEq/L/hr or 20 mEq/L/day. It is important to ensure that during treatment of hyponatremia the S_{Na} is raised only to the normal range. Central pontine myelinolysis has been correlated both with too rapid correction of hyponatremia and with its overcorrection in patients with chronic hyponatremia.

Hypovolemic Hyponatremia

Initial therapy should include discontinuation of diuretics, correction of nonrenal fluid losses, and expansion of the effective circulating volume with 0.9% NaCl to replace one-third of the sodium deficit over 6 hr and the remainder over 24–48 hr. Total body sodium deficit for a man (for a woman substitute 0.5 for 0.6 to calculate TBW) can be estimated from the following equation:

$$\text{sodium deficit (mEq)} = 0.6 \times \text{LBM (kg)} \times (140 - S_{Na})$$

Euvolemic Hyponatremia

The hyponatremia can usually be treated by water restriction to 1 L/day. The volume of excess water that needs to be excreted to normalize S_{Na} can be calculated as

$$\text{excess water (L)} = \text{current TBW} - \text{normal TBW}$$

where current TBW = $0.6 \times$ current lean body mass and

$$\text{normal TBW} = \frac{(0.6 \times \text{current LBM}) \times \text{current } S_{Na}}{\text{normal } S_{Na}}$$

When the cause of SIADH is not reversible, *demeclocycline* (600–1200 mg/day) or *lithium carbonate* (300 mg po three times daily) can be used to induce a state of nephrogenic diabetes insipidus.

Hypervolemic Hyponatremia

Initial therapy should include salt and fluid restriction if the hyponatremia is due to the primary disease. Therapy to improve cardiac output (if reduced) should also be optimized. Patients with renal failure may require dialytic therapy to remove the excess fluid.

HYPEROSMOLAR HYPONATREMIA

Hypertonic infusions of glucose, mannitol, or glycine can cause osmotic shifts of intracellular fluid to ECF with reduction in S_{Na}:

For every 100 mg/dL glucose greater than 100 mg/dL, S_{Na} will fall by 1.6 mEq/L.

HYPERNATREMIA

Hypernatremia (S_{Na} > 145 mEq/L) is less frequent than hyponatremia but occurs in about 1% of hospitalized elderly patients.

Pathophysiology

Hypernatremia implies a relative deficiency of TBW compared with total body sodium. In general, this results from excessive water loss or from excessive sodium retention (e.g., administration of hypertonic NaCl or $NaHCO_3$). Normally, a small increase in S_{osm} stimulates ADH secretion and thereby increases renal water retention. Because hypertonicity also stimulates thirst, even patients who are ADH deficient (central diabetes insipidus) can maintain their S_{osm} if they can drink.

Etiology

Hypernatremia can be readily classified according to the total body sodium content and the state of hydration.

Decreased Total Body Sodium

Loss of hypotonic body fluids results in effective circulating volume depletion and hypernatremia. The usual signs of hypovolemia are present. Hypotonic fluid losses can occur from extrarenal and renal sources.

Extrarenal Sources. Skin or gastrointestinal losses (e.g., vomiting, nasogastric suction, osmotic diarrhea) are common. The renal response leads to a high U_{osm} (>800 mOsm/kg H_2O) and a low U_{Na} (<10 mEq/L).

Renal Sources. Hypotonic polyuria can be produced by (*a*) diuretics; (*b*) osmotic diuresis caused by glucose, mannitol, or urea (e.g., postobstructive diuresis); or (*c*) nonoliguric ATN. The urine may be either hypotonic or isotonic, and the U_{Na} is usually >20 mEq/L. More commonly, osmotic agents shift fluid to the ECF compartment resulting in *hypo*natremia.

Normal Total Body Sodium

Losses of free water can result in hypernatremia. Evidence of volume contraction is lacking unless the water losses are extreme. The usual causes include extrarenal and renal water loss.

Extrarenal Water Loss. Both skin and pulmonary losses of water can result in hypernatremia. In addition, water can be drawn from the ECF into damaged cells (e.g., rhabdomyolysis) with similar consequences. The U_{osm} is high, and U_{Na} is a function of sodium intake.

Renal Water Loss. This more common cause of excess water loss is usually due to partial or complete failure to synthesize or secrete ADH (central diabetes insipidus) or to diminished or absent renal response to its action (nephrogenic diabetes insipidus). These disorders are characterized by an inability to concentrate the urine maximally, the result of both ADH deficiency (or resistance) and washout of the medullary osmotic gradient by chronic polyuria. Approximately half of the cases of central diabetes insipidus are idiopathic (usually diagnosed in childhood). The remainder are caused by head trauma, hypoxic or ischemic encephalopathy, and central nervous system neoplasms. Patients with nephrogenic diabetes insipidus have impaired urinary concentrating ability despite maximal synthesis and release of ADH. Nephrogenic diabetes insipidus results from (*a*) a failure of the countercurrent mechanism to generate a hypertonic medullary and papillary interstitium and/or (*b*) a failure of ADH to increase the water permeability of the collecting duct. Nephrogenic diabetes insipidus may be congenital but more commonly is acquired. Chronic diseases of the renal medulla (e.g., medullary cystic disease, pyelonephritis), poor protein or salt intake, hypercalcemia, hypokalemia, various systemic diseases (e.g., amyloidosis, multiple myeloma), and numerous drugs (e.g., demeclocycline, lithium, glyburide) have been implicated as causes of nephrogenic diabetes insipidus.

Increased Total Body Sodium

This is usually an iatrogenic complication resulting from administration of hypertonic sodium-containing solutions (e.g., $NaHCO_3$ given to patients with metabolic acidosis) or from

Table 10.1
Fluid Deprivation Test

During the test, urine output, weight, and vital signs must be strictly monitored to prevent severe volume contraction; weight loss should not exceed 3–5%

Patients with mild polyuria (<10 L/day) should have fluids withheld the night preceding the test (e.g., 6 PM); patients with severe polyuria (>10 L/day) should be fluid deprived only during the day (e.g., 6 AM) to allow close observation; time to achieve a maximal U_{osm} varies from 4 to 18 hr

S_{osm} should approach 295 mOsm/kg H_2O after fluid deprivation and before ADH administration

U_{osm} is measured at baseline and hourly until two values vary by <30 mOsm/kg H_2O or 3–5% of body weight is lost

Five units subcutaneous aqueous vasopressin or 10 µg intranasal DDAVP are administered, and 1 hr later a final U_{osm} is measured

DDAVP, deamino-8-D-arginine vasopressin.

inappropriate repletion of hypotonic insensible fluid losses with 0.9% saline in critically ill patients.

Clinical Presentation and Diagnosis

Signs and symptoms of hypernatremia include lethargy, restlessness, hyperreflexia, spasticity, and seizures, which may progress to coma and death. Patients with central or nephrogenic diabetes insipidus may have profound polyuria and polydipsia. Cerebral dehydration leads to capillary and venous congestion, cerebrovascular tears, venous sinus thrombosis, and subcortical-subarachnoid hemorrhages. Mortality in infants and children is 43% in acute and 7–29% in chronic hypernatremia, whereas adults with acute hypernatremia have mortality rates as high as 60%.

Central diabetes insipidus can be distinguished from nephrogenic diabetes insipidus by the *fluid deprivation test* followed by exogenous ADH administration (Table 10.1). Patients with severe central diabetes insipidus have baseline S_{osm} and S_{Na} that are high normal, and their urinary concentrating ability improves after ADH treatment but not after water deprivation. In patients with severe nephrogenic diabetes insipidus, baseline S_{osm} is also increased, but they fail to respond to either ADH treatment or water deprivation. A more direct approach to distinguish central diabetes insipidus is to measure plasma or urine ADH levels simultaneously with S_{osm} after either fluid restriction or hypertonic saline infusion. Patients with central diabetes insipidus will have subnormal levels of ADH for the level of S_{osm}, whereas patients with nephrogenic diabetes insipidus will exhibit normal or elevated ratios.

Treatment

Decreased Total Body Sodium

Initially patients should receive isotonic NaCl until the effective circulating volume has been restored. Thereafter, hypotonic solutions (D_5W or 0.45% NaCl) can be used.

Normal Total Body Sodium

Pure water loss should be replaced with D_5W. Free water deficit (FWD) can be calculated as follows:

$$\text{FWD (L)} = (0.6 \times \text{current LBM}) \times \frac{\text{current } S_{Na} - 140}{140}$$

Normally the free water deficit should be replaced over 48 hr with frequent monitoring of the S_{Na} and S_{osm}. The S_{osm} should decrease by approximately 1–2 mOsm/kg H_2O/hr. Faster rates of correction can cause seizures.

The treatment of choice for central diabetes insipidus is intranasal deamino-8-D-arginine vasopressin (DDAVP), a synthetic analogue of ADH, 10–20 µg twice daily. Therapy for acquired nephrogenic diabetes insipidus should be directed toward the primary disorder. Thiazide diuretics and a low salt intake will decrease the polyuria.

Increased Total Body Sodium

Hypertonic sodium-containing solutions should be discontinued and diuretics administered to promote excretion of the excess salt and water.

Suggested Readings

Anderson RJ. Hospital-associated hyponatremia. Kidney Int 1986; 29:1237–1247.

Arieff AI. Hyponatremia associated with permanent brain damage. Adv Intern Med 1987;32:325–344.

Berl T. Treating hyponatremia: damned if we do and damned if we don't. Kidney Int 1990;37:1006–1018.

Marsden PA, Halperin ML. Pathophysiological approach to patients presenting with hypernatremia. Am J Nephrol 1985;5:229–235.

Robertson GL, Berl T. Pathophysiology of water metabolism. In: Brenner BM, Rector FC Jr, eds. The kidney. Philadelphia: Saunders, 1991: 677–736.

Schrier RW. Body fluid volume regulation in health and disease: a unifying hypothesis. Ann Intern Med 1990;113:155–159.

Chapter 11

Potassium Disorders

Charles S. Wingo

Hypokalemia (serum potassium (S_K) < 3.5 mEq/L or mmol/L) and hyperkalemia (S_K > 5.0 mEq/L) are both common and potentially lethal.

PHYSIOLOGY

Of the normal daily potassium intake of 50–150 mEq, approximately 90% is eliminated in the urine. However, with compromised renal function, up to 30% of daily potassium intake may be eliminated in the feces. When diarrhea is present, enteric losses of potassium can be substantial. Because only 2% of total body potassium is in the extracellular fluid and 98% is intracellular, factors causing transcellular potassium shifts can lead to large changes in S_K.

Insulin promotes cellular potassium uptake through stimulation of Na^+-K^+-ATPase. Hyperkalemia stimulates insulin release, whereas hypokalemia has an inhibitory effect.

Catecholamines, particularly the β_2 agonists such as terbutaline, stimulate Na^+-K^+-ATPase and can cause hypokalemia. In contrast, β-blockers such as propranolol can cause hyperkalemia.

Aldosterone stimulates cellular potassium uptake and facilitates renal potassium excretion. This hormone stimulates Na^+-K^+-ATPase in the renal collecting duct, colon, sweat glands, and muscles. Aldosterone deficiency can cause mild hyperkalemia, which may become severe if renal function is impaired or if sodium intake is restricted.

Metabolic acidosis promotes hyperkalemia, whereas *alkalosis* promotes hypokalemia. Administration of acids such as HCl or

NH_4Cl increases S_K, but organic acids (lactic, β-hydroxybutyric) and respiratory acid-base disorders have smaller effects on S_K.

RENAL REGULATION OF POTASSIUM

Renal potassium excretion is primarily due to active transport in the collecting duct. This segment has the capacity for active potassium secretion and active potassium absorption. Active potassium secretion occurs largely in the cortical collecting duct and its proximal extension, the initial collecting tubule. It depends on sodium absorption and requires the active cellular uptake of potassium from the peritubular fluid. Conductive sodium entry at the luminal membrane is necessary for sodium extrusion in exchange for potassium uptake by basolaterally oriented Na^+-K^+-ATPase. Potassium is secreted passively at the luminal membrane via either potassium channels or coupled to chloride secretion. Potassium secretion is stimulated by hyperkalemia, a reduction in luminal chloride concentration, increased tubular fluid flow, increased distal sodium delivery, and diuretics. Dietary potassium loading and chronic hyperaldosteronism each stimulate potassium secretion by the cortical collecting duct.

The kidney conserves potassium when potassium intake is reduced by active potassium reabsorption largely in the medullary collecting duct but also in the cortical collecting duct. This process is mediated by a luminal proton-potassium pump, an H^+,K^+-ATPase.

HYPOKALEMIA

Evaluation

Evaluation should begin with a careful history and physical examination. Particular attention should be given to the drug history and assessment of the patient's volume status and blood pressure. Table 11.1 provides a differential diagnosis for hypokalemia.

The clinical manifestations of hypokalemia are usually present at concentrations below 2.5 mEq/L or with a rapid fall in S_K (Table 11.2).

A diagnostic approach to hypokalemia is detailed in Figure 11.1. Measurements of blood pressure and blood and urinary

Table 11.1
Differential Diagnosis of Hypokalemia

Artifactual (high white blood cell count, leukemia)
Redistribution (cellular shift)
    β-Adrenergic agonists (epinephrine, terbutaline)
    Alkalosis
    Theophylline toxicity
    Refeeding (intravenous hyperalimentation)
    Insulin administration
    Periodic paralysis (familial, thyrotoxic)
    Barium poisoning
    Mineralocorticoid excess (both renal and extrarenal effects, see below)
Inadequate dietary intake
Gastrointestinal losses
    Diarrhea and chronic laxative abuse
    Ureterosigmoidostomy (urinary diversion)
    Villous adenoma
    Gastrointestinal fistulas
Renal losses
    Metabolic alkalosis (vomiting or nasogastric drainage)
    Diuretics
    Hypomagnesemia (frequently associated with diuretics)
    Antibiotic/antifungal/chemotherapeutic agents
        Penicillins (e.g., carbenicillin)
        Amphotericin B (renal tubular acidosis)
        Aminoglycosides
        Cis-platin
    Glucocorticoids (causes both increased cellular potassium loss and increased excretion)
    Cushing's syndrome
    Mineralocorticoid excess (enhanced renal potassium clearance)
        Adrenal adenoma or bilateral adrenal hyperplasia
        Glycyrrhizic acid intoxication (licorice ingestion)
        Adrenal enzyme deficiency syndromes
    Renal tubular acidosis (drug-induced, classic distal and proximal)
    Acute renal failure syndromes (typically observed with recovery of renal function)
        Diuretic phase of acute tubular necrosis
        Postobstructive diuresis
        Interstitial nephritis
    Bartter's syndrome
    Acute leukemia (lysozymuria)

Table 11.2
Clinical Manifestations of Hypokalemia

Cardiac
  Predisposition to digitalis glycoside toxicity
  Ventricular irritability
  Abnormal ECG (flattened T waves, U waves, and ST segment depression)
  Coronary artery spasm
Neuromuscular
  Skeletal (weakness, cramps, tetany, paralysis, and rhabdomyolysis)
  Gastrointestinal (constipation, ileus)
  Encephalopathy (in patients with liver disease)
Renal
  Polyuria (nephrogenic diabetes insipidus), polydipsia
  Increased ammoniagenesis
  Decreased renal blood flow (increased renal vascular resistance)
Endocrine and metabolic
  Carbohydrate intolerance
  Decreased plasma aldosterone concentration

electrolytes are of central importance. Serum magnesium and arterial blood gases may provide critical information. Additional studies include plasma renin, aldosterone, and cortisol. One should first determine whether hypokalemia is artifactual, the result of redistribution of potassium, or a representation of true potassium depletion. Artifactual values may be seen in leukemic patients with a white blood cell count of 100,000–250,000; to avoid spurious values, plasma from leukemic patients should be separated quickly.

True hypokalemia can be due to either renal or extrarenal mechanisms. In the latter case frank renal conservation is present. In this case renal potassium excretion is <20 mEq/day unless aggressive potassium replacement has begun. If urinary potassium excretion equals or exceeds potassium intake in the face of hypokalemia, a renal mechanism is, at least in part, responsible for the hypokalemia.

Hypokalemia in the hypertensive patient can be due to diuretics, potassium depletion, and primary mineralocorticoid excess (e.g., hyperaldosteronism). Glucocorticoid excess (e.g., Cushing's syndrome) is less frequently associated with hypokalemia. Whereas thiazides and loop diuretics are a common cause of hypokalemia, these agents seldom produce severe hypokale-

Hypokalemia

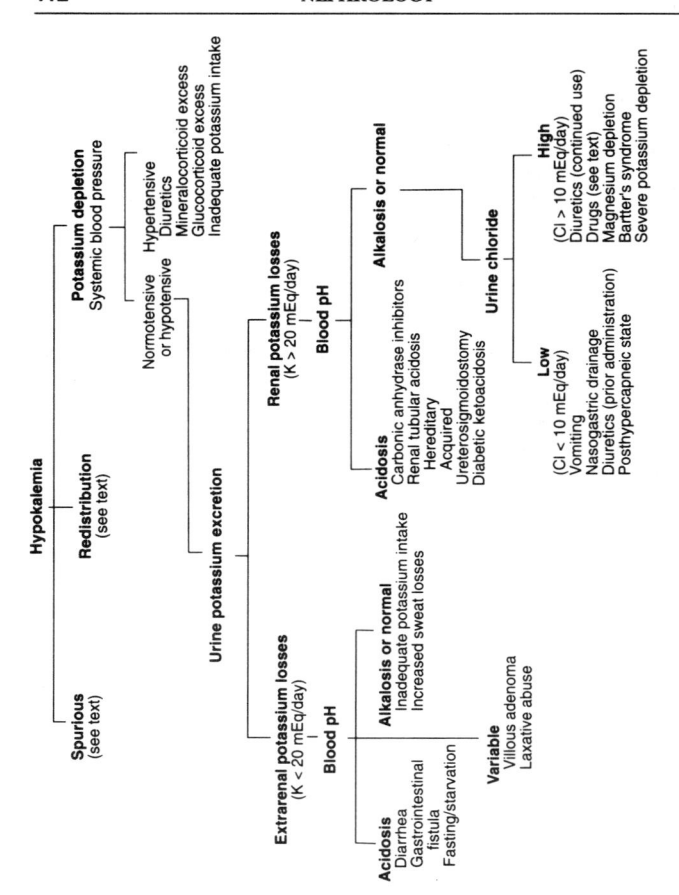

- **Spurious** (see text)
- **Redistribution** (see text)
- **Potassium depletion**
  - Systemic blood pressure
    - Hypertensive
      - Diuretics
      - Mineralocorticoid excess
      - Glucocorticoid excess
      - Inadequate potassium intake
    - Normotensive or hypotensive
      - Urine potassium excretion
        - **Extrarenal potassium losses** (K < 20 mEq/day)
          - Blood pH
            - Acidosis
              - Diarrhea
              - Gastrointestinal fistula
              - Fasting/starvation
            - Alkalosis or normal
              - Inadequate potassium intake
              - Increased sweat losses
            - Variable
              - Villous adenoma
              - Laxative abuse
        - **Renal potassium losses** (K > 20 mEq/day)
          - Blood pH
            - Acidosis
              - Carbonic anhydrase inhibitors
              - Renal tubular acidosis
                - Hereditary
                - Acquired
              - Ureterosigmoidostomy
              - Diabetic ketoacidosis
            - Alkalosis or normal
              - Urine chloride
                - Low (Cl < 10 mEq/day)
                  - Vomiting
                  - Nasogastric drainage
                  - Diuretics (prior administration)
                  - Posthypercapneic state
                - High (Cl > 10 mEq/day)
                  - Diuretics (continued use)
                  - Drugs (see text)
                  - Magnesium depletion
                  - Bartter's syndrome
                  - Severe potassium depletion

Figure 11.1. Diagnostic approach in hypokalemic patients.

mia (S_K < 3.0 mEq/L) without other compounding factors such as a large sodium and reduced potassium intake, magnesium depletion, or hyperaldosteronism. Plasma renin activity helps to distinguish the hypertensive patient with diuretic-induced hypokalemia from the individual with excessive mineralocorticoid activity. Plasma renin activity is nearly always increased with diuretic-induced hypokalemia but is invariably suppressed in uncomplicated hyperaldosteronism.

Treatment

S_K is not an exact indicator of the total body potassium deficit, but severe hypokalemia with serum potassium levels below 3.0 mEq/L generally reflect potassium deficits of >300 mEq, whereas serum potassium levels of <2.0 mEq/L may reflect deficits of more than 1000 mEq. Four factors should be considered in the correction of hypokalemia:

1. *Acid-base status: Correction of coexisting metabolic acidosis*, particularly diabetic ketoacidosis, can cause the S_K to decrease further.
2. *Intravenous glucose administration* can cause potassium levels to decrease. In life-threatening hypokalemia, initial potassium replacement should be given in glucose-free solutions.
3. *Overzealous administration of potassium* can cause hyperkalemia, especially with impaired renal function or with long-standing potassium depletion. In the latter case aldosterone secretion is suppressed; hence, extrarenal potassium uptake is impaired. Urine output should be adequate before potassium replacement, and S_K should be checked periodically.
4. *Coexisting hypomagnesemia* can prevent correction of hypokalemia.

Intravenous potassium is reserved for patients unable to take potassium orally or in life-threatening situations (e.g., paralysis, digitalis intoxication (with arrhythmias), hypokalemic-induced hepatic coma) and those with electrocardiogram (ECG) abnormalities. Oral therapy (20–120 mEq/day) rarely causes "overshoot" hyperkalemia in the presence of nearly normal renal function. Over-the-counter salt substitutes are an economical source of potassium and contain 15–40 mEq/teaspoon. KCl is the appropriate replacement therapy for potassium depletion and should be used when there is chloride depletion and metabolic alkalosis. Liquid or enteric-coated preparations can cause gastrointestinal irritation or ulceration. Wax matrix KCl tablets are generally preferable.

Intravenous potassium can be given safely at rates of 10 mEq/hr by peripheral vein without ECG monitoring and in concentrations of up to 30 mEq/L (to avoid pain or phlebitis). If the serum potassium is <2.5 mEq/L in association with ECG abnormalities or severe neuromuscular complications, doses of 40 mEq/hr can be given through a central venous catheter with continuous ECG monitoring; *however, doses of this magnitude are rarely necessary.* Frequent determinations of S_K are the best guide to replacement therapy (every 4–6 hr).

Treatment of chronic hypokalemia includes the use of oral potassium supplements or the potassium-sparing diuretics: spironolactone (50–100 mg daily), triamterene (50–100 mg once or twice daily), or amiloride (5–10 mg daily). Combined use of potassium supplements and potassium-sparing diuretics is usually contraindicated.

HYPERKALEMIA

Evaluation

An S_K above 5.0 mEq/L may reflect true hyperkalemia or may be spurious (pseudohyperkalemia; see Table 11.3). Key points in the history include diet, medications, individual or family history of renal disease, and assessment of urine volume or evidence of obstruction. Helpful clinical symptoms or signs include weakness, paresthesias, and flaccid paralysis. *However, these findings may be absent despite the presence of life threatening hyperkalemia.* Any ECG finding of hyperkalemia is potentially life threatening because progression to ventricular fibrillation may be rapid and unpredictable (Table 11.4).

Diagnosis

First, eliminate spurious hyperkalemia by drawing a fresh blood sample through a large-bore needle (to avoid hemolysis) without prolonged tourniquet time for plasma potassium determination

Table 11.3
Causes of Hyperkalemia

Spurious
  Hemolysis
  Thrombocytosis
  Leukocytosis
  Ischemic blood drawing
  Infectious mononucleosis
  Familial pseudohyperkalemia
Redistribution
  Increased cellular potassium release
    Exercise
    Tissue necrosis or trauma (rhabdomyolysis, hematoma, etc.)
    Hyperkalemic periodic paralysis, succinylcholine
    Hyperosmolality
  Decreased cellular potassium uptake
    Insulin deficiency (e.g., diabetic ketoacidosis)
    Aldosterone deficiency or blockade (spirolactone)
    β-Adrenergic blockers (e.g., propranolol)
    Digitalis poisoning
  Other
    Exogenous potassium administration (particularly intravenously)
    Arginine and lysine administration
    Fluoride intoxication
    Acidosis
Decreased renal clearance
  Acute or chronic renal failure
  Hyperkalemic renal tubular acidosis
  Drug-induced hyperkalemia (see Table 11.5)
  Mineralocorticoid deficiency (acquired and hereditary forms)
  Hyperkalemic hypertensive syndrome

Table 11.4
ECG Findings in Hyperkalemia

Peaking or tenting of T waves
Flattening of P waves
Prolongation of PR interval
Widening of QRS complex (to sine wave)
Ventricular fibrillation, asystole, or both

(heparized tube). The white blood cell and platelet count should be evaluated also. If the clinical and initial laboratory findings suggest the need for urgent treatment, ECG confirmation of hyperkalemia may often be quicker than confirmation by measurement of plasma potassium. Moreover, this approach allows monitoring of the effectiveness of therapy.

Pseudohyperkalemia occurs from potassium released during clotting when the platelet count is >1,000,000 or the white blood cell count is >200,000. In such cases the discrepancy between serum potassium and plasma potassium values may exceed 1.0 mEq/L. Rarely, pseudohyperkalemia may be due to "leaky" erythrocytes of either acquired (infectious mononucleosis) or hereditary etiology.

In the absence of pseudohyperkalemia or potassium redistribution (Table 11.3), a S_K above 5.0 mEq/L reflects reduced renal potassium clearance. Diminished renal potassium clearance is frequently observed when renal function is severely compromised (GFR < 20 mL/min) or with modest renal insufficiency (GFR = 20–60 mL/min) and impaired collecting duct function. In the latter case, patients may exhibit hyperkalemic renal tubular acidosis (HRTA). Conditions frequently present in patients with hyperkalemia include diabetic nephropathy, interstitial nephritis, and drug-induced hyperkalemia (Table 11.5). Most of these patients have some degree of intrinsic renal parenchymal disease. In contrast, less common causes of dimin-

Table 11.5
Drug-Induced Hyperkalemia

Common
  Potassium-sparing diuretics
  Nonsteroidal antiinflammatory drugs
  Cyclosporine
  Heparin
  Angiotensin-converting enzyme inhibitors
  Pentamidine
  Sulfamethoxazole-trimethoprim (high dose therapy)
Uncommon
  β-Adrenergic antagonists
  Succinylcholine
  Digitalis poisoning

ished renal potassium clearance such as defective adrenal mineralocorticoid production and the rare hyperkalemic hypertensive syndrome are not due to intrinsic renal parenchymal disease.

HRTA may reflect either increased potassium reabsorption or diminished potassium secretion in the collecting duct. These patients usually have modest renal insufficiency, and both hypertension and edema are frequently present. Patients with true hyporeninemic hypoaldosteronism represent a subset of HRTA with impaired potassium secretion. In hyporeninemic hypoaldosteronism, plasma renin and plasma aldosterone values are decreased, but plasma cortisol values are normal. Mineralocorticoid replacement therapy should restore S_K to normal in patients with hyporeninemic hypoaldosteronism. However, this approach may aggravate fluid retention and hypertension that is present in most patients with HRTA. For this reason, HRTA is usually best managed with the combination of a loop diuretic and $NaHCO_3$ therapy.

Patients with adrenal cortical insufficiency (Addison's disease) may exhibit mild degrees of hyperkalemia, but impairment of renal sodium conservation is usually the predominant clinical finding. These individuals typically have hyperpigmentation, hypotension, hyponatremia, salt (NaCl) wasting, and acidosis. However, hyperkalemia can be severe during periods of volume depletion or in an addisonian crisis. Treatment consists of saline administration and both glucocorticoid and mineralocorticoid replacement therapy.

Table 11.6 lists laboratory and diagnostic tests that are helpful in establishing the etiology of hyperkalemia. Frequent causes of hyperkalemia include drugs, intravenous potassium administration, and renal disease. The presence of "dirty-brown casts" in the urine sediment may suggest the diagnosis of acute tubular nephrosis. Bladder catheterization (to eliminate bladder neck obstruction) and renal ultrasonography (to eliminate hydronephrosis or small kidneys of end-stage renal disease) are important considerations.

Treatment

Hyperkalemia is life threatening because of its effects on cardiac conduction. Drug therapy for the acute treatment of hyperkale-

Table 11.6
Laboratory and Diagnostic Tests to Evaluate Hyperkalemia

Urinalysis
Bladder catheterization
Renal ultrasound
ECG
Urine and serum electrolytes
Serum creatinine and blood urea nitrogen
Arterial blood gases and pH
White blood cell count
Platelet count
Hematocrit (if low, may indicate chronic renal failure)

Table 11.7
Drug Therapy for Hyperkalemia

Drug	Dose	Onset of Action (min)
Calcium gluconate or chloride	10–30 mL (10% solution) iv	1–2
$NaHCO_3$	50 mEq iv	15–30
Glucose/insulin	25–50 g glucose iv/5 units regular insulin (repeat every 15 min)	15–30
Kayexalate	Enema 50–100 g or oral 40 g (see text)	60–120

mia is listed in Table 11.7. Simultaneous use of several or all of these measures may be indicated if ECG abnormalities exist. With the exception of Na^+-K^+ exchange resins, none of the treatments remove potassium from the body and should be considered as temporary measures. Severe hyperkalemia often requires emergent dialysis.

Calcium rapidly antagonizes the effects of potassium on cardiac conduction, but the effect lasts for only 15–20 min. The dose listed below can be repeated once, but further doses are generally ineffective. Calcium should not be administered in solutions that contain bicarbonate because of precipitation of calcium carbonate in the infusion line. Sodium bicarbonate

($NaHCO_3$) administration can be repeated every 15 min if ECG changes persist. However, $NaHCO_3$ ampules are hypertonic and can cause hypernatremia, volume expansion, and circulatory overload. Moreover, the high osmolality of these solutions can result in cellular potassium loss (secondary to solvent drag) that mitigates the correction of the hyperkalemia. Alternatively, 2 ampules $NaHCO_3$ can be mixed with 1 L $D_{10}W$ and 25–50 units regular insulin. This solution can be infused at 300–500 mL for the first 30 min and the rate titrated to S_K values thereafter.

Sodium polystyrene sulfonate (Kayexalate) is a Na^+-K^+ exchange resin that binds approximately 1 mEq potassium/g resin orally and 0.5 mEq potassium/g resin by enema. Oral doses are usually given in a hyperosmotic sorbitol solution (20%) to promote rapid gastrointestinal transit and should be repeated every 2–4 hr until S_K is normal. If the patient is nauseated, retention enemas are preferred.

Approximately 50–100 g of the resin in water are placed through a Foley catheter inserted rectally; the balloon is inflated to ensure retention for 30–60 min. Enemas should be repeated every 2–4 hr as needed. Both oral and rectal administration can precipitate circulatory overload secondary to sodium absorption.

Dialysis should be employed where hyperkalemia is complicated by volume overload, severe uremia, or acidosis (see Chapter 22). Hemodialysis can remove potassium at a rate of 25–30 mEq/hr, whereas peritoneal dialysis can remove 10–15 mEq/hr.

Treatment of chronic hyperkalemia (chronic renal failure, HRTA) first entails dietary restriction of potassium to 40–60 mEq/day. Loop diuretics are beneficial, especially in patients who have edema and hypertension, but potassium-sparing diuretics (amiloride, triamterene, spironolactone) are clearly contraindicated. Oral bicarbonate therapy can also be employed with initial doses of $NaHCO_3$ of 650 mg three times a day and increased as needed to maintain a serum total CO_2 of 22–24 mEq/L. Sodium polystyrene sulfonate can be used orally in doses of 15–60 g four times a day. Finally, fludrocortisone acetate (Florinef) can be given in initial doses of 0.1–0.3 mg daily in patients without evidence of volume expansion, hypertension, or circulatory overload. Hypertension and sodium retention complicate its use.

Suggested Readings

Gabow PA, Peterson LN. Disorders of potassium metabolism. In: Schrier RW, ed. Renal and electrolyte disorders. Boston: Little, Brown, 1986:207–249.

Magner PO, Robinson L, Halperin RM, Zettle R, Halperin ML. The plasma potassium concentration in metabolic acidosis: a reevaluation. Am J Kidney Dis 1988;11:220–224.

Narins RG, Jones ER, Stom MC, Rudnick MR, Bastl CP. Diagnostic strategies in disorders of fluid, electrolyte and acid-base homeostasis. Am J Med 1982;72:496–519.

Ponce SP, Jennings AE, Madias NE, Harrington JT. Drug-induced hyperkalemia. Medicine 1985;64:357–370.

Stokes JB. Ion transport by the collecting duct. Semin Nephrol 1993;13:202–212.

Tannen RL. Potassium disorders. In: Kokko JP, Tannen RL, eds. Fluids and electrolytes, 2nd ed. Philadelphia: Saunders, 1990:195–256.

Wingo CS, Armitage FE. Potassium transport in the kidney: regulation and physiological relevance of H^+,K^+-ATPase. Semin Nephrol 1993;13:213–224.

Wright FS, Giebisch G. Regulation of potassium excretion. In: Seldin DW, Giebisch G, eds. The kidney: physiology and pathophysiology. 2nd ed. New York: Raven, 1992:2209–2247.

Chapter 12

Acid-Base Disorders

Charles S. Wingo

Acidosis is the manifestation of a disease process that, if left unopposed, results in acidemia (blood pH < 7.35). (As with all laboratory values, slight differences may exist for the range of normal values among different laboratories. Hence, laboratory data should be interpreted with knowledge of correct ranges of normal values for that laboratory.) *Alkalosis* is the manifestation of a disease process that, if left unopposed, results in alkalemia (blood pH > 7.45). Acidosis can be subdivided into metabolic (a primary reduction in plasma bicarbonate concentration) and respiratory (a primary increase in CO_2 partial pressure (pCO_2)). Likewise, alkalosis can be divided into metabolic (a primary increase in plasma bicarbonate concentration) and respiratory (a primary decrease in pCO_2). Simple acid-base disorders are due to a *single* primary change in either pCO_2 or bicarbonate concentration. In most cases, simple acid-base disorders result in an abnormal blood pH. Certain terms that are frequently confused are defined below.

- pH: a measure of acidity, equal to $-\log[H^+]$.
- pCO_2: partial pressure (mmHg or Torr) of CO_2 in a solution; concentration of CO_2 in blood ($[CO_2]$, in mM) is equal to $pCO_2 \times 0.03$, e.g., approximately 1.2 mM for a pCO_2 of 40 mmHg.
- Total CO_2: moles of CO_2 that can be released from a solution by adding a strong acid; plasma bicarbonate concentration approximates plasma total CO_2.

The simple acid-base disorders are listed in Table 12.1 with the primary causes and compensatory changes.

Table 12.1
Simple Acid-Base Disturbances and Predicted Compensations

Disorder	Mechanism	Primary Change	Compensatory Change	Expected Compensatory Response[a]
Metabolic acidosis	Excessive acid production or retention	↓[HCO_3^-]	↓pCO_2	$pCO_2 = 1.5 \times$ [HCO_3^-] $+ 8$ (± 2)
	Excessive base loss			or
				$pCO_2 =$ last two digits of pH
Metabolic alkalosis	Excessive base intake or retention	↑[HCO_3^-]	↑pCO_2	$pCO_2 = 0.9 \times$ [HCO_3^-] $+ 16$ (± 5)
	Excessive acid loss			or
				$pCO_2 =$ last two digits of pH
Respiratory acidosis		↑pCO_2	↑[HCO_3^-]	
Acute	Decreased CO_2 elimination			[H^+] $= 0.75 \times pCO_2 + 9$ (± 4)
				Δ[HCO_3^-] $= 0.1 \times \Delta pCO_2$
Chronic	Decreased CO_2 elimination			[H^+] $= 0.3 \times pCO_2 + 28$ (± 3)
				Δ[HCO_3^-] $= 0.4 \times \Delta pCO_2$
Respiratory alkalosis		↓pCO_2	↓[HCO_3^-]	
Acute	Increased CO_2 elimination			[H^+] $= 0.75 \times pCO_2 + 9$ ($\pm$)4
				Δ[HCO_3^-] $= 0.2 \times \Delta pCO_2$
Chronic	Increased CO_2 elimination			[H^+] $= 0.3 \times pCO_2 + 28$ ($\pm$)4
				Δ[HCO_3^-] $= 0.5 \times \Delta pCO_2$

[a]These following equations can predict expected steady-state relations between a primary and a compensatory change. For example, a decrease in [HCO_3^-] to 15 mEq/L (metabolic acidosis) will produce a secondary change in pCO_2. With 95% confidence pCO_2 will be $pCO_2 = 1.5 \times 15 + 8$ (± 2) $= 30.5 \pm 2$ or 28.5 to 32.5 mmHg. By coincidence the last two pH digits approximate the predicted pCO_2.

PATHOPHYSIOLOGY

Acid-base homeostasis is maintained within a narrow range through a series of reversible chemical buffers and physiologic pulmonary and renal compensations. Intracellular and extracellular buffers that counteract changes in pH include CO_2/bicarbonate, phosphate, protein (particularly hemoglobin), and bone. Although all body buffers participate in acid-base regulation, it is convenient to think in terms of the bicarbonate buffer system because all extracellular buffers are essentially in equilibrium. This relationship may be expressed in terms of the Henderson-Hasselbach equation as follows:

$$pH = 6.10 + \log\{[HCO_3^-]/(pCO_2 \times 0.03)\} = 7.62 + \log\{[HCO_3^-]/pCO_2\}$$

It is frequently more convenient to utilize the linear (Henderson) form:

$$[H^+] = \frac{24 \times pCO_2}{[HCO_3^-]}$$

The normal blood pH of 7.40 ± 0.05 is equivalent to a hydrogen ion concentration of 40 ± 5 nM. Between pH 7.20 and 7.50, each 0.1 increase in pH results in a decreased hydrogen ion concentration of approximately 10 nM.

Compensation to Primary Acid-Base Disorders

Physiological compensation to changes in systemic pH involves changes in both alveolar ventilation (pCO_2) and renal acid excretion. Complete respiratory compensation to metabolic acidosis requires 12–24 hr. The kidney reacts more slowly to changes in systemic pH to alter net acid excretion. Net acid excretion is defined as the rate of ammonium plus titratable acid excretion minus the rate of bicarbonate excretion and organic acid excretion. Renal excretion of an alkali load may require 24–48 hr, whereas full renal elimination of an acid load may require as much as 72 hr.

Approach to Acid-Base Disorders

Evaluating a patient with an acid-base disturbance requires consideration of both the clinical presentation and the laboratory data. A carefully taken history can simplify a complex set of blood gas and electrolyte data. The arterial blood gas is the cornerstone of diagnosis of most acid-base disturbances, but several caveats should be considered.

- Systemic pH, pCO_2, bicarbonate, and electrolytes should be evaluated simultaneously, and the calculated bicarbonate from the blood gas should approximate the total CO_2.
- A blood gas value represents a specific point in time; identical values can be obtained for different acid-base disturbances moving in opposite directions.
- Nomograms may lead to the wrong diagnosis if the clinical presentation is ignored.
- Physiologic compensation to a primary acid-base disorder seldom normalizes systemic pH.

METABOLIC ACIDOSIS

Metabolic acidosis represents a primary decrease in plasma bicarbonate concentration, which decreases blood pH. There are four mechanisms: (*a*) net acid production or net acid intake abruptly increases to exceed renal net acid excretion (e.g., ketoacidosis, lactic acidosis, ammonium chloride loading); (*b*) renal net acid excretion fails to match net acid production plus net acid intake (e.g., renal tubular acidosis (RTA), carbonic anhydrase inhibitors); (*c*) bicarbonate may be lost via the gastrointestinal tract (e.g., diarrhea, fistula); (*d*) extracellular fluid can be diluted by a non–bicarbonate-containing solution (e.g., rapid saline administration).

The *compensatory response* to metabolic acidosis is an increase in ventilation that returns pH toward normal. When fully compensated, the pCO_2 closely approximates the last two digits of the serum pH. If this is not the case, a mixed acid-base disturbance should be considered.

Clinical Presentation

Nausea, vomiting, and abdominal pain are frequent with metabolic acidosis, particularly diabetic ketoacidosis. Respiratory compensation produces rapid, deep (Kussmaul) respirations. Severe acidosis can be associated with decreased myocardial contractility, hypotension, pulmonary edema, and tissue hypoxia. The arterial blood gas reveals a reduced pH and plasma bicarbonate concentration and usually a reduced pCO_2.

The anion gap helps in determining the etiology of a metabolic acidosis.

$$\text{anion gap} = [Na^+] - ([Cl^+] + [HCO_3^-])$$

A normal anion gap ranges between 8 and 16 mM, provided that plasma albumin and globulin concentrations are normal. Table 12.2 provides the differential diagnosis of an elevated anion gap acidosis, key clinical features, supporting laboratory data, and a brief outline of treatment options.

Normal anion gap metabolic acidosis with increased serum chloride concentration is generally due to gastrointestinal tract or renal bicarbonate wasting.

Therapy for these disorders involves treatment of the primary process. Uremic acidosis typically has an increased anion gap and should be treated with oral bicarbonate therapy. If a nonrenal mechanism of acidosis (e.g., diabetic ketoacidosis) is present and renal function is near normal, alkali therapy is generally not indicated (unless serum pH is <7.10) because the metabolism of the organic anions to bicarbonate will usually restore plasma bicarbonate to normal. Most formulas overestimate the base requirement unless acid production is continuous (e.g., lactic acidosis). Therefore, the base deficit should be calculated using the accompanying formula, but after half the bicarbonate has been administered, the need for bicarbonate therapy should be reassessed.

$$\text{bicarbonate deficit (mEq)} = 0.4 \times \text{weight (kg)} \times ([HCO_3^-]_{desired} - [HCO_3^-]_{observed})$$

Recent evidence indicates that administration of bicarbonate to patients with lactic acidosis may actually stimulate the production of lactate.

Renal Tubular Acidosis

RTA is a hyperchloremic, normal anion gap, metabolic acidosis caused by the inability of the kidney to maintain a normal plasma bicarbonate concentration. Other causes of normal anion gap

Table 12.2
Differential Diagnosis of Elevated Anion Gap Metabolic Acidosis

	Etiology	Clinical Features	Laboratory	Treatment
K	Diabetic ketoacidosis	Fruity breath	Increased glucose > 300 mg/dL; serum or urine ketones	Intravenous insulin and saline
U	Uremia	Oliguria, uremic breath; pericarditis	Increased BUN and creatinine; low urine output	Consider dialysis
S	Salicylate intoxication	Tinnitus; hyperventilation	Positive urine ferric chloride test; increased serum salicylate	Diuresis and alkalinization of urine; hemodialysis
S	Starvation ketosis	None	Serum or urine ketones	Refeeding
M	Methanol	"Blind drunk"	Elevated osmolal gap	Ethanol infusion
A	Alcohol ketoacidosis	Ethanol abuse, often with binge drinking	Increased alcohol level; serum lactate increased	Glucose and saline; phosphorous and potassium
U	Unmeasured osmoles Ethylene glycol; paraldehydes	May have accompanying renal failure	Elevated osmolal gap; calcium oxalate crystals in urine	Consider dialysis
L	Lactic acidosis	Shock, tissue hypoperfusion	Lactate level	Correct underlying cause

Table 12.3
Differential Diagnosis of Normal Anion Gap Metabolic Acidosis

Gastrointestinal tract bicarbonate loss from diarrhea, pancreatic or biliary fistulas, or an immature ileostomy yields fluid losses with a higher bicarbonate concentration than that of serum and produces potassium depletion

Ureterosigmoidostomy with urine retention in the colon causes chloride and water reabsorption with bicarbonate secretion

Ingestion of chloride salts or chloride-containing anion exchange resins (i.e., $CaCl_2$, $MgCl_2$, or cholestyramine) causes chloride to exchange for bicarbonate across the gastrointestinal tract

Renal tubular acidosis may be associated with frank renal bicarbonate loss or failure to match net acid excretion to net acid intake and production

---

acidosis are listed in Table 12.3. The kidney normally excretes the daily acid load that represents, in part, the end products of sulfur (e.g., cystine, methionine) and phosphorous (e.g., phospholipid) metabolism. This metabolism produces mineral acids (e.g., H_2SO_4 and H_3PO_4) that would otherwise reduce the plasma bicarbonate concentration if they are not excreted by the kidney.

Classic distal (type I) RTA is characterized by a metabolic acidosis caused by defective collecting duct acidification. Serum potassium is low or normal, and the urine cannot be maximally acidified (pH < 5.5) even with profound acidemia. This disorder can occur as an autosomal dominant inherited disease. Acquired forms are frequently associated with autoimmune diseases (e.g., systemic lupus erythematosus, pernicious anemia, or Sjögren's syndrome), nephrocalcinosis (e.g., hyperparathyroidism), or toxins (e.g., amphotericin B, lithium, or toluene). Type III RTA is a variant of distal RTA that occurs in children with excessive bicarbonate wasting.

Patients often present with musculoskeletal weakness or with nephrolithiasis. Severe distal RTA can present in childhood as a medical emergency with acute hypokalemic paralysis, coma, shock, or even death if the plasma bicarbonate concentration is below 5 mEq/L.

The pathogenesis of distal RTA is not established, but laboratory studies suggest that defects in the normal function of a H^+, K^+-activated ATPase may explain certain cases of distal

RTA. Patients with incomplete distal RTA are not frankly acidemic and may not be detected without a formal test of urine acidification. These patients fail to reduce urine pH to less than 5.5 on administration of an NH_4Cl load.

Small amounts (1–2 mEq/kg/24 hr) of oral bicarbonate are usually sufficient to correct the acidosis and increase serum bicarbonate to >22 mEq/L. Bicarbonate therapy may improve the hypokalemia. Sources of bicarbonate include the following.

- Sodium bicarbonate:
    325 mg and 650 mg tablets
    325 mg ≈ 4 mEq base
- Shohl's solution (Bicitra):
    5 mL = 500 mg sodium citrate dihydrate/334 mg citric acid
    1 mL = 1 mEq base and 1 mEq sodium
- Polycitra:
    5 mL = 550 mg potassium citrate + 500 mg sodium citrate and 334 mg citric acid
    1 mL = 2 mEq base, 1 mEq potassium, and 1 mEq sodium
- Polycitra-K:
    5 mL = 1100 mg potassium citrate/334 mg citric acid
    1 mL = 2 mEq base and 2 mEq potassium

Other potassium citrate preparations include K-Lyte (25 mEq potassium), K-Lyte DS (50 mEq potassium), and Urocit-K (5 mEq potassium).

Proximal (type II) RTA is characterized by excessive bicarbonaturia in the absence of severe acidosis. However, in this disorder the urine pH is <5.5 during severe acidosis. Type II RTA is due to a proximal tubular defect and can be observed with acetazolamide administration or with Fanconi's syndrome. In the latter case bicarbonaturia, phosphaturia, and aminoaciduria are present. Medullary cystic disease, multiple myeloma, the nephrotic syndrome, or transplantation can also lead to a proximal RTA.

Proximal RTA is the result of impaired reabsorption of bicarbonate in the proximal tubule. Plasma bicarbonate concentration decreases because of increased fractional bicarbonate excretion. Eventually, the plasma bicarbonate concentration decreases sufficiently to limit the amount of bicarbonate presented to the distal nephron and the collecting duct. Under these conditions the reduced filtered load of bicarbonate is within the capacity of the proximal and distal nephron to reabsorb most of the filtered bicarbonate. This permits normal acidification by the collecting duct to reduce urine pH maximally. Patients with proximal RTA typically have only a mild to moderate acidosis. The plasma bicarbonate concentration is typically >15 mEq/L.

Proximal RTA usually occurs in children and presents as failure to thrive, growth retardation, vomiting, volume depletion, and lethargy. X-rays may reveal features suggestive of rickets in children and osteopenia in adults. Serum potassium is low or normal.

The fractional excretion of bicarbonate can be used to distinguish between proximal and distal RTA when the plasma bicarbonate concentration is normal and is defined as:

$$\frac{U[HCO_3^-]}{P[HCO_3^-]} \times \frac{P_{creatinine}}{U_{creatinine}}$$

Fractional excretion of bicarbonate is <5% in distal RTA but exceeds 15% if the plasma bicarbonate concentration is >20 mEq/L in proximal RTA. In proximal RTA the urine pH will be >5.5 unless the acidosis is severe.

Proximal RTA can be difficult to treat, often requiring 10–25 mEq/kg/24 hr of oral bicarbonate. Large doses of alkali are required because of the large fractional excretion of bicarbonate owing to the proximal tubular defect. Increased distal delivery of bicarbonate promotes secretion of potassium and can lead to severe hypokalemia. Thus, significant amounts of the alkali therapy should be given as the potassium salt. Osteomalacia may require vitamin D and calcium supplements, whereas rickets can be corrected with vitamin D and 1.6 g/day of sodium phosphate.

Hyperkalemic (type IV) RTA frequently coexists with chronic renal insufficiency. Less frequently, this disorder is observed in the presence of normal renal function. In the latter case, a defect in aldosterone production or action is usually responsible for both the hyperkalemia and the acidosis. Mild hyperkalemia and acidosis are frequently observed with chronic renal disease but in patients with hyperkalemic RTA the degree of hyperkalemia is out of proportion to the degree of renal insufficiency (glomerular filtration rate 20–60 mL/min). Hyperkalemia leads to an impairment in ammonium excretion and, hence, renal net acid excretion. Such individuals, however, can reduce urine pH to <5.5. Hyperkalemia reflects either impaired potassium secretion (primarily in the cortical collecting duct) or enhanced potassium reabsorption (primarily in the medullary collecting duct). Some of these cases reflect impaired aldosterone production (syndrome of hyporeninemic hypoaldosteronism) and respond well to mineralocorticoid replacement therapy (fludrocortisone acetate (Flornef) 0.1–0.2 mg/day). However, it is equally frequent to find hyperkalemic RTA in the presence of hypertension and extracellular fluid volume expansion (edema), features that are not typically associated with mineralocorticoid deficiency when renal function is normal. In this latter group mineralocorticoid therapy usually fails to restore serum potassium or plasma bicarbonate to normal but may worsen the hypertension and NaCl retention. Hyperkalemic RTA is especially common in diabetic nephropathy, interstitial nephritis, obstructive uropathy, and after renal transplantation. Most patients with hyperkalemic RTA are best treated with a loop diuretic (e.g., furosemide) and sodium alkali therapy (1–2 mEq/kg/24 hr) if necessary. Chapter 11 provides a further discussion of hyperkalemic RTA.

RESPIRATORY ACIDOSIS

Respiratory acidosis represents a primary increase in pCO_2, which decreases systemic pH. The increased pCO_2 is generally due to failure of CO_2 excretion from decreased alveolar ventilation rather than increased CO_2 production. Respiratory acidosis frequently occurs with diseases involving the central nervous system, lungs, and heart. Sedatives and opiates that depress central nervous system centers of respiration are common iatrogenic causes of respiratory acidosis. Severe electrolyte abnormalities (hypokalemia, hypophosphatemia), impaired mechanical ventilation, and bronchopulmonary diseases are causes of respiratory acidosis (Table 12.4).

The increased CO_2 results in an increased carbonic acid concentration that is buffered primarily by intracellular buffers, such as hemoglobin or phosphate, resulting in a small increase in plasma bicarbonate concentration. The kidneys compensate by increasing net acid excretion, which generates new bicarbon-

Table 12.4
Causes of Respiratory Acidosis

Decreased alveolar ventilation and CO_2 removal
  Obstruction (e.g., bronchospasm, emphysema, or aspiration)
  Primary depression of respiratory center (e.g., drugs, trauma, neoplasm or infection)
  Mechanical or structural defect (e.g., pneumothorax, hemothorax, or adult respiratory distress syndrome)
  Mechanical or neuromuscular defect (e.g., primary muscular disease, neuromuscular diseases, drugs, botulism or tetanus)
  Decreased stimulation of respiratory center (sleep apnea)
Decreased capillary exchange of CO_2
  Cardiac arrest
  Circulatory shock
  Severe pulmonary edema
  Massive pulmonary embolus

ate that is returned to the blood. Enhanced urinary acidification increases urinary chloride excretion that in turn reduces plasma chloride concentration. The renal response usually takes longer than 24 hr to develop fully.

Patients may present with respiratory distress, dyspnea, or obtundation. They may complain of headaches or show signs of increased intracranial pressure caused by cerebral vasodilation produced by CO_2. The pCO_2 is increased, and the blood pH is decreased. The treatment is restoration of adequate ventilation.

METABOLIC ALKALOSIS

Metabolic alkalosis is due to a primary increase in plasma bicarbonate concentration, resulting in an increase in blood pH. This increase in plasma bicarbonate concentration can result from addition of bicarbonate or its precursors to the extracellular fluid or loss of fluid with a chloride-to-bicarbonate ratio greater than that of serum. Metabolic alkalosis is usually due to chloride or potassium depletion. Uncomplicated potassium depletion in humans produces only a mild metabolic alkalosis unless there is concomitant hyperaldosteronism.

The administration of bicarbonate or bicarbonate precursors, such as lactate, citrate, or acetate, increases the plasma bicarbonate concentration, but if the glomerular filtration rate is normal, most of the bicarbonate load is excreted. The ability of the kidney to rapidly excrete an alkali load depends on several factors, but a role for distal delivery of chloride to a site of bicarbonate secretion within the cortical collecting duct appears critical for alkali excretion. Bicarbonate secretion in the cortical collecting duct has been shown to occur via a chloride-bicarbonate exchanger on the apical membrane of type B intercalated cells of the cortical collecting duct.

Metabolic alkalosis is frequently related to a loss of chloride salts or hydrochloric acid. Certain diuretics and gastrointestinal diseases can induce a greater loss of chloride than bicarbonate. This leads to extracellular fluid volume contraction and an increase in bicarbonate concentration. Alveolar hypoventilation is the compensatory respiratory response to this primary disturbance that increases pCO_2; however, this compensation is usually limited to a rise in pCO_2 to 55–60 mmHg, because hypoxia stimulates ventilation. The volume depletion increases renal bicarbonate retention by decreasing the glomerular filtration rate, increasing the proximal and distal tubule proton secretion and reducing the luminal chloride delivery to the collecting duct, which limits chloride-bicarbonate exchange. In contrast, excessive mineralocorticoid activity stimulates renal generation of bicarbonate. In this condition the increase in plasma bicarbonate reflects the generation and retention of bicarbonate by the kidney as a consequence of increased net acid excretion.

Clinical Presentation

The clinical presentation of most common causes of metabolic alkalosis can be divided into conditions with and those without volume depletion. Metabolic alkalosis associated with volume depletion is invariably due to chloride depletion. Such individuals may exhibit orthostatic hypotension, tachycardia, azotemia, and other features of reduced effective circulating volume. Unless a renal mechanism is responsible for the volume and chloride depletion (e.g., diuretics), these patients will exhibit intense chloride conservation, and urinary chloride concentration will be <10 mEq/L. Common causes of chloride-responsive metabolic alkalosis are given in Table 12.5.

In contrast the most common cause of volume resistant metabolic alkalosis is excessive mineralocorticoid action. Blood pressure is usually increased, and volume depletion is not

Table 12.5
Causes of Metabolic Alkalosis

Chloride responsive metabolic alkalosis: frequently observed with extracellular fluid contraction (urine [Cl$^-$] < 10 mEq/L without diuretics)
  Vomiting/nasogastric suction
  Villous adenoma
  Diuretic therapy (urine [Cl$^-$] > 10 mEq/L)
  Posthypercapnia state
Chloride-resistant metabolic alkalosis: frequently observed with excessive mineralocorticoid effect and hypokalemia (urine [Cl$^-$] > 20 mEq/L and typically reflects intake)
  Primary hyperaldosteronism (Conn's syndrome)
  Bilateral adrenal hyperplasia
  Other causes of excessive mineralocorticoid effect
    Glycyrrhizic acid (licorice)
    Cushing's syndrome or disease
    Congenital adrenocorticoid excess or ectopic ACTH
    Diseases associated with high plasma renin activity
  Potassium depletion
  Bartter's syndrome
Milk-alkali syndrome
Acute alkali load

present. Urinary chloride excretion typically reflects intake and is usually > 20 mEq/L.

Hypokalemia is a consistent feature of metabolic alkalosis unless frank renal insufficiency is present. The hypokalemia and decreased ionized calcium may contribute to muscle cramps, weakness, and hyperreflexia. Plasma bicarbonate concentration and pH are increased, and the compensatory alveolar hypoventilation increases pCO_2 but decreases O_2 partial pressure that can lead to signs of hypoxia. Severe alkalemia can lead to cardiac arrhythmias.

Therapy

Chloride-responsive metabolic alkalosis will correct with administration of NaCl chloride (saline), but coexisting depletion of potassium, magnesium, and phosphate must be sought and corrected if detected. Chloride-resistant alkalosis is usually due to mineralocorticoid excess and coexisting hypokalemia. Both of these disorders must be corrected for acid-base balance to be restored to normal. Spironolactone can be used to treat hyperaldosteronism.

Table 12.6
Causes of Respiratory Alkalosis

Increased central nervous system drive for respiration
  Anxiety
  Central nervous system infection, infarction, trauma
  Drugs: salicylates, nicotine, aminophylline
  Fever, sepsis: especially Gram-negative sepsis
  Pregnancy, progesterone
  Liver disease
Increased stimulation of chemoreceptors
  Anemia
  Carbon monoxide toxicity
  Pulmonary edema, pneumonia
  Pulmonary emboli
  Reduced inspired O_2 tension: high altitude
Increased mechanical ventilation
  Iatrogenic

RESPIRATORY ALKALOSIS

Respiratory alkalosis results from a primary decrease in pCO_2 caused by increased alveolar ventilation. Pain, anxiety, hypoxia, severe anemia, progesterone and other drugs, endotoxin, and primary pulmonary disease can increase ventilation and lead to hypocapnia (Table 12.6). The initial response to alkalemia is buffering with intracellular protons. The renal compensation, which occurs over several days, decreases net acid excretion and plasma bicarbonate concentration and restores pH toward normal. Patients may often present with hyperventilation, perioral and extremity paresthesias, muscle cramps, hyperreflexia, seizures, or cardiac arrhythmias.

The arterial blood gas measurement reveals a decreased pCO_2 and an increased pH. Plasma bicarbonate concentration will be decreased, and serum chloride concentration is usually increased. Some electrolyte changes of chronic respiratory alkalosis may mimic a nonanion gap acidosis. The only effective therapy is to eliminate the cause of the hyperventilation.

MIXED ACID-BASE DISORDERS

Patients may present with two or even three primary acid-base disorders. The first step in diagnosis is to define the primary disorder and the pulmonary or renal compensation (Table 12.1). Identification of the primary disturbance can be made from the pH. A pH below 7.35 indicates a primary acidosis, whereas a pH above 7.45 indicates a primary alkalosis. "Overcompensation" does not occur for primary acid-base disturbances.

A reduced plasma bicarbonate concentration indicates a metabolic acidosis or respiratory alkalosis. A bicarbonate concentration below 15 is typically due to metabolic acidosis. A bicarbonate concentration of >45 occurs most commonly with metabolic alkalosis. Use of the formulas in Table 12.1 assumes adequate time for compensation.

The most common clinical settings for mixed acid-base disorders appear in Table 12.7. A severe acidemia can result from a combined metabolic and respiratory acidosis. Even though pCO_2 and bicarbonate concentration may not be severely changed, the pH will be <7.35 and the pCO_2 >45 mmHg. In metabolic acidosis and respiratory alkalosis the bicarbonate concentration and pCO_2 are both reduced, but pCO_2 will be lower than predicted for the respiratory compensation of the metabolic acidosis.

A mixed *metabolic acidosis* and *metabolic alkalosis* can be difficult to diagnose because both disorders affect the plasma bicarbonate concentration primarily. The pH and bicarbonate concentration can be increased, decreased, or normal. An elevated anion gap with an increased or normal bicarbonate concentration suggests this diagnosis. Many causes of metabolic acidosis are accompanied by vomiting, so this mixed disorder is not uncommon.

A combined metabolic alkalosis and *respiratory acidosis* is characterized by an increased bicarbonate concentration and increased pCO_2. By using the formulas in Table 12.1, the elevation in bicarbonate concentration will be greater than predicted for compensation caused by respiratory acidosis.

Severe alkalemia can result from a combined metabolic and respiratory alkalosis. A mixed disorder is present if a respiratory alkalosis is not accompanied by the appropriate decrease in bicarbonate concentration or metabolic alkalosis is not accompanied by the appropriate increase in pCO_2. This combination occurs frequently in critically ill patients owing to excessive mechanical ventilation and diuretic use.

Finally, a triple acid-base disturbance can exist. This is due to combined metabolic acidosis and metabolic alkalosis accompanied by either respiratory acidosis or respiratory alkalosis. It

Table 12.7
Common Causes of Mixed Acid-Base Disorders

Disorder	Example	Clinical Features
Metabolic acidosis/respiratory acidosis	Cardiopulmonary arrest Severe pulmonary edema	Lactic acidosis with decreased ventilation
Metabolic acidosis/respiratory alkalosis	Salicylate intoxication	Elevated anion gap acidosis and central respiratory stimulation
	Sepsis, severe liver disease	Lactic acidosis with respiratory stimulation
Metabolic acidosis/metabolic alkalosis	Renal failure with vomiting Alcoholic or diabetic ketoacidosis with vomiting Critically ill patients on gastric suction	Sepsis, renal failure, or diabetic ketoacidosis accompanied by gastric suction
Metabolic alkalosis/respiratory acidosis	Chronic obstructive pulmonary disease with vomiting Adult respiratory distress syndrome with gastric suction	Often caused by theophylline toxicity Found in patients with cor pulmonale Can be exacerbated with chloride depletion from low NaCl intake
Metabolic alkalosis/respiratory alkalosis	Inappropriate mechanical ventilation with gastric suction Pregnancy with vomiting	Frequently seen in intensive care units Pregnancy normally induces a chronic respiratory alkalosis

frequently occurs in an alcoholic or diabetic patient with vomiting (metabolic alkalosis), lactic or ketoacidosis (metabolic acidosis), and a respiratory alkalosis caused by sepsis or liver disease.

Suggested Readings

Battle DC, Hiton M, Cohen E, Gutterman C, Gupta K. The use of the urinary anion gap in the diagnosis of hyperchloremic metabolic acidosis. N Engl J Med 1988;318:594–599.

Emmett M, Narins R. Clinical use of the anion gap. Medicine 1977;56:38–54.

Galla JH, Luke RG. Pathophysiology of metabolic alkalosis. Hosp Pract 1987;22:95–118.

Hamm LL, Hering-Smith KS. Acid-base transport in the collecting duct. Semin Nephrol 1993;13:246–255.

Narins R, Emmett M. Simple and mixed acid-base disorders: a practical approach. Medicine 1980;59:161–187.

Chapter 13

Calcium, Phosphorus, and Magnesium Disorders

John C. Peterson

CALCIUM

Total serum calcium concentration (S_{Ca}) normally is 8.8–10.4 mg/dL (2.2–2.6 mmol/L). It consists of (*a*) protein-bound calcium (40%), (*b*) complexed calcium (15%), and (*c*) ionized calcium (45%), which ranges from 4.0 to 4.8 mg/dL (1.0–1.2 mmol/L). Serum albumin and phosphate should always be measured with S_{Ca}.

Factors Altering Calcium Concentration

Serum Albumin

A decrease of 1 g/dL in serum albumin decreases *total* S_{Ca} by 0.8 mg/dL.

Tourniquet

Transudation of plasma water (but not plasma protein) into the tissues elevates the *total* S_{Ca}.

pH

The binding of calcium to protein increases with pH. A change of 0.1 pH units causes an opposite change of 0.12 mg/dL in the *ionized* calcium.

Parathyroid Hormone

All patients with primary hyperparathyroidism (in the absence of a confounding clinical problem such as renal failure or severe vitamin D deficiency) have elevated *ionized* calcium.

Serum Phosphate

Increments in serum phosphate first lower *ionized* calcium, then *total* S_{Ca} as calcium phosphate is deposited in bone.

Calcium Homeostasis

Parathyroid hormone (PTH) and/or 1,25-vitamin D_3 increase S_{Ca}, whereas calcitonin reduces S_{Ca}.

Parathyroid Hormone

PTH causes osteoclastic bone resorption, enhances distal tubular reabsorption of calcium, increases fractional excretion of phosphorus, and stimulates formation of 1,25-vitamin D_3.

1,25-Vitamin D_3

This form of vitamin D_3 stimulates osteoclastic bone resorption and gastrointestinal absorption of calcium and augments tubular reabsorption of calcium.

Calcitonin

Calcitonin inhibits osteoclastic bone reabsorption and enhances calcium excretion but does not change *normal* calcium levels.

HYPERCALCEMIA

Hypercalcemia is defined as total S_{Ca} of >10.5 mg/dL (2.63 mmol/L) or an ionized calcium of >4.8 mg/dL (1.2 mmol/L).

Pathophysiology

The skeleton has the ability to buffer changes in S_{Ca}. After a calcium infusion, S_{Ca} returns to normal when only 10–15% of the infused load has been excreted; thus, hypercalcemia is a perturbation of the dynamic equilibrium between osteolytic and osteoblastic factors.

TABLE 13.1
Clinical Features Associated with Specific Diseases

Hyperparathyroidism: nephrolithiasis, hyperchloremic acidosis, hypophosphatemia, pseudogout, osteitis fibrosa cystica on bone x-rays

Sarcoidosis: hilar adenopathy on chest x-ray, rash, lymphadenopathy, conduction abnormalities on electrocardiogram

Malignancy: S_{Ca} above 15 mg/dL (3.75 mmol/L), anorexia, weight loss

Thyrotoxicosis: hyperreflexia, systolic hypertension

Etiology and Pathogenesis

Ninety percent of the cases of hypercalcemia are due to primary hyperparathyroidism, malignancy, or granulomatous diseases. The major clinical features of these diseases are displayed in Table 13.1.

Primary Hyperparathyroidism

This occurs more frequently in postmenopausal women. Approximately 75% of the patients have single adenomas, 25% have multiglandular adenomatosis or hyperplasia, and 1–2% have parathyroid carcinoma. The hypercalcemia is due to increased bone resorption, increased gastrointestinal absorption of calcium caused indirectly through PTH stimulation of 1,25-vitamin D_3, and increased renal reabsorption of calcium. Asymptomatic hypercalcemia is the most common presentation.

Malignancy

The incidence of hypercalcemia with neoplasms is 10–20%. The most common neoplasms are breast and lung cancer and multiple myeloma. Malignant hypercalcemia results from local destruction of bone by metastatic lesions, recruitment of osteoclasts by tumor-produced humoral factors, and, very rarely, tumor secretion of PTH.

Granulomatous Diseases

Sarcoidosis, tuberculosis, and histoplasmosis elevate 1,25-vitamin D_3 levels via activated monocytes.

Thyroid Disease

Thyroid hormone accelerates osteolysis, and 10–20% of thyrotoxic patients have hypercalcemia with suppressed PTH levels. Hypothyroidism can also cause hypercalcemia, presumably by reducing bone turnover.

Vitamin D Intoxication

This condition is seen most commonly in dialysis patients or women undergoing treatment for osteoporosis.

Immobilization

Immobilization may produce hypercalcemia if bone turnover is accelerated (e.g., Paget's disease).

End-Stage Renal Failure

These patients (especially dialysis patients) are at risk for hypercalcemia caused by vitamin D toxicity, severe secondary hyperparathyroidism, or aluminum toxicity, which inhibits bone mineralization.

Postrenal Transplant

Hypercalcemia is caused by parathyroid gland hyperplasia that developed during renal insufficiency and usually abates within 6 months after transplantation.

Acute Renal Failure

Hypercalcemia may occur in the polyuric recovery phase of acute tubular necrosis due to elevated PTH and 1,25-vitamin D_3 levels or dissolution of ectopic (usually muscle) calcium phosphate deposits.

Milk-Alkali Syndrome

This is caused by ingestion of large amounts of calcium (>5 g/day) and alkali. Alkalosis increases protein binding of calcium and stimulates tubular calcium reabsorption.

Thiazide Diuretics

Thiazides can worsen hypercalcemia in patients with primary hyperparathyroidism, whereas normal individuals have only a mild or transient hypercalcemia. Thiazides increase calcium reabsorption in the proximal tubule and early distal tubule.

Clinical Presentation

- Confusion, stupor, and coma
- Anorexia, nausea, and vomiting
- Constipation
- Polyuria and polydipsia
- Hypertension
- Nephrolithiasis
- Decreased renal function
- Peptic ulcer disease
- Metastatic calcification
- Electrocardiogram changes (shortened conduction intervals)

Diagnostic Tests

The PTH intact hormone assay most accurately reflects the time-integrated level of PTH secretion and is the preferred assay. PTH levels in patients with hypercalcemia of malignancy are normal or low, whereas levels in patients with primary hyperparathyroidism are generally elevated. Figure 13.1 describes an algorithm for the differential diagnosis of hypercalcemia.

Treatment

Hypercalcemia requires immediate therapy when

- Central nervous system symptoms are present;
- Total S_{Ca} is >13 mg/dL (3.25 mmol/L);
- The product of calcium and phosphorus exceeds 80 (risk of metastatic calcification is high).

The safest acute therapy is saline and a furosemide diuresis.

- Priming dose of 1–2 L of isotonic saline iv over 1 hr;
- Furosemide 40–80 mg iv every 2–3 hr;

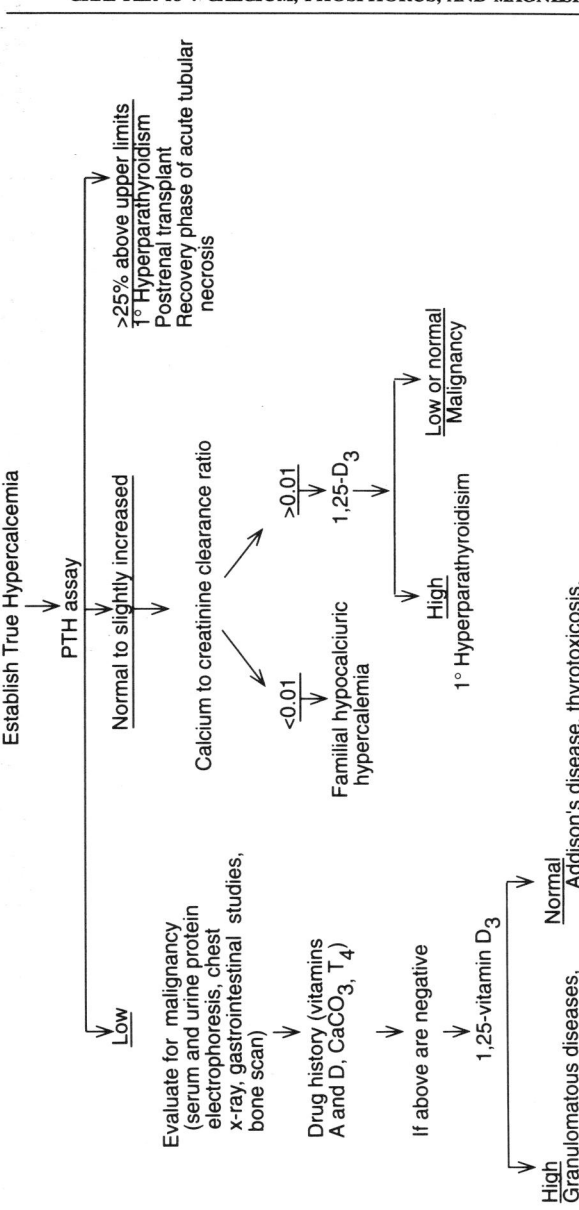

Figure 13.1. Evaluation of hypercalcemia. (Modified from Levine M, Kleeman CR. Hypercalcemia: pathophysiology and treatment. Hosp Pract 1987;22:93–110.)

- Measure urine volume hourly and urine sodium, potassium, and magnesium every 4–6 hr;
- Replace urinary losses of sodium with isotonic saline and KCl;
- If diuresis is to be continued for more than 24–48 hr, replace magnesium losses with intermittent doses of 1 g $MgSO_4$ added to intravenous fluids.

After 48 hr, institution of maintenance therapy is needed. Calcitonin and mithramycin are rapid in onset but require intravenous administration and may cause tachyphylaxis and thrombocytopenia, respectively. Disodium etidronate (7.5 mg/kg iv daily for 3 days, then 20 mg/kg/day orally for 30 days) has the advantages of oral dosing and onset of action within 2 days with no reported adverse effects.

HYPOCALCEMIA

Hypocalcemia is defined as a total S_{Ca} below 8.5 mg/dL (2.13 mmol/L) with a normal serum albumin concentration.

Etiology

Hypomagnesemia

Hypomagnesemia decreases secretion of PTH and leads to resistance to PTH action on bone.

Acute Respiratory Alkalosis

An increase in blood pH results in increased protein binding of calcium and decreased *ionized* calcium.

Vitamin D Deficiency

Vitamin D deficiency can result from decreased dietary intake or malabsorption, decreased production of 25-OH D_3 because of liver disease or 1,25-vitamin D_3 because of chronic renal failure, and accelerated loss of 25-OH D_3 because of the nephrotic syndrome or abnormalities of the enterohepatic circulation.

PTH Deficiency

PTH deficiency can result from absence of functional tissue owing to surgical removal, replacement by tumor, or infiltration with amyloid. Pseudohypoparathyroidism is the result of end-organ resistance to PTH.

"Chemical" Removal of Calcium from Serum

Hyperphosphatemia of any cause will lead to formation of $CaPO_4$ with deposition in soft tissue. Pancreatitis results in retroperitoneal saponification. Osteoblastic metastases and severe secondary hyperparathyroidism after parathyroidectomy cause increased calcium uptake by bone.

Clinical Presentation

Manifestations include tetany, muscle spasms, cramps, carpopedal spasm, and seizures. Latent tetany can be detected by a light tap over the facial nerve resulting in an ipsilateral facial twitch (Chvostek's sign) or by inflation of a sphygmomanometer above the systolic pressure for more than 3 min, resulting in carpal spasm (Trousseau's sign).

Hypocalcemia can cause congestive heart failure, hypotension, prolongation of the Q-T interval, ventricular conduction abnormalities, and resistance to digitalis.

Differential Diagnosis

The first step is verification of true hypocalcemia (i.e., reduction of *ionized* calcium). Serum albumin and pH must be measured to exclude pseudohypocalcemia and acute respiratory alkalosis. The next step is to exclude hypomagnesemia. The third step is to evaluate the PTH level: if low or normal, hypoparathyroidism is present; if high, the serum phosphorus is measured. A low phosphorus level signifies vitamin D deficiency, pancreatitis, or metastatic bone disease. A high phosphorus level is seen with rhabdomyolysis, chronic renal failure, and pseudohypoparathyroidism.

Treatment

Acute symptomatic hypocalcemia requires immediate therapy with 10–15 mEq (200–300 mg) iv calcium to forestall laryngeal spasm and/or seizures. This can be supplied by one 10-mL ampule of $CaCl_2$ (272 mg calcium per 10-mL vial) or preferably by 10–20 mL calcium gluconate (90 mg calcium per 10-mL ampule), which is less irritating. The infusion rate should not exceed 2 mL/min. Patients on digoxin require electrocardiogram monitoring. Intravenous calcium should not be mixed with bicarbonate because $CaCO_3$ will precipitate. In severe hypocalcemia, continuous intravenous infusion of calcium may be necessary, i.e., 15–20 mg/kg body weight over 4–8 hr (30–40 mL of 10% calcium gluconate in 500–1000 mL of 5% dextrose over 4–8 hr) to prevent tetany. Thereafter, start oral calcium supplements (and vitamin D if indicated) as $CaCO_3$ and calcium lactate (1–2 g calcium three times a day by mouth).

PHOSPHORUS

The normal concentration of serum phosphate in adults is 2.8–4.5 mg/dL (0.9–1.6 mmol/L). It exists mainly as a free ion.

The kidney has the major influence on phosphorus balance; 85–90% of the filtered load is reabsorbed in the proximal tubule and the final 10% in the distal nephron. Factors that increase urinary phosphate excretion include PTH (inhibits proximal and distal nephron phosphate reabsorption), cortisol, absence of growth hormone, high dietary phosphorus intake, and vitamin D. The latter increases tubular phosphate reabsorption acutely, but chronically, phosphaturia may occur secondary to an increased filtered load.

HYPOPHOSPHATEMIA

Incidence

In hospitalized patients, 10–15% develop moderate hypophosphatemia (1.0–2.5 mg/dL) as shown in Table 13.2.

Clinical Presentation

Patients are usually asymptomatic unless serum phosphorus is <1.0 mg/dL. Hypophosphatemic effects on organ systems are detailed in Table 13.3.

Differential Diagnosis

The key to diagnosis is the urinary phosphorus excretion. Values below 100 mg/day imply gastrointestinal losses or redistribution. If urinary phosphorus exceeds 100 mg/day, tubular defects (glycosuria, aminoaciduria, or bicarbonaturia) associated with

TABLE 13.2
Etiology of Hypophosphatemia

Excessive external losses
  Decreased gastrointestinal absorption: prolonged malnutrition, malabsorption, vitamin deficiency (vitamin D-dependent rickets), chronic diarrhea, aluminum-containing antacids
  Primary renal losses: primary hyperparathyroidism, secondary hyperparathyroidism (including postrenal transplantation), extracellular fluid expansion, diuretics (acetazolamide), Fanconi's syndrome, postobstructive diuresis, diuretic phase of recovery from acute tubular necrosis, glycosuria (especially with chronic diabetic ketoacidosis)
Redistribution
  Respiratory alkalosis
  Recovery from malnutrition
  Parenteral hyperalimentation
  Alcohol withdrawal
  Severe burns

TABLE 13.3
Organ Systems Affected by Hypophosphatemia

Red blood cells: decreased deformability causes hemolysis, reduced 2,3-diphosphoglycerate content decreases O_2 delivery
White blood cells: decreased phagocytic and chemotactic responses predisposing to bacterial and fungal infections
Muscle: skeletal myopathy (elevated creatine phosphokinase) can cause respiratory failure; cardiomyopathy is frequent
Bone: osteolysis can progress to osteomalacia
Central nervous system: metabolic encephalopathy with diffuse slowing on electroencephalogram

Fanconi's syndrome should be considered. If these are absent, a S_{Ca} will discriminate between primary hyperparathyroidism (elevated calcium), secondary hyperparathyroidism, or vitamin D-resistant rickets (low calcium).

Treatment

The goal of therapy is to provide 1000 mg (32 mmol) of elemental phosphorus daily.

With hyperalimentation, 450 mg of elemental phosphorus should be given with each 1000 Kcal infused. The dose of intravenous phosphorus should not exceed 2 mg elemental phosphorus/kg body weight per each 6-hr period to prevent metastatic calcium phosphate crystallization. Serial treatments should be given to restore the serum phosphorus to 2.5 mg/dL.

HYPERPHOSPHATEMIA

Hyperphosphatemia is a serum phosphorus level above 5 mg/dL (1.6 mEq/L).

Etiology

- Decreased glomerular filtration rate (usually <20 mL/min)
- Increased tubular reabsorption
    Hypoparathyroidism (including pseudohypoparathyroidism)
    Acromegaly
    Thyrotoxicosis
    EHDP (ethane-1-hydroxy-1, 1-diphosphanate), a potent stimulator of phosphorus reabsorption, which is approved for use in Paget's disease of bone
- Massive release of phosphorus into the extracellular fluid
    Endogenous
        Tumor lysis (cytotoxic therapy)
        Rhabdomyolysis
    Exogenous
        Vitamin D administration (especially use of 1,25-vitamin D_3 in patients with chronic renal failure)
        Phosphate enemas

Clinical Presentation

The main symptoms are due to hypocalcemia caused by precipitation of calcium phosphate. In addition, phosphate decreases renal conversion of 25-vitamin D_3 to 1,25-vitamin D_3 and thereby decreases gastrointestinal absorption of calcium.

Treatment

Because phosphorus is ubiquitous in food, dietary restriction to <800 mg/day is impractical, and phosphate binders are required to decrease gastrointestinal absorption. Because aluminum-containing antacids have been associated with aluminum toxicity in patients with chronic renal failure, calcium acetate or $CaCO_3$ is preferred. The goal is to maintain the serum phosphorus below 4.5 mg/dL.

For *acute hyperphosphatemia*, saline infusion will increase renal clearance. The addition of 1 ampule of 50% dextrose in 1 L of H_2O combined with 10 units of regular insulin can partition phosphorus into cells. Hemo- or peritoneal dialysis can remove large quantities of inorganic phosphorus.

MAGNESIUM

The serum magnesium concentration is maintained between 1.8 and 2.3 mg/dL (0.75–0.95 mmol/L). Only 15% is protein bound.

With a normal daily intake of 300 mg (12.5 mmol) of magnesium, 30–40% is absorbed. Renal excretion is generally 5% of the filtered load (100 mg/day) but can be reduced **(0.5%)** by hypomagnesemia or increased (40–80%) by hypermagnesemia. The thick ascending limb of Henle's loop is responsible for most magnesium reabsorption.

HYPERMAGNESEMIA

Hypermagnesemia is defined as a serum magnesium above 2.3 mg/dL (1.9 mEq/L). Hypermagnesemia is rare in patients with normal renal function unless massive loads of magnesium are given.

Etiology

Causes include chronic renal failure, acute renal failure, $MgSO_4$ administration (toxemia of pregnancy), and magnesium-containing antacids or enemas (especially with renal insufficiency or failure).

Signs and Symptoms

Hypermagnesemia blocks neuromuscular transmission and cardiac conduction and alters central nervous system function. Reflexes decrease at a serum magnesium above 5–6 mg/dL

(2.1–2.5 mmol/L). Higher levels cause confusion, lethargy, hypotension, respiratory and cardiac depression, and ultimately death.

Treatment

Effects of hypermagnesemia are antagonized by intravenous calcium. This should be used only transiently before removal of excess magnesium by hemodialysis.

HYPOMAGNESEMIA

Hypomagnesemia is defined as a serum magnesium below 1.8 mg/dL (0.75 mmol/L).

Etiology

The causes of hypomagnesemia include decreased intake, e.g., starvation or magnesium-free enteral feedings, decreased gastrointestinal absorption (nasogastric suction or malabsorption), and increased renal losses, e.g., chronic alcoholics, diuretic therapy, postobstructive diuresis, the polyuric phase of acute tubular necrosis, diabetic ketoacidosis, hypercalcemia, primary hyperaldosteronism, Bartter's syndrome, and drug therapy with aminoglycosides, cisplatin, and cyclosporin.

Pathophysiology

Chronic alcoholism is the most common cause of hypomagnesemia. Acute intake of alcohol increases urinary excretion of magnesium, and when coupled with poor dietary intake of magnesium containing foods (green, leafy vegetables), hypomagnesemia results.

Hypomagnesemia can produce hypokalemia and hypocalcemia. Magnesium depletion causes excessive urinary loss of potassium, which is correctable only after magnesium replacement.

Patients with hypomagnesemia may have muscular fasciculations and Chvostek's and Trousseau's signs. Electrocardiographic changes mimic those of hypokalemia. Calcium and potassium should always be measured when hypomagnesemia is suspected. Digitalis toxicity is markedly potentiated by hypomagnesemia.

Treatment

Hypomagnesemic tetany requires intravenous $MgSO_4$ (each gram of $MgSO_4$ contains 8.12 mEq or 98 mg magnesium). With normal renal function, mix 6 g (24 mmol) $MgSO_4$ in 1000 mL D_5W and infuse continuously over 6 hr. Thereafter, adjust the infusion to the serum magnesium level.

For prolonged oral supplementation, MgO (1 g contains 600 mg of magnesium), 250–500 mg by mouth four times daily is well tolerated.

Suggested Readings

Bilezikian JP. Management of acute hypercalcemia. N Engl J Med 1992;326:1196–1203.

Levine MM, Kleeman CR. Hypercalcemia: pathophysiology and treatment. Hosp Pract 1987;22:93–110.

Singer FR, Ritch PS, Lad TE, et al. Treatment of hypercalcemia of malignancy with intravenous etidronate: a controlled multicenter trial. Arch Intern Med 1991;151:471–476.

Slatopolsky E, Klahr S. Disorders of calcium, phosphorus and magnesium metabolism. In: Schrier RS, Gottschalk CW, eds. Diseases of the kidney, 4th ed. Boston: Little, Brown, 1993:2599–2644.

Whang R, Whang DD, Ryan P. Refractory potassium repletion: a consequence of magnesium deficiency. Arch Intern Med 1992;152:40–45.

Chapter 14

Renal Stone Disease

I. David Weiner

Renal stone disease affects approximately 4% of the general population, with a male-to-female ratio of 4:1, and it is associated with significant morbidity due to pain. Prompt diagnosis and therapy are required to minimize pain and prevent complications such as infection, obstructive uropathy, and renal damage.

PATHOPHYSIOLOGY

Kidney stones occur as a result of the interaction of three factors. These include the supersaturation of stone-forming compounds in the urine, the presence of physical or chemical stimuli in urine that promote stone formation, and inadequate amounts of compounds in urine that inhibit stone formation. Therefore, stone formation can be due to any combination of

- Low urine volume (e.g., hot climates);
- High urine excretion of calcium, uric acid, or oxalate;
- Abnormal urine pH (e.g., uric acid and cystine are less soluble in acid urine, whereas struvite and calcium phosphate are less soluble in alkaline urine);
- Nidus for crystal precipitation (e.g., sodium urate crystallization promotes calcium oxalate stone formation);
- Deficiency of inhibitors of stone formation such as citrate and magnesium.

CLINICAL PRESENTATION

There are several clinical presentations of stone disease.

Calcium oxalate **Uric acid** **Cystine**

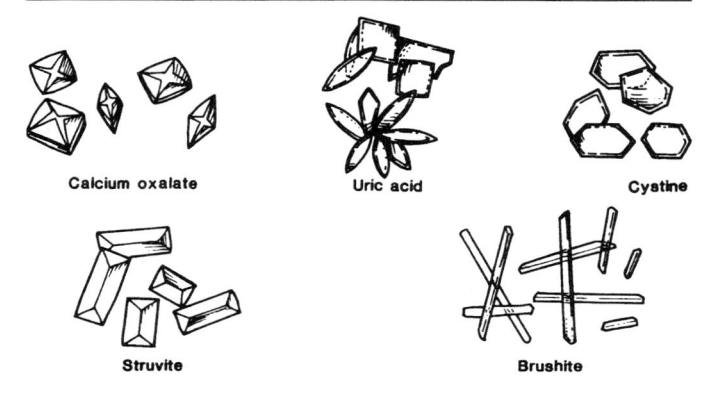

Struvite **Brushite**

Figure 14.1. Urine crystal morphology.

- *Pain* is typically of sudden onset and is quite intense. It may be either steady or colicky and typically radiates to the groin. The pain may be associated with nausea and vomiting.
- *Hematuria* may occur from trauma caused by the stones.
- *Infection* of the stone may lead to either recurrent symptomatic urinary tract infections or to asymptomatic infections that can lead to progressive renal dysfunction.
- *Obstruction* of the renal pelvis or the ureter may occur. Untreated obstruction, even if partial, can lead to irreversible loss of renal function.
- *Asymptomatic stones* may be discovered on an abdominal radiograph or ultrasound obtained for other reasons.

DIAGNOSIS

- *History* should emphasize diet, drug ingestion, and familial disorders.
- *Urinalysis* usually reveals either gross or microscopic hematuria. If pyuria is present, then infection should be excluded by a urine culture. Crystalluria may permit a presumptive identification of stone type (Fig. 14.1).
- *Plain abdominal radiograph* may show radiodense stones (85% of all stones) containing either calcium, struvite, or cystine but may miss radiolucent uric acid stones. An

Table 14.1
Easily Treatable Causes of Stone Disease

Test	Diagnosis
Serum calcium and phosphate	Primary hyperparathyroidism
Serum electrolytes	Distal renal tubular acidosis
Urinalysis	Infection, cystinosis, oxalosis
Stone analysis	Type of stone
Radiologic finding	
Nephrocalcinosis	Distal renal tubular acidosis
Radiolucent stones	Uric acid nephrolithiasis
Staghorn calculi	Struvite stone
"Soft, soap-like" stones	Cystinosis

intravenous pyelogram may determine if an opacity seen on plain x-ray is within the collecting system or may disclose radiolucent stones.
- *Ultrasonography* is used to identify stones and obstruction.
- *Crystallographic stone analysis* is critical for establishing the chemical nature of a stone and guiding therapy. Patients should strain their urine until the stone is passed.

ETIOLOGY OF NEPHROLITHIASIS

All patients should be screened for easily treatable causes of stone disease, as shown in Table 14.1. Disorders found on initial screening should receive diagnosis and specific treatment.

Many patients will not have a disorder found on initial screening. Those with recurrent nephrolithiasis should consider investigation of other causes of stone disease. Most stones contain calcium; causes of calcium-containing stones include hypercalciuria, hypocitraturia, hyperuricosuria, and hyperoxaluria. The relative frequency of these disorders is shown in Table 14.2 (numbers equal more than 100% because many patients have more than one cause of stone disease). Cystinosis and uric acid stones are less frequent causes of stone disease.

Evaluation of these possibilities is a two-step process. First, three 24-hr urine samples are collected for measurement of calcium, citrate, oxalate, cystine, uric acid, sodium, and creatinine content. Second, the patient should fast overnight, then

Table 14.2
Metabolic Abnormalities Found in Stone-Forming Patients

Abnormality	Frequency (%)
Hypercalciuria	55
Absorptive, types 1 and 2	40
Absorptive, type 3	5
Renal	10
Hypocitraturia	50
Hyperuricosuric calcium urolithiasis	40
Hyperoxaluria	15
Primary hyperparathyroidism	8
Infection stones (struvite)	5

collect a 2-hr urine sample for calcium and creatinine measurement. The patient then ingests 1 g of calcium gluconate, followed by a 4-hr urine collection, again for determination of total calcium and creatinine content.

Hypercalciuria

The most common abnormality predisposing to stone formation is hypercalciuria. Hypercalciuria can be due to primary renal calcium wasting or secondary to excessive gastrointestinal tract absorption. The most common cause is intestinal calcium hyperabsorption, resulting in increased urinary calcium excretion and a normal serum calcium (absorptive hypercalciuria, types 1 and 2). Absorptive hypercalciuria can also be due to hypophosphatemia, which stimulates production of 1,25-vitamin D_3, increasing gastrointestinal tract calcium absorption and thereby urinary calcium excretion (absorptive hypercalciuria, type 3). Less frequent is a primary decrease in renal tubular reabsorption of calcium, leading to renal hypercalciuria. Table 14.3 summarizes the diagnostic tests used to differentiate between these conditions.

Many systemic diseases can cause hypercalciuria. Primary hyperparathyroidism accounts for 8% of calcium stones and is potentially curative with surgical therapy. Other causes include sarcoidosis, excess vitamin D and calcium intake, immobilization, and the milk-alkali syndrome.

Table 14.3
Diagnostic Tests in Hypercalciuric Nephrolithiasis

| | Hypercalciuria | | | |
| | Absorptive | | | |
Laboratory Finding	Type 1	Type 2	Type 3	Renal
Elevated 24-hr urine calcium >4 mg/kg/day	+	+	+	+
Fasting urine calcium >0.11 mg/100 mL creatinine clearance	−	−	−	+
Urine calcium after oral calcium load >0.20 mg calcium/mg urine creatinine	+	−	−	+
Hypophosphatemia	−	−	+	−

Hypocitraturia

Urinary citrate both increases the solubility of calcium and slows the growth of calcium oxalate stones. Consequently, hypocitraturia is an important cause of recurrent stone disease. Hypocitraturia can result from distal renal tubular acidosis, chronic diarrhea, or thiazide diuretics.

Hyperuricosuric Calcium Urolithiasis

Hyperuricosuria can predispose to calcium-containing stone formation. When the concentration of sodium urate is sufficiently high, it can crystalize out of solution and act as a nidus for calcium oxalate crystal growth.

Hyperoxaluria

Hyperoxaluria (>60 mg/day) is present in 15% of patients with recurrent stone disease. Primary hyperoxaluria is a rare, autosomal recessive inborn error of metabolism that leads to markedly elevated urinary oxalate excretion, recurrent stone formation, and renal failure in childhood. Secondary hyperoxaluria is much more common (Table 14.4).

Struvite (Magnesium Ammonium Phosphate) Stones

Urinary tract infections with urea-splitting bacteria (i.e., *Proteus, Pseudomonas, Klebsiella,* and, rarely, *Escherichia coli*) can increase

Table 14.4
Secondary Causes of Hyperoxaluria

Gastrointestinal	Other
Bacterial overgrowth	Dietary oxalate excess
Jejunoileal bypass	Ascorbic acid ingestion
Ileal resection	Pyridoxine deficiency
Chronic pancreatitis	Ethylene glycol intoxication
Biliary disorders	Methoxyfluranes
Inflammatory bowel disease	

urine pH, leading to the development of struvite stones. Over 50% of struvite stones occur in association with other risk factors for stone formation.

Uric Acid Stones

Uric acid stones are the most common cause of radiolucent kidney stones. They can form when there is hyperuricosuria and a persistently acid urine. Many patients have normal plasma uric acid levels. Myeloproliferative syndromes, chemotherapeutic treatment of Burkitt's lymphoma and acute leukemia, and Lesch-Nyhan syndrome can cause hyperuricosuria with stone formation or urate nephropathy.

Cystine Stones

Cystinuria is due to an inherited tubular defect of cystine, ornithine, arginine, and lysine transport. Cystine is poorly soluble, especially in acid urine. Urinalysis reveals hexagonal crystals in 50% of patients. The urinary nitroprusside screening test is positive with 75–175 mg cystine/g creatinine. Confirmation is made by measurement of 24-hr urinary cystine excretion exceeding 60 mg/g creatinine.

ACUTE MANAGEMENT OF STONE DISEASE

Acute therapy of stone disease is aimed toward relief of pain, treatment of infection, and removal of the stone. Pain relief usually requires narcotic analgesics. Intravenous fluid is necessary in nauseated or dehydrated patients. It also increases urine flow to facilitate stone passage. Antibiotics are required if infection is present. Patients may need to be hospitalized for the following:

- Intractable pain and vomiting;
- Severe urinary tract infection or sepsis;
- Complete ureteral obstruction;
- Partial obstruction of a solitary kidney.

The likelihood that a stone will pass spontaneously is related to size; 93% of stones smaller than 4 mm will pass, whereas stones larger than 8 mm rarely pass. Extracorporeal shock-wave lithotripsy is frequently effective when stones do not pass spontaneously.

CHRONIC MANAGEMENT OF STONE DISEASE

An important part of therapy in all patients with recurrent stones is to increase urine output. For most patients, a urine volume of 2 L/day will markedly decrease the recurrence of stone disease.

All patients with stone disease should be screened for easily treatable causes, as described under "Etiology of Nephrolithiasis." As many as 50% of patients will have no further stones in the subsequent 10 years. Further evaluation is generally not required for patients with a single episode of nephrolithiasis. In contrast, those with recurrent stones and most children can benefit from further evaluation and appropriate therapy. Therapy is then directed at metabolic abnormalities if present.

Hypercalciuria

Dietary Considerations

- Reduce dietary intake of calcium when excessive. If hyperoxaluria is present, calcium intake should not be restricted because oxalate absorption may increase.
- If hyperoxaluria is present, restrict dietary intake of spinach, cranberries, tea, cocoa, and nuts.
- In presence of hypercalciuria, restrict NaCl to 6 g/day (increased sodium excretion is associated with increased calcium excretion).
- With hyperuricosuria, restrict meat intake to 8–10 oz/day.

Drug Therapy of Hypercalciuric Patients

- *Thiazide diuretics* (e.g., hydrochlorothiazide, 25–50 mg twice a day) decrease urinary calcium excretion by 40–60% and lower urinary oxalate excretion. Dietary sodium should be restricted, otherwise thiazide therapy is ineffective. Potassium citrate should be given to prevent thiazide-induced hypocitraturia. Thiazide diuretics are effective in renal hypercalciuria and mild absorptive hypercalciuria (type 2).
- *Cellulose sodium phosphate* (5 g three times a day with meals) binds intestinal calcium and is useful in the treatment of absorptive hypercalciuria, type 1. Hyperoxaluria and hypomagnesuria can occur; dietary oxalate restriction and magnesium supplements are frequently needed.
- *Neutral sodium phosphate* (500 mg four times a day) increases pyrophosphate excretion, corrects hypophosphatemia, and decreases calcium excretion in absorptive hypercalciuria, type 3.
- *Allopurinol* is useful in patients with hyperuricosuria to inhibit uric acid production.

Hypocitraturia

Citrate, administered as the potassium salt, can correct hypocitraturia. The sodium salt should not be used because sodium loads increase urinary calcium excretion.

Struvite Stones

- Treat with an appropriate antimicrobial agent for at least 6 weeks.
- Consider surgical intervention or extracorporeal shockwave lithotripsy.
- Other metabolic abnormalities are present in 50% of patients with struvite stones and need to be treated also.

Uric Acid Stones

- Alkalinize the urine to decrease uric acid precipitation ($NaHCO_3$ or potassium citrate, 1–3 mEq/kg/day in four doses).

Avoid purine-rich foods.

Use allopurinol if hyperuricosuria is present (>1000 mg/day).

Cystine Stones

- Maintain urine output of 4 L/day to keep cystine in solution.
- Alkalinization of the urine to a pH of >7.5 can be tried. However, this is difficult and requires 15–25 g/day of $NaHCO_3$.
- Dietary restriction of methionine will decrease cystine excretion.
- D-Penicillamine forms soluble mixed disulfide bonds with cystine. It may be used when other measures fail.

FOLLOW-UP

The effect of therapy should be monitored by measurement of urinary and plasma chemistries 1–2 months after initiating treatment and then yearly. Yearly x-rays should be obtained. New stones or growth in the size of existing stones suggests therapy is ineffective and should be reevaluated.

Suggested Readings

Barcelo P, Wuhl O, Servitge E, Rousaud A, Pak CY. Randomized double-blind study of potassium citrate in idiopathic hypocitraturic calcium nephrolithiasis. J Urol 1993;150:1761–1764.

Cicerello E, Merlo F, Gambaro G, et al. Effect of alkaline citrate therapy on clearance of residual stone fragments after extracorporeal shock wave lithotripsy in sterile calcium and infection nephrolithiasis patients. J Urol 1994;151:5–9.

Coe FL, Parks JH, Asplin JR. The pathogenesis and treatment of kidney stones. N Engl J Med 1992;327:1141–1152.

Preminger GM. Renal calculi pathogenesis, diagnosis and management. Semin Nephrol 1992;12:200–216.

Smith LH. Diet and hyperoxaluria in the syndrome of idiopathic calcium oxalate urolithiasis. Am J Kidney Dis 1991;17:370–375.

Chapter 15

Urinary Tract Infection

John C. Peterson

Urinary tract infections (UTI) are among the most common problems in clinical practice. UTIs can be divided into upper (pyelonephritis) and lower (cystitis, urethritis, prostatitis) tract involvement. Recurrent infection by the same organism within 2 weeks of therapy is termed *relapse*. *Reinfection* refers to recurrence of infection with a different pathogen or beyond 2 weeks of therapy. The diagnosis of acute urethral syndrome refers to a presentation of dysuria, often with lower UTI.

INCIDENCE

Among adults, UTIs occur most frequently in women, with a female-to-male ratio of 10:1 to 50:1. The annual incidence of UTIs among sexually active women is 3–10%. This incidence doubles during pregnancy and is higher still in those with a previous history of a UTI. UTIs in males can complicate structural abnormalities or prostatism.

ETIOLOGY

Escherichia coli accounts for 80–90% of uncomplicated UTIs in the ambulatory patient. *Staphylococcus saprophyticus* is responsible for 10–15% of UTIs in young women. In complicated UTIs or in the hospitalized patient, other Gram-negative organisms and enterococci assume greater importance. *S. aureus* bacteriuria is uncommon and implies hematogenous renal involvement. The acute urethral syndrome has been associated with *Chlamydia, Neisseria gonorrhoeae, Trichomonas vaginitis,* or bacterial vaginosis.

PATHOPHYSIOLOGY

Sterility of the urine, bladder, and upper tract is maintained by host defenses including colonization of the periurethral region by nonpathogenic flora, shedding of epithelial cells, mechanical flushing by micturition, secretion of proteins by the bladder and renal tubules to prevent adhesion, antibacterial effects of intrinsic urinary factors (urea, pH), prostatic secretions, and local polymorphonuclear leukocytes. When these defense mechanisms are breached by urine stasis, calculi, foreign material, vesicoureteral reflux, instrumentation or coitus, UTI may develop. In addition, bacteriuria may occur in pregnancy due to functional impairment of ureteral tone and enlarged bladder capacity.

Lower UTIs develop when enteric pathogens are introduced retrograde into the bladder, leading to cystitis or other lower tract infections. Bacteria may infect the upper tract in ascending fashion, leading to pyelonephritis depending on the virulence of the organism and the functional status of the defense mechanisms (vide supra). Pyelonephritis may also occur by hematogenous dissemination of organisms such as *S. aureus* and *Mycobacterium tuberculosis*.

Acute pyelonephritis develops in discrete foci and spreads from the renal pelvis to the cortex. The kidney is grossly edematous, and small subcapsular abscesses may be present. Microscopically, there is an acute focal inflammatory cell infiltration interspersed with normal histology. White cell casts may be seen within the tubules. In *chronic pyelonephritis*, there is cortical scarring and calyceal dilatation. The infiltration consists of lymphocytes, plasma cells, and eosinophils along with tubular atrophy and interstitial fibrosis.

BACTERIOLOGIC AND RADIOGRAPHIC EVALUATION

Urinalysis and quantitative urine culture with antibiotic sensitivities should be obtained to confirm infection and guide therapy; empiric treatment of symptomatic young women without culture has also been advocated with close follow-up for evidence of recurrence or reinfection. Testing for urine nitrites and leukocyte esterase by dipstick is a useful screening test with sensitivities of 70–95% and specificities of 65–85%. The finding of bacteria by high-power field in an uncentrifuged urine sample correlates well with 10^5 organisms/mL urine on culture. Examination of the urine sediment may reveal white blood cell casts suggesting renal parenchymal involvement.

Significant bacteriuria is defined as the isolation of 10^5 organisms/mL of urine collected by clean catch technique or by recovery of 10^2 organisms/mL by sterile catheterization. Recovery of low bacterial counts or polymicrobial bacteriuria may imply improper collection unless the patient is clinically symptomatic.

Urologic studies are indicated on women with relapsing UTIs or men with UTIs. Such tests in an unselected population will reveal structural abnormalities in less than 1%. Table 15.1 lists the findings in various conditions.

CLINICAL PRESENTATION AND MANAGEMENT OF SPECIFIC UTI SYNDROMES

Asymptomatic Bacteriuria

True asymptomatic bacteriuria has >10^5 organisms/mL of urine on several cultures. In most adults, asymptomatic bacteriuria has a benign prognosis and may not require specific treatment. Exceptions include patients with abnormalities of the urinary tract, diabetes, immunocompromised status, history of pyelonephritis, and pregnancy. In nonpregnant adults with asymptomatic bacteriuria, single dose or short course (3–7 days) therapy is usually successful.

Approximately 20–30% of pregnant women with untreated asymptomatic bacteriuria will develop pyelonephritis and should be treated and monitored for recurrence. Tetracycline, trimethoprim, and chloramphenicol should not be used in pregnancy; sulfonamides should be avoided in the third trimester.

Acute Urethral Syndrome

Acute urethral syndrome occurs in young women with dysuria and pyuria. Urine culture reveals <10^4 organisms/mL of urine. Empiric single dose or short course antibiotic therapy may be effective. Lower urinary tract symptoms and pyuria, but negative cultures, may suggest the presence of tuberculosis, sexually transmitted disease, or a gynecologic disorder requiring further evaluation. Women having only dysuria (no pyuria, negative cultures) should be treated with urinary analgesics.

Table 15.1
Findings by Renal Imaging in Complicated Urinary Tract Infections

Condition	Intravenous Pyelography	Ultrasonography	Computed Tomography
Acute pyelonephritis uncomplicated	Normal in 75% ↑ Renal size Prolonged nephrogram[a]	↑ Renal size Variable parenchymal echogenicity No hydronephrosis	↑ Renal size ↓ Corticomedullary definition ↓ Function
Chronic pyelonephritis	↓ Cortical width ↓ Function Focal scarring and caliectasis	↓ Renal size Lobar hypertrophy with "pseudotumor"	↓ Renal size ↓ Function "Pseudotumor"
Renal-perinephric abscess	Mass effect Distortion of renal contour and calyces Absent psoas margin	Thick-walled cystic mass with external echoes	Thick-walled cystic mass ↓ Attenuation of contents
UTI with obstruction	↓ Function Mass effect	Dilated collecting system with echogenic debris	Dilated collecting system ↓ Function Contents of variable density
Renal tuberculosis	Punctuate calcifications Calyceal deformity Autoamputation	Nonspecific findings	Scattered areas of decreased attenuation

Modified from Benson M, LiPuma JP, Resick MI. Urol Clin North Am 1986;13:605–625.
[a] ↓ Function indicates prolonged nephrogram and delayed excretion of contrast agent.

Table 15.2
Single Dose Regimens

Drug	Dose	Cure Rate
Trimethoprim, 160 mg/sulfamethoxazole, 800 mg (Bactrim DS)	2 tablets	76–95%
Amoxicillin	3 g	50–85%

Cystitis and Pyelonephritis

Although the separation of UTIs into lower or upper tract infections is conceptually attractive, this distinction is clinically difficult. Some 30–50% of women with cystitis and $>10^5$ organisms/mL of urine have concomitant silent upper tract infection. Nevertheless, this distinction is important with regard to duration of treatment.

Cystitis is suggested by the presence of dysuria, frequency, pelvic pain, pyuria, bacteriuria, or hematuria. The presence of flank pain, high fevers, prostration, nausea, vomiting, hypotension, leukocytosis, or pyuria with white cell casts in addition to lower tract findings suggests acute pyelonephritis.

Treatment of lower UTIs includes single dose therapy (Table 15.2) or short course treatment for 3–7 days. Single dose regimens have the advantages of convenience, lower cost, and high compliance but are ineffective for upper UTIs or silent pyelonephritis. Single dose regimens are not suitable for males, patients with complicated UTIs, or individuals not available for follow-up evaluation.

Patients who relapse after single dose therapy should have a quantitative culture performed and treatment with short course (3–7 days) antibiotics. Patients who relapse after short course therapy with appropriate antibiotics should be treated for an additional 2–6 weeks and investigated for underlying factors predisposing to UTI. Prophylactic therapy may be indicated for frequent reinfections.

Reliable patients with uncomplicated acute pyelonephritis and adequate follow-up may be treated as outpatients. Patients with complicated pyelonephritis require hospitalization and parenteral antibiotics until afebrile for 48 hr, then oral antibiotics for at least 2 weeks. Therapy is guided by susceptibility testing. Patients who fail to respond within a few days while on appropriate therapy or who present with sepsis should undergo prompt evaluation for complicating obstructive uropathy, infected renal calculi (see Chapter 14), and intrarenal or perinephric abscess. Posttreatment urine cultures should be obtained 2 weeks after completion of therapy and again at 6–12 weeks to screen for relapse and reinfection, respectively.

An intrarenal abscess may complicate acute pyelonephritis or may arise by hematogenous infection with *S. aureus*, *M. tuberculosis* or *Candida* species. Patients with obstructive abnormalities, vesicoureteral reflux, renal calculi, and diabetes mellitus are at particular risk. Intrarenal or perinephric abscess may mimic pyelonephritis and requires timely radiographic investigation. Appropriate antibiotic therapy can successfully resolve most intrarenal abscesses. Perinephric abscess always requires drainage in addition to antibiotic therapy, because mortality with this complication is 20–50%.

Catheter-Related UTI

Chronic indwelling urinary catheters are the most common cause of Gram-negative bacteriuria in hospitalized patients. They should be used only where necessary and removed as soon as possible because they inevitably lead to bacteriuria. Intermittent and suprapubic catheterization are alternatives. Antibiotic therapy is reserved for symptomatic infections. Long-term suppressive therapy in patients with indwelling catheters leads to selection of resistant pathogens and is generally not indicated. Candiduria may occur in this setting, and treatment includes removal of the indwelling catheter and administration of fluconazole or intravesical amphotericin B.

Prostatitis

Acute bacterial prostatitis presents with symptoms of lower UTI, perineal pain, or obstruction. Examination reveals a tender and swollen prostate. Urinalysis usually reveals pyuria and bacteriuria with typical uropathogens on culture. Treatment is similar to UTIs but is extended for 30 days. When urine cultures fail to identify a causative organism, nonbacterial causes such as *Ureaplasma urealyticum*, *Chlamydia*, or tuberculosis should be considered. A trial of antibiotic therapy with trimethoprim-sulfamethoxazole or tetracycline may be employed when urine cultures fail to identify an infecting organism.

Chronic bacterial prostatitis is an important cause of recurrent UTI in males. Inflammatory cells and bacteria may be expressed in prostatic fluid. Trimethoprim-sulfamethoxazale can be given for 4–16 weeks; however, cure rates are poor. Refractory cases may require long-term antibiotic suppression or total prostatovesiculectomy.

UTI in Chronic Renal Disease

UTIs in the presence of chronic renal insufficiency require careful antibiotic selection, dosage adjustment, and avoidance of nephrotoxic agents (e.g., aminoglycosides) and of nitrofurantoin because of the potential for peripheral neuropathy.

Patients with infected cysts may require long-term antibiotic therapy with drugs such as trimethoprim, clindamycin, or fluoroquinalones that penetrate into cyst fluid. Dialysis patients may accumulate a reservoir of urine in the bladder that can become infected. In the evaluation of febrile dialysis patients, a single diagnostic bladder catheterization to exclude UTI should not be overlooked.

Suggested Readings

Andriole VT, Patterson, TF. Epidemiology, natural history and management of urinary tract infections in pregnancy. Med Clin North Am 1991;75:359–373.

Benson M, LiPuma JP, Resnick MI. The role of imaging studies in urinary tract infection. Urol Clin North Am 1986;13:605–625.

Hooton T, Stamm W. Management of acute uncomplicated urinary tract infection in adults. Med Clin North Am 1991;75:339–358.

Lipsky BJ. Urinary tract infections in men. Ann Intern Med 1989; 110:138–150.

Roberts JA. Etiology and pathophysiology of pyelonephritis. Am J Kidney Dis 1991;17:1–9.

Svanborg C, De Man P, Sandberg T. Renal involvement in urinary tract infection. Kidney Int 1991;39:541–549.

Chapter 16

Tubulointerstitial Nephritis

Nicolas J. Guzman

Tubulointerstitial nephritis (TIN) is an inflammatory disorder of the renal interstitium that is commonly accompanied by tubular inflammation. Occasionally, the latter may be primary with involvement of the interstitium occurring as a secondary event. TIN that accompanies primary glomerular or vascular diseases and allograft rejection will be discussed elsewhere. Approximately half of the cases of acute TIN are drug related.

INCIDENCE

TIN is responsible for 11–14% of the cases of acute renal failure (ARF), whereas chronic TIN is an infrequent cause of end-stage renal failure.

ETIOLOGY

Infections

- Acute:
  Bacterial
    Acute pyelonephritis
    Rocky Mountain spotted fever
  Viral
    Cytomegalovirus
- Chronic:
  Bacterial
    Chronic obstructive pyelonephritis
    Tuberculosis

Fungal
  Histoplasmosis
Parasitic infection
  Schistosomiasis
  Malaria (*Plasmodium falciparum*)
Xanthogranulomatous pyelonephritis
Malacoplakia
Sarcoid nephropathy

Drugs

Analgesic nephropathy
Lithium nephropathy

Metabolic Causes

Hypokalemic nephropathy
Hypercalcemic nephropathy
Urate nephropathy
Oxalate nephropathy

Other Causes

Heavy metals
Reflux nephropathy
Obstructive uropathy
Neoplastic diseases
  Plasma cell dyscrasias
  Myeloma kidney
  Light chain deposition disease
  Lymphoproliferative diseases
  Leukemia

CLINICAL MANIFESTATIONS

Except for the acute diffuse forms of TIN (e.g., drug hypersensitivity), the early stages of the disease are characterized by a normal or mildly decreased glomerular filtration rate and proteinuria of <2 g/24 hr. The urinary sediment usually contains white blood cells, red blood cells, and occasionally white blood cell casts. Eosinophils may be seen on Wright's or Hansel's stain of the urinary sediment in patients with drug-induced hypersensitivity TIN. Peripheral eosinophilia is, however, a more consistent finding. As inflammation progresses, the glomeruli may also be involved, resulting in progressive renal insufficiency, worsening proteinuria and hematuria, oliguria, and hypertension. At these more advanced stages of the disease, the clinical picture is difficult to differentiate from that of a primary glomerular disease, and the diagnosis will often have to be made by kidney biopsy.

In its early stages, TIN can present as any combination of three patterns of renal dysfunction: proximal tubular dysfunction manifested as renal tubular acidosis (type II) with or without Fanconi's syndrome; distal tubular dysfunction manifested as renal tubular acidosis (type I), salt wasting, or hyperkalemia; and renal medullary dysfunction resulting in decreased concentrating ability with polyuria and nocturia.

ACUTE TUBULOINTERSTITIAL NEPHRITIS

The two most common causes of acute TIN are bacterial pyelonephritis (see Chapter 15) and drug-induced hypersensitivity TIN. Other forms of acute TIN, such as TIN associated with systemic infections (reactive TIN) and idiopathic TIN, are uncommon and will not be discussed here.

Acute Drug-Induced Hypersensitivity TIN

The number of drugs reported to cause acute TIN is large and continues to increase (Table 16.1). Drugs implicated more frequently include the β-lactam antibiotics, particularly methicillin, and the nonsteroidal antiinflammatory drugs (NSAID), particularly propionic acid derivatives such as ibuprofen, fenoprofen, and naproxen. The risk of developing acute TIN increases with prolonged therapy. The mean duration of therapy before the onset of methicillin-induced TIN is 15 days, but it has been seen as early as 2 days and as late as 44 days. The absence of prior penicillin allergy is no protection against the development of TIN.

Pathophysiology

Drug-induced acute TIN occurs as a result of both humoral and cell-mediated hypersensitivity reactions mounted against a hapten (drug or drug metabolite) protein complex. The response is

Table 16.1
Drugs Commonly Associated with Acute Hypersensitivity TIN

Antibiotics	Nonsteroidal antiinflammatory agents
β-Lactam antibiotics (e.g., penicillins, cephalosporins)	Indomethacin
Ethambutol	Phenylbutazone
Tetracyclines	Fenoprofen
Sulfonamides	Mefenamic acid
Vancomycin	Ibuprofen
Trimethoprim-sulfamethoxazole	Aspirin
Erythromycin	Naproxen
Rifampin	Tolmetin
Ciprofloxacin	Others
Diuretics	Cimetidine
Furosemide	Phenytoin
Bumetanide	α-Methyl-dopa
Thiazides	Carbamazepine
	Allopurinol

not dose related and recurs rapidly after drug rechallenge. Within a class of related drugs, structural similarity can lead to immunological cross-reactivity. For example, the presence of a sulfa group in both furosemide and bumetanide precludes their use in patients who have demonstrated hypersensitivity to either drug.

Histologically, light microscopy reveals focal interstitial infiltrates of mononuclear cells, predominantly lymphocytes, accompanied by edema and variable numbers of eosinophils. Acute tubular necrosis is common, but the medulla, glomeruli, and vessels are usually spared. A smaller number of patients will present with one or more of three variations: (*a*) a granulomatous response usually associated with allopurinol, thiazides, sulfonamides, oxacillin, and polymyxin; (*b*) minimal change nephrotic syndrome associated with nonsteroidal antiinflammatory drugs; and (*c*) a predominant tubular injury as in rifampin-induced TIN.

Clinical Manifestations

Acute drug-induced TIN presents with signs and symptoms characteristic of an allergic reaction as shown in Table 16.2. Blood eosinophilia is usually transient. Eosinophiluria is a common finding in acute TIN but is also frequently seen in other kidney diseases. ARF occurs more frequently in the elderly

Table 16.2
Clinical Features of Acute Drug-Induced TIN

Signs and Symptoms	Laboratory Findings
Fever (85–100%)	Hematuria (95%)
Maculopapular rash (25–50%)	Eosinophilia (80%)
Arthralgias	Sterile pyuria
Uremic symptoms	Low grade proteinuria
	Eosinophiluria
	White blood cell casts

(20–50%). Even in the absence of all of the above clinical features, acute drug-induced TIN should be suspected in all patients with ARF of unknown etiology.

Investigations

A detailed history of drug intake and previous allergic reactions should be obtained. Careful examination of the urinary sediment is essential. Ultrasound examination may reveal kidney enlargement. Radioactive gallium scanning during acute TIN shows intense uptake of the isotope by the kidneys and is reported to be useful in differentiating acute TIN from acute tubular necrosis in which gallium uptake by the kidneys is not increased. A kidney biopsy should be performed in those patients in whom the diagnosis is unclear.

Treatment and Prognosis

The offending agent should be discontinued to prevent progressive renal insufficiency. Acute dialysis therapy is necessary in up to 35% of patients. Although corticosteroids have been reported to be beneficial in some patients, controlled clinical trials are not yet available.

Most patients will have complete recovery of renal function within 1 year, and only a few will have permanent functional impairment. Prolonged ARF lasting longer than 3 weeks and advanced age at onset are adverse prognostic indicators.

Nonsteroidal Antiinflammatory Drugs

NSAIDs can cause various adverse renal effects including sodium retention, hyporeninemic hypoaldosteronism with hyperkalemia, ARF, nephrotic syndrome, and acute TIN. Patients with this entity tend to be older and generally have taken the drugs for a prolonged time (1–2 years). They may or may not present with signs and symptoms characteristic of a hypersensitivity reaction. Most patients with NSAID-induced minimal change nephrotic syndrome do not have evidence of hypersensitivity. These syndromes are rapidly reversed upon discontinuation of the offending drug.

Rifampin can cause three different patterns of renal injury: (*a*) classic acute TIN; (*b*) direct proximal tubular injury with little interstitial involvement (probably because of a toxic mechanism); and (*c*) minimal change nephrotic syndrome. The clinical pattern of rifampin-induced TIN is unique, with the abrupt onset of renal failure occurring upon rechallenge with the drug. Most cases have occurred during intermittent therapy (two to three times per week) or after resumption of therapy following a drug-free interval. The clinical presentation is highly suggestive of a hypersensitivity reaction, with fever, chills, myalgias, arthralgias, skin rashes, eosinophilia, eosinophiluria, and oliguric ARF. The toxic form presents as a more gradual decline in renal function associated with granular casts. In either case, renal function improves over several weeks once the drug is discontinued.

CHRONIC DRUG-INDUCED TUBULOINTERSTITIAL NEPHRITIS

The most common form of chronic drug-induced TIN is analgesic nephropathy. The ingestion of large amounts of analgesics over prolonged periods can lead to both chronic TIN and papillary necrosis.

Incidence

The incidence of analgesic nephropathy in the United States varies significantly among different geographic areas. Studies on patients with end-stage renal failure in Washington DC and Philadelphia showed an incidence of analgesic abuse of 2.8 and 1.7%, respectively. In North Carolina, however, where there was a high incidence of the use of over-the-counter, phenacetin-containing powders, analgesic nephropathy was found in up to 13% of patients with end-stage renal failure.

Pathophysiology

Although papillary necrosis is seen most commonly after ingestion of mixtures of aspirin and phenacetin, TIN can occur with prolonged use of various combinations of aspirin, phenacetin, acetaminophen, aminopyrine, phenazone, and salicylamide. Renal injury is dose dependent. The accepted criterion for the diagnosis of analgesic nephropathy in a patient with TIN is a cumulative analgesic intake of 3 kg or more or ingestion of 1 g/day for 3 years. Phenacetin metabolites (e.g., acetaminophen) and aspirin are concentrated in the kidney, particularly in the papillae, where dehydration further increases their concentration. Acetaminophen is metabolized in the renal papillae to reactive metabolites that cause toxic injury by covalently binding to macromolecules or by lipid peroxidation.

On pathological examination, the early stages of analgesic nephropathy are characterized by patchy necrosis of interstitial cells, loops of Henle, and capillaries of the inner medulla. As the disease progresses, there is necrosis of the tip of the papillae and outer medulla and early focal atrophy of cortical tubules. Later stages are characterized by total necrosis of the inner medulla and papillae and cortical atrophy.

Clinical Manifestations

Analgesic nephropathy occurs most frequently in women with a history of chronic headaches, arthritis, or muscular pain. When questioned, they often deny or underestimate the actual intake. Nocturia caused by the inability to concentrate urine is a common early symptom. Gross hematuria, sometimes associated with sloughed papillary fragments in the urine and renal colic, is an occasional presenting symptom. Patients commonly present with moderate hypertension and anemia. The latter is usually compounded by occult gastrointestinal blood loss from analgesic-induced gastritis or peptic ulcer. Both persistent sterile pyuria and bouts of bacterial pyelonephritis occur frequently. Proteinuria (<1 g/24 hr) and renal tubular acidosis are common. Occasionally, there is diminished citrate secretion leading to nephrocalcinosis.

Investigations

Most patients (90%) with analgesic nephropathy have an abnormal intravenous pyelogram. Initially, calyces appear widened, and incipient papillary detachment may lead to leakage of contrast material into the renal parenchyma. Papillary necrosis, followed by detachment of the necrotic papillae, results in cavity formation. Blunting of the calyces and reduction in kidney size occur in advanced disease.

Treatment

Cessation of analgesic abuse, control of hypertension, and treatment of urinary tract infections are essential. Early diagnosis and treatment of obstruction is also critical to avoid progressive renal insufficiency. The prognosis in patients treated early is usually good, and renal function can stabilize or improve with time. Persistent analgesic abuse invariably leads to chronic renal insufficiency and end-stage renal failure.

Suggested Readings

Fried T. Acute interstitial nephritis. Postgrad Med 1993;93:105–120.

Hoitsma AJ, Wetzels JF, Koene RA. Drug-induced nephrotoxicity: etiology, clinical features and management. Drug Saf 1991;6:131–47.

Kleinknecht D, Vanhille PH, Morel-Maroger L, et al. Acute interstitial nephritis due to drug hypersensitivity. Adv Nephrol 1983;12:277–308.

Murray T, Goldberg M. Chronic interstitial nephritis. Etiologic factors. Ann Intern Med 1975;82:453–459.

Murray T, Goldberg M. Analgesic-associated nephropathy in the USA. Kidney Int 1978;13:64–71.

Porile JL, Bakris GL, Garella S. Acute interstitial nephritis with glomerulopathy due to nonsteroidal anti-inflammatory agents: a review of its clinical spectrum and effects of steroid therapy. J Clin Pharmacol 1990;30:468–475.

Whelton A, Hamilton CW. Nonsteroidal anti-inflammatory drugs: effects on kidney function. J Clin Pharmacol 1991;31:588–598.

Chapter 17

Renal Cystic Disease

Christopher S. Wilcox

Renal cysts are fluid-filled cavities with epithelial linings. Simple renal cysts increase in frequency with age but are of little clinical importance. Ultrasound examination of renal cysts reveals a homogeneous pattern without internal echoes. Computed tomography (CT) scanning shows an attenuation value close to water, no enhancement with intravenous contrast, no measurable thickness or irregularity of the cyst wall, and a smooth interface with the renal parenchyma.

Three cystic diseases that occur in adults cause significant complications: autosomal dominant polycystic kidney disease (adult type) (ADPKD), medullary sponge kidney disease, and medullary cystic kidney disease (Table 17.1). Additionally, an autosomal recessive polycystic kidney disease is encountered predominantly in children and presents with renal failure.

ETIOLOGY

Renal cysts develop from tubules with which they may retain continuity. Therefore, they usually increase slowly in size by accumulation of glomerular filtrate or secreted solutes and fluid. The etiology of renal cysts may involve tubular obstruction elevating luminal pressure, increased elasticity of the tubular basement membrane, or proliferation of epithelial cells with production of excessive basement membrane.

Table 17.1
Clinical Features of Major Renal Cyst Diseases

	Simple renal cysts	Autosomal dominant polycystic kidney diseases	Medullary sponge kidney	Medullary cystic kidney disease
Incidence	1:10	1:600	1:5000	Rare
Median age at presentation	Variable	20–40 years	40–60 years	Variable
Inheritance	None	Autosomal dominant	None	Mainly autosomal dominant
Cyst location	Variable	Proximal and distal tubules	Collecting duct	Corticomedullary junction
Flank pain or hematuria	Rare	Frequent	With stones or infection	None
Major complications	Rare	Hypertension UTIs Renal stones Aneurysms	UTIs Renal stones	Salt wasting Polyuria
Renal failure	Absent	Frequent	Rare	Inevitable

UTI, urinary tract infection.

AUTOSOMAL DOMINANT POLYCYSTIC KIDNEY DISEASE

Clinical Presentation and Diagnosis

Inheritance by an autosomal-dominant trait with nearly complete penetrance implies that each patient should have one affected parent and that the disease will be present on average in half the siblings. However, there is considerable variability of expression. The most common mutant gene is closely linked to the α-globulin gene locus on the short arm of chromosome 16.

A family history of ADPKD is obtained in 75% of patients. Most have episodes of abdominal or flank pain, often associated with gross or microscopic hematuria. More than half have hypertension, and many have urinary tract infections or renal stone disease. Both kidneys are usually enlarged and have an irregular surface that can often be palpated by abdominal examination. Some 20% have hepatic cysts. Urinalysis typically

Table 17.2
Diagnostic Criteria for ADPKD

Primary criteria
  Five or more fluid-filled cysts scattered diffusely throughout renal cortex and medulla of both kidneys
  Definite history of polycystic kidney disease in genetically related family members
Secondary criteria
  Cysts of liver
  Cysts of pancreas
  Aneurysms of cerebral arteries
  Renal insufficiency

---

shows modest proteinuria (<200 mg/day). Hematocrit may be higher than expected for the degree of renal failure because of increased erythropoietin secretion.

The diagnosis rests on a typical spectrum of clinical findings. The most sensitive test for confirming the diagnosis is CT scanning with contrast. However, renal ultrasound can detect cysts down to 0.5 cm and is nearly as sensitive as CT scanning. Because of its lower cost and the absence of exposure to x-rays or radiocontrast agents, ultrasound is often preferred for diagnosis or screening (Table 17.2).

Treatment of Complications

Pain

Patients may have episodes of disabling abdominal or flank pain often related to rupture of a blood vessel into a cyst or around the kidney. The pain usually responds to bed rest and analgesics.

Hematuria

This can be caused by rupture of a cyst or by renal stones, cyst infection, or malignant transformation. Hematuria should prompt a search to determine the cause.

Renal Infection

Bacterial cyst infection is difficult to diagnose and eradicate. Urinalysis may be normal, because cyst fluid does not communicate directly with the urine. Helpful signs include pain, fever, diaphoresis, bacteremia, and leukocytosis. Infected cysts may have an increased wall thickness by CT scanning. Infecting organisms include *Escherichia coli*, *Staphylococci*, and *Bacteroides*. Some infected cysts respond to high-dose, relatively prolonged (2–3 weeks) therapy with a conventional antibiotic regimen such as a broad-spectrum penicillin or cephalosporin plus an aminoglycoside. However, other infected cysts are quite impenetrable except by lipid-soluble antibiotics such as clindamycin, chloramphenicol, ciprofloxacin, or trimethoprim-sulfamethoxazole.

Hypertension

Most patients develop hypertension. Activation of the renin-angiotensin system and salt retention are implicated, especially with the development of renal insufficiency. Usually, hypertension responds to α- or β-blockers or calcium antagonists.

Cerebral Aneurysms

Some 10–35% of patients have a cerebral aneurysm. Where the diameter is below 1 cm, rupture is unusual; larger aneurysms can produce intracranial hemorrhage. Currently, magnetic resonance imaging followed by arteriography to diagnose cerebral aneurysms is not universally recommended in the absence of symptoms. The knowledge that aneurysms are common mandates meticulous treatment of hypertension.

Nephrolithiasis

Some 10–20% of patients have nephrolithiasis, typically calcium oxalate. Patients should maintain a high fluid intake sufficient to produce 2 L of urine daily. Established renal stone disease requires careful evaluation and treatment as discussed in Chapter 14, because it can accentuate the decline in renal function and predisposes to infection.

Renal Insufficiency

Renal failure eventually develops in most patients, although occasionally this may be delayed into old age. It is helpful to plot the reciprocal of serum creatinine concentration ($1/S_{cr}$) against time. A steepening of the slope of the line may indicate the need for more aggressive treatment of hypertension or a search for a complication such as unrecognized renal stones. Measures that may delay progression of renal failure include meticulous treatment of hypertension, use of an angiotensin-converting enzyme inhibitor for antihypertensive therapy, and prescription of a low-protein intake.

Patients with ADPKD respond well to *chronic hemodialysis*. *Peritoneal dialysis* is less satisfactory because the enlarged kidneys may limit the abdominal space available for fluids. *Renal transplantation* is offered routinely. It is critical to evaluate living related donors very carefully to ensure that they do not have an early form of the disease.

Counseling

A nephrologist should direct counseling and screening of family members once a patient with ADPKD has been identified.

Prognosis

The creatinine clearance halves (i.e., the serum creatinine doubles) on average every 36 months once renal insufficiency has developed. No therapy unequivocally prolongs renal function.

MEDULLARY SPONGE KIDNEY

Pathology

Although probably present at birth, manifestations are usually delayed until age 40–60 years. There is marked enlargement of the medullary and papillary portions of the collecting ducts, which may affect one or more papillae. Unless there are complications from stone disease or infection, renal function is well maintained.

Clinical Presentation

The disease usually presents with hematuria (gross or microscopic), recurrent urinary tract infections, or nephrolithiasis. There may be a defect in urine concentrating ability, a distal-type renal tubular acidosis with a reduced ability to lower urinary pH below 5.5, or nephrocalcinosis. Diagnosis is by intravenous pyelography, which demonstrates the dilated terminal collecting ducts.

Therapy

Renal tubular acidosis requires alkali therapy. Patients with nephrolithiasis typically have hypercalciuria, which, with the renal tubular acidosis, accounts for the high incidence of stone disease. Asymptomatic patients should drink sufficiently to excrete 2 L of urine daily. Hypercalciuric patients require thiazides.

MEDULLARY CYSTIC DISEASE

Pathology

Multiple small cysts develop at the corticomedullary junction. The kidneys are small, the cortex is reduced, and the glomeruli are sclerotic.

Clinical Presentation

Progressive renal failure may be seen in childhood but can present in the adult. Patients often have polyuria, polydipsia, and sodium wasting. There is no specific therapy, although the free water clearance and sodium-losing conditions require careful management. The disease progresses to end-stage. Diagnosis is by open biopsy.

ACQUIRED CYSTIC KIDNEY DISEASE

About half of the patients receiving dialysis for more than 4 years develop multiple cysts in their remnant kidneys that may contribute to erythrocytosis or hypertension. These cysts can contain neoplastic foci arising from the cyst lining that resemble a renal adenoma or adenocarcinoma.

The diagnosis is usually made by ultrasound or CT scanning. Fortunately, the neoplastic potential of these cysts is not usually expressed by invasion or metastasis, although this can occur. Cystic kidneys can be removed surgically or ablated radiologically using intraarterial injection of alcohol. Cysts, once detected, can be followed by regular CT scanning with contrast, and any change suggestive of neoplasia should trigger consideration of nephrectomy or renal ablation.

Suggested Readings

Gabow P. Autosomal dominant polycystic kidney disease; more than a renal disease. Am J Kidney Dis 1990;16:403–413.

Gehring JJ, Gottheiner TI, Swenson RS. Acquired cystic disease of the end-stage kidney. Am J Med 1985;79:609–620.

Kaehny WD, Gabow PA. Polycystic kidney disease. Contemp Issues Nephrol 1991;15:49–72.

Sklar AH, Caruana RJ, Lammers JE, Strauser GD. Renal infections in autosomal-dominant polycystic kidney disease. Am J Kidney Dis 1987;10:81–88.

Welling LW, Grantham JJ. Cystic and developmental diseases of the kidney. In: Brenner BM, Rector FC, eds. The kidney, 4th ed. Philadelphia: Saunders, 1991:1657–1694.

Welling LW, Grantham JJ. Cystic diseases of the kidney. In: Tisher CC, Brenner BM, eds. Renal pathology with clinical and functional correlations, 2nd ed. Philadelphia: Lippincott, 1994:1312–1354.

Chapter 18

AIDS and Kidney Disease

C. Craig Tisher

In most patients the kidney is not the major organ involved in acquired immune deficiency syndrome (AIDS). However, acute and chronic renal failure and significant fluid and electrolyte disturbances are observed in affected patients and often require intervention by a nephrologist. The magnitude of the problem is difficult to assess because detailed epidemiologic data are limited. However, more than 300,000 patients with AIDS have been reported to the Centers for Disease Control and Prevention, and it is estimated that more than 1 million individuals are human immunodeficiency virus (HIV) positive. It is clear that as the number of patients with HIV seropositivity, AIDS-related complex (ARC), and AIDS increases, the number of individuals who develop renal failure will increase in parallel.

Kidney involvement falls into three categories: (*a*) acute renal failure (ARF); (*b*) chronic renal failure, most often associated with proteinuria and histologic lesions of focal and segmental glomerulosclerosis, so-called HIV-associated nephropathy; and (*c*) patients with renal failure on maintenance hemodialysis who subsequently develop AIDS.

ACUTE RENAL FAILURE

ARF is a frequent complication in patients with HIV infection, especially those with the clinical picture of AIDS. Diagnosis is essentially the same as in any patient who manifests a rising blood urea nitrogen or serum creatinine (see Chapter 8). Sepsis with hypotension and drug nephrotoxicity secondary to pentamidine, antibiotics, and radiocontrast agents explain the ARF in most patients. Other potentially nephrotoxic agents commonly employed to treat many of the infectious complications in HIV-infected patients include rifampin, dapsone, trimethoprim-sulfamethoxazole, and amphotericin B. Occasionally, ARF may be secondary to a drug-induced allergic tubulointerstitial nephritis or to hyperuricemia resulting from the use of certain chemotherapeutic agents in the treatment of AIDS-related malignancies.

There is little doubt that ARF contributes to the mortality and morbidity in these patients, although sepsis remains the leading cause of death. If these patients are hemodynamically stable, hemodialysis can be beneficial, and the decision to treat should be made using the same clinical criteria as in non–HIV-infected patients.

CHRONIC RENAL FAILURE

There has been considerable controversy regarding the existence of a specific HIV-associated nephropathy. The clinicopathologic features that include proteinuria in the nephrotic range, rapidly advancing renal failure, and the histologic lesions of focal and segmental glomerulosclerosis are also observed in patients with prolonged heroin use in the absence of HIV infections. Because many HIV-positive patients are also intravenous heroin users, especially in large metropolitan areas where the disease is more prevalent, it has been difficult to distinguish between these two potential etiologies. However, with more clinical experience gained by examining nonaddicted patients with HIV infection, it is becoming increasingly apparent that HIV-associated nephropathy should be considered a separate entity.

The results of chronic dialysis treatment in patients with end-stage renal failure complicating AIDS generally have been dismal. Many are too debilitated to be treated as outpatients, and they die of other complications of their illness within a few weeks. Often they become cachectic on hemodialysis despite intensive nutritional support and die of a combination of uremia, malnutrition, and infections. Although the decision to treat in this group of patients must be individualized, there is growing evidence that maintenance hemodialysis is not effective in prolonging survival.

In contrast to the experience in patients with AIDS and end-stage renal failure, those patients with chronic renal failure who have ARC or are seropositive for HIV appear to have a better prognosis with maintenance dialysis. Although the experience is limited to small numbers of patients, both continuous ambulatory peritoneal dialysis and hemodialysis, including self-dialysis at home, have met with some success. Again, treatment decisions must be individualized.

Another group of patients has been described who develop AIDS after becoming uremic and beginning dialysis. The typical patient has a history of intravenous drug use that often contributed to the chronic renal failure initially. Although intravenous drug addicts maintained on chronic hemodialysis exhibit a relatively stable course, the additional complications of AIDS are generally fatal within a few weeks.

FLUID AND ELECTROLYTE DISORDERS

Hyponatremia is the most common electrolyte disturbance observed in HIV-infected patients and is due to various causes. These include adrenal insufficiency with renal salt wasting, excessive vomiting and diarrhea often complicated by inappropriate fluid replacement with hypotonic solutions, and altered hormonal control of water excretion. Hypo- and hyperkalemia are also observed, the latter often in association with nonanion gap hyperchloremic metabolic acidosis. Both hypo- and hypercalcemia are found, although the latter entity is rare.

TRANSPLANTATION

Patients with AIDS and chronic renal failure are not candidates for renal transplantation in most transplant centers. The requirement for use of immunosuppressive drugs simply precludes serious consideration.

There are now several reported instances in which an organ donor has served as a source for transmission of an HIV infection. The recipients who have contracted AIDS via a graft or through contaminated blood products have generally experienced a rapid downhill course. Therefore, prospective donors with positive enzyme-linked immunosorbent assay screens are excluded in most transplant centers, regardless of the results of the Western blot. In addition, organ donation is avoided in certain high-risk groups for AIDS including hemophiliacs, intravenous drug addicts, and homosexuals.

DIALYSIS PROCEDURES IN HIV-INFECTED PATIENTS

Because of the potential lethal nature of HIV infections, there has been great concern among health care workers regarding the establishment of necessary and proper precautions for dialysis of patients who are known to be HIV positive. At present, the Centers for Disease Control and Prevention recommend that those procedures currently employed in dialysis units to prevent hepatitis B transmission are adequate to prevent transmission of the HIV. These include blood precautions, restriction of nondisposable supplies to a single patient unless the items are sterilized between uses, and cleaning and disinfection of dialysis machines and surrounding surfaces. It has also been suggested that to minimize blood spray from a dislodged needle, a transparent plastic bag should be placed over the patient's arm during dialysis.

In those patients being treated for end-stage renal failure with peritoneal dialysis, it is recommended that bleach be added to each bag of dialysate effluent before disposal of the bags.

Protection of the staff is critical. Even though the current experience with HIV-infected patients suggests that the risk of the infection to medical workers exposed to AIDS is extremely low, the lethal nature of the disease dictates extreme caution. Therefore, the policies developed by San Francisco General Hospital (see Humphreys and Schoenfeld under "Suggested Readings") for their personnel remain quite appropriate (Table 18.1).

Considerable controversy exists regarding the value of routine screening for HIV antibodies in patients with end-stage renal failure, especially for those not in the high-risk categories. It is argued that the low transmission rate of HIV in dialysis units and the apparent success of current precautions to prevent transmission of viral infections render routine screening unnecessary. In many states, routine screening is not permitted without the consent of the patient. As noted under "Transplantation,"

Table 18.1
Precautions When Caring for HIV-Infected Patients

Dispose of needles and syringes in puncture-resistant containers without breaking or recapping the needle

Dispose of needles immediately after use; do not throw needles into regular trash; home dialysis patients should be provided with containers that are brought to the hospital for disposal with other contaminated waste

Wear gloves for contact with blood or body substances

Wear gloves to cover cuts, abrasions, ulcers, rash, or skin infections on your hands while working

Wash hands as soon as possible after contact with blood or body substances or after touching objects that have been in contact with blood or body substances

Wear protective eyewear when performing procedures that may result in splashes to the face (e.g., operative procedures, venous catheter placement, dialyzer reuse, endoscopies)

Wear a mask when patient is coughing and diagnosis of tuberculosis has not been excluded or when performing a procedure that may result in splashes of blood or body fluids to the face and mucous membranes; wear a mask when specified for communicable diseases that require respiratory precautions

Wear a gown in anticipation of spills of blood or body fluids onto your clothing or when in contact with wounds or infected sites

Contact your supervisor when you have had a needle stick or other exposure or splash

---

where permitted, all prospective transplant donors should be tested. Otherwise, routine screening in patients who fall outside the high-risk categories is not advocated. Results of voluntary testing for HIV seropositivity in metropolitan chronic hemodialysis patients reveal that in high-risk patients, the prevalence of seropositivity is high (30–40%), whereas in patients without such risk factors (intravenous drug use, male homosexuality, Haitian background, blood transfusion), the risk is negligible. The findings provide additional evidence that transmission of HIV in chronic hemodialysis units must be a rare event. Another survey of voluntary testing involving several dialysis centers that included far fewer patients in high-risk categories for AIDS reported an HIV-seropositive rate of 0.77%, which is somewhat higher than that in blood donors.

Suggested Readings

Bourgoignie JJ. Renal complications of human immunodeficiency virus type I. Kidney Int 1990;37:1571–1584.

Bourgoignie JJ, Pardo V. The nephropathy in human immunodeficiency virus (HIV-1) infection. Kidney Int 1991;40(suppl 35):S19–S23.

Chirgwin K, Rao TKS, Landesman SH, Friedman EA. Seroprevalence of antibody to human immunodeficiency virus (HIV) in patients treated by maintenance hemodialysis (MH) [Abstract]. Kidney Int 1989;35:242.

Favero MS. Recommended precautions for patients undergoing hemodialysis who have AIDS or non-A, non-B hepatitis. Infect Control 1985;6:301–305.

Humphreys MH, Schoenfeld PY. AIDS and renal disease. Kidney 1987;20:7–12.

Kumar P, Pearson JE, Martin HD, et al. Transmission of human immunodeficiency virus by transplantation of a renal allograft, with development of the acquired immunodeficiency syndrome. Ann Intern Med 1987;106:244–245.

Marcus R, Solomon SL, Favero MS, et al. Human immunodeficiency virus (HIV) antibody in patients undergoing chronic hemodialysis [Abstract]. Kidney Int 1989;35:255.

Rao TKS. Clinical features of human immunodeficiency virus associated nephropathy. Kidney Int 1991;40(suppl 35):S13–S18.

Stone HD, Appel RG. Human immunodeficiency virus-associated nephropathy: Current concepts. Am J Med Sci 1994;307:212–217.

Chapter 19

Approach to the Hypertensive Patient

Christopher S. Wilcox

Hypertension is a level of blood pressure (BP) sufficiently high to increase the risk of stroke or renal or cardiovascular disease. BP above 140/90 mmHg in a young adult, 150/90 mmHg in middle age, or 160/95 mmHg in the elderly is usually considered abnormal.

Severity of hypertension can be determined as follows.

- Borderline: diastolic BP 90–94 mmHg;
- Mild: diastolic BP 95–104 mmHg;
- Moderate: diastolic BP 105–114 mmHg;
- Severe: diastolic BP above 115 mmHg.

Treatment of mild hypertension is not urgent. Moderate hypertension requires treatment within weeks and severe hypertension within hours.

ISOLATED SYSTOLIC HYPERTENSION

Systolic hypertension in the young usually is due to a high cardiac output and rapid left ventricular ejection, whereas in the elderly it is due to the loss of elasticity in the large arteries and implies advanced atherosclerosis. This explains why it carries an unfavorable prognosis for stroke and myocardial infarction in the elderly.

INCIDENCE

The incidence of hypertension is about 5% in young adults, 20% by age 50–60 years, and 50% by age 80. The incidence is higher in African-Americans and increases in those with diabetes mellitus or renal insufficiency.

RISKS

Hypertension increases the risk of the following:

- Myocardial infarction;
- Stroke;
- Renal failure (notably nephrosclerosis);
- Cardiac failure;
- Arterial aneurysm;
- Peripheral vascular disease.

Risk of vascular complication is increased by the following:

- Smoking;
- Age (elderly have worse prognosis);
- Previous organ injury (e.g., stroke);
- Coincident arterial disease (e.g., atherosclerosis, aneurysm, diabetes mellitus);
- Race (African-American patients have a worse prognosis);
- Left ventricular hypertrophy (LVH);
- Hypercholesterolemia;
- Obesity/underactivity;
- Family history of vascular disease.

Hypertension accelerates damage caused by other diseases affecting the heart and kidneys. For instance, the decline in renal function in diabetic nephropathy is greater with inadequately treated hypertension.

CLASSIFICATION

Each patient with hypertension should be classified according to the pathologic type (benign, accelerated, or malignant) and the major cause (essential or secondary).

Benign Hypertension

Benign hypertension is usually asymptomatic and progresses slowly. Pathological changes in large and small arteries include concentric medial hypertrophy without necrosis. Pathological examination often shows hypertrophy of the heart and fibrosis and sclerosis of the kidneys.

Accelerated Hypertension

Accelerated hypertension implies a recent increase in BP over previous levels associated with evidence of vascular damage in the fundi but without papilledema.

Malignant Hypertension

Malignant hypertension now accounts for less than 1% of all hypertension. The hallmarks are papilledema, retinal hemorrhages, and exudates. BP usually exceeds 200/120 mmHg. It is often accompanied by headache and fluctuating neurologic signs caused by increased intracranial pressure and patchy ischemia. This can progress to seizures, fixed neurologic deficits, coma, and death. Most patients have proteinuria and rapidly progressive renal failure. Some have a microangiopathic hemolytic anemia.

Pathologic changes in arterioles include fibrinoid necrosis, proliferation of the intima, and narrowing or obliteration of the lumen. The end organs show ischemia or necrosis. Malignant hypertension often develops abruptly in a patient with long-standing hypertension, which may have a secondary cause such as renal artery stenosis. The life expectancy for patients with untreated malignant hypertension is 3–4 months. Because renal function deteriorates rapidly, treatment is urgent (see Chapter 21).

Essential Hypertension

This encompasses the majority (90–98%) of patients in whom no discernible cause is apparent. Most (60%) have a family history of hypertension that usually presents between 20 and 55 years of age.

Secondary Hypertension

Secondary hypertension encompasses the 2–10% of hypertensive patients who have an identifiable cause (see Chapter 20).

ESSENTIAL HYPERTENSION

Certain etiologic factors have been defined in essential hypertension.

Genetic

The risk of developing hypertension is increased 6-fold if one parent is hypertensive and 10-fold if an identical twin is hypertensive.

Diet

Excessive intake of the following dietary constituents is associated with increased BP: sodium chloride, unsaturated fats, caffeine, and alcohol (more than two drinks per day). Lower BP is associated with high intakes of calcium, potassium, and fish oils.

Renin-Angiotensin-Aldosterone Axis

There is an abnormal spread of renin values in hypertensive patients. About 40% are in the low-renin category. This group includes many African-Americans and elderly hypertensives who often have salt-sensitive hypertension. About 10% are in the high-renin category but do not have renovascular hypertension; they are often young. Even among the normal-renin category, about half have abnormal angiotensin II regulation of aldosterone secretion, renal blood flow, or sodium balance. Thus, the renin axis is abnormal in hypertension, but its role is subtle and incompletely understood.

Sympathetic Nervous System

Plasma levels of norepinephrine and epinephrine are normal or mildly elevated in most hypertensives. However, a subgroup clearly has increased sympathetic tone (hyperdynamic circulation, raised heart rate, elevated catecholamine levels). Baroreceptor function is impaired in hypertension, especially in the elderly. This permits greater fluctuations of BP.

Renal Function

Early in the development of hypertension, renal blood flow is reduced while the glomerular filtration rate is maintained. The ensuing rise in the filtration fraction promotes renal salt retention. In some hypertensives, renal function deteriorates, creating a vicious cycle whereby a decline in renal function impairs salt excretion, which raises BP and perpetuates further renal damage.

Lifestyle

BP is increased by emotional stress, fear, or anxiety. Repeated episodes may lead to established hypertension. Obesity and smoking raise BP, whereas regular exercise lowers it.

Clinical Presentation

There are no specific symptoms. Headaches occur in severe hypertension; they are usually occipital, throbbing, and present on awakening. Examination of all hypertensive patients should include measurement of BP and pulse by the physician while the patient is lying down and after 2 min of standing. An orthostatic fall in BP implies blocked cardiovascular reflexes (e.g., drugs, autonomic neuropathy, pheochromocytoma) or volume depletion (heart rate rises with standing). Initially, measure BP in both arms and examine the timing of femoral and radial pulses (marked differences in pulse pressure or a delayed femoral pulse suggest aortic atherosclerosis or coarctation). In children or adolescents, measure BP in the leg to exclude coarctation of the aorta. Examine and palpate the brachial artery; a tortuous, stiff vessel (locomotor brachialis) implies severe atherosclerosis. Examine the fundi for evidence of hypertensive and atherosclerotic changes. More severe changes imply prolonged duration of disease and a poor prognosis. Grade IV retinal changes are seen in malignant hypertension (Table 19.1).

The following questions should be answered in the routine history and examination of each patient suspected of hypertension.

Does the patient have hypertension? Several measurements of BP are necessary, because patients are often anxious at the first visit. Patients should record their BP at home. The self-recorded BP should be checked against a clinic measurement to ensure accuracy of the patient's measurement. The following can overestimate BP: fear, pain, anxiety, a rigid arterial wall (checked by palpation at wrist during BP measurement), or a large arm (use a large cuff).

Is BP stable, labile, or accelerated? Labile hypertension is seen in the prehypertensive phase and in the elderly. An accelerated course or rapid increase in drug requirements suggests malignant hypertension or an underlying secondary cause (e.g., renovascular hypertension).

Has there been organ damage? Assess impact on the *heart* (heart failure, hypertrophy, ischemia, extra heart sounds, pulmonary rales, a raised jugular venous pressure), *kidney* (proteinuria, hematuria), *vessels* (peripheral pulses and bruits, abdominal aneurysms), and *fundi* (Table 19.1).

Is there a secondary cause? Most patients with essential hypertension have a positive family history and present between age 20 and 55 years. Therefore, the absence of these factors suggests a secondary cause. For further discussion see Chapter 20.

Are there dietary factors contributing to hypertension? Assess the level of sodium intake from measurements of 24-hr renal sodium excretion; measure creatinine excretion on the same sample to assess the adequacy of collection. Patients on a "no added salt" diet should achieve a daily sodium excretion of 120 mmol (equals 120 mEq) or less. Alcohol intake (more than two drinks per day) contributes to hypertension.

What are the coincident risk factors for vascular disease? These include hyperlipemia, smoking, glucose intolerance, electrocardiogram abnormalities, and obesity.

LABORATORY TESTS

The following are ordered routinely in the author's clinic in patients with hypertension to assess the effect on end organs and to screen for some secondary causes:

- Urinalysis (protein, glucose, and blood; microscopy);
- Electrolytes, calcium, blood urea nitrogen, and serum creatinine;
- Fasting blood sugar and cholesterol;
- Electrocardiogram.

Additional tests that are often helpful include:

- 24-hr urine for sodium excretion, creatinine clearance, and total protein excretion (important where proteinuria is detected on dipstick or serum creatinine concentration is increased);
- Chest x-ray.

These routine tests will not identify some secondary causes, especially renovascular hypertension and pheochromocytoma.

SPECIAL INVESTIGATIONS

The following have value in selected patients.

Table 19.1
Classification of Hypertensive Retinopathy

Class	Arterial-to-Venous Ratio[a]	Focal Arteriolar Spasm[b]	Hemorrhages and Exudates	Papilledema	Arteriolar Light Reflex
Normal	3:4	1:1	0	0	Fine yellow line, blood column seen
Grade I	1:2	1:1	0	0	Broad yellow line, blood column seen
Grade II	1:3	2:3	0	0	Broad "copper wiring" line, no blood column seen
Grade III	1:4	1:3	+	0	Broad "silver wire" line, no blood column seen
Grade IV	Fine	Obliteration	+	+	Fibrous cords, no blood column seen

[a]Ratio of arterial to venous diameters.
[b]Ratio of diameters of regions of spasm to more proximal segments.

Intravenous Pyelogram, Computed Tomography, or Renal Ultrasound

These are indicated where the kidneys are palpated on examination (suggesting polycystic kidney disease or tumor) or anatomical abnormalities of the collecting system are suspected, e.g., patients with recurrent urinary tract infection, unexplained pyuria or hematuria, symptoms of prostatism, or previous renal stone disease. Renal ultrasound is helpful to assess renal size (decreased in unilateral renal artery stenosis or renal parenchymal disease), to exclude obstructive uropathy, or to assess renal cyst disease.

Radionuclide Scanning

[^{131}I]-Hippuran is a tracer for renal plasma flow, whereas [^{99m}Tc]-diethylenetriamine pentaacetic acid is a tracer for glomerular filtration rate.

[^{99m}Mercaptoacetotriglycine$_3$] is handled similar to Hippuran. These tests are used in the work-up of suspected renovascular hypertension (see Chapter 20) and before renal reconstructive surgery or nephrectomy to assess function in the residual kidney.

Renal Arteriography

Aortography and selective renal arteriography are the definitive procedures for visualizing renal artery stenosis. They are also valuable in the work-up of polyarteritis nodosa (classic type for demonstration of renal aneurysms) and in the diagnosis of renal infarction or tumor. A digital-subtraction arteriogram that decreases the dye load is useful where the risk of contrast-induced renal failure is increased due to impaired renal function, volume depletion, or diabetes mellitus.

Echocardiogram

The echocardiogram documents ventricular wall thickness and ejection fraction. It also reveals diastolic dysfunction as seen in severe hypertension.

Suggested Readings

Fifth report of the joint national committee on detection, evaluation, and treatment of high blood pressure. Arch Intern Med 1993;153: 154–183.

Genest J, Kuchel O, Hamet P, Canten M, eds. Hypertension: physiology and treatment, 2nd ed. Minneapolis: McGraw-Hill, 1983.

Kaplan NM. Clinical hypertension, 5th ed. Baltimore: Williams & Wilkins, 1990.

Laragh JH, Brenner BM, eds. Hypertension: pathophysiology, diagnosis and management. New York: Raven, 1990.

Smith MC, Dunn MJ. Hypertension due to renal parenchymal disease. In: Brenner BM, Rector FC, eds. The kidney, 4th ed. Philadelphia: Saunders, 1991:1968–1996.

Chapter 20

Secondary Forms of Hypertension

Christopher S. Wilcox

Approximately 10% of patients with hypertension will have a secondary cause. The low prevalence of secondary causes mandates a discrete screening program to limit expensive testing (Table 20.1).

The prevalence of secondary hypertension increases among patients with severe hypertension. Specific clinical and laboratory findings should prompt appropriate screening tests, which must be highly sensitive (few false-negatives) to avoid missing patients with a secondary cause.

RENAL PARENCHYMAL DISEASE

Any decrease in renal function may cause hypertension. Conversely, hypertension itself may cause nephrosclerosis, especially in African-Americans. Hypertension accounts for 24% of cases of end-stage renal failure. It accelerates the progression of renal injury, especially in patients with diabetes mellitus or heavy proteinuria. This category of hypertension is due predominantly to excessive salt and water retention, but overproduction of renin and angiotensin are of predominant importance in some. Consequently, the mainstays of therapy in the former are salt restriction and diuretic therapy. In the latter, therapy is aimed at decreasing plasma renin activity (PRA) or angiotensin II generation with β-blockers or angiotensin-converting enzyme inhibitors. Calcium antagonists are effective in both categories.

Table 20.1
Secondary Causes of Hypertension

Cause	Prevalence (%)
Renal parenchymal disease	5
Renovascular disease	0.5–5
Primary aldosteronism	<0.5
Pheochromocytoma	<0.2
Cushing's syndrome	<0.2
Drug related	0.1–1

Table 20.2
Renal Lesions Causing Renovascular Hypertension

Intrinsic Renal Lesions	Extrinsic Lesions
Atherosclerosis	Retroperitoneal tumors
Fibromuscular dysplasia	Retroperitoneal fibrosis
Vasculitis	Emboli
Renal cysts	Urinary tract obstruction
Renal capsular hematoma	Abdominal aortic aneurysm

RENOVASCULAR HYPERTENSION

Renal artery stenosis is a narrowing (usually greater than 75% to be functionally significant) of one or both renal arteries or their branches. Renovascular hypertension (RVHTN) is that caused by renal hypoperfusion, usually secondary to renal artery stenosis. Renovascular disease is a generic concept that encompasses renal artery stenosis, RVHTN, and renal vascular diseases (Table 20.2).

Pathophysiology

Renal hypoperfusion or a reduction in extracellular fluid volume elicits release of renin from the myoepithelial cells of the afferent arteriole. Renin catalyzes the transformation of angiotensinogen to angiotensin I (AI) while angiotensin-converting enzyme, located predominantly on the vascular endothelium, catalyzes formation of angiotensin II (AII) from AI. AII is a potent vasoconstrictor and potentiates renal sodium and water retention both directly and by stimulating aldosterone secretion.

If only one kidney is hypoperfused, the sodium-retaining effects of the reduced renal perfusion pressure and the increased AII and aldosterone secretion are counterbalanced by a pressure natriuresis in the contralateral kidney. However, where there is no normal kidney (e.g., patients with bilateral renal artery stenosis or stenosis of a transplanted, solitary, or dominant kidney), hypertension becomes primarily volume dependent. Such patients may have episodes of "overflow" pulmonary edema caused by inappropriate renal salt retention. The natural history of atherosclerotic disease is a progressive decrease in renal blood flow, which ultimately results in complete loss of renal function.

Clinical Features

Clinical features suggestive of RVHTN follow:

- Onset of HTN before age 20 or after age 55;
- Accelerated or malignant hypertension;
- Signs and symptoms of arteriosclerotic disease;
- Smoking history;
- Azotemia, especially developing with angiotensin-converting enzyme inhibitor therapy;
- Abdominal bruit (especially diastolic or in the flank);
- Recurrent pulmonary edema (suggests bilateral renal artery stenosis);
- Asymmetric kidneys with a size differential of >1.5 cm;
- Hypokalemia or alkalosis (suggesting hyperaldosteronism).

Screening Tests

The captopril stimulation test is suggested:

- Reserved for patients with findings suggestive of RVHTN;
- Exclude patients with renal failure (serum creatinine > 2.5 mg/dL), cardiovascular instability, edema, or allergy to angiotensin-converting enzyme inhibitors;
- Discontinue antihypertensives and diuretics 10 days before the test or replace with labetalol and/or nifedipine;
- Withhold antihypertensives on the day of the test;
- Draw samples for PRA before and 60 min after captopril;
- Administer 50 mg of crushed captopril with water while patient is seated, and monitor blood pressure before and during test;

Criteria for a positive test depend on the PRA assay used (see Muller et al., 1986 under "Suggested Readings"). With the Baxter-Travenol or Smith-Kline-French radioimmunoassay, a positive test is a postcaptopril PRA > 5.7 ng/mL/hr.

Diagnostic Tests

The rapid sequence intravenous pyelogram, Hippuran renogram, or renal vein renins are not sufficiently accurate for routine use. Although captopril renography can quantify individual kidney function, controversy remains regarding the utility of these tests for screening (see "Screening Tests"). Presently, they are used in conjunction with aortography to assess the functional significance of a renal artery stenosis lesion. Intravenous digital subtraction angiography can be useful to screen for renal artery stenosis; however, this test may not provide sufficient detail of the anatomy to make therapeutic decisions.

Captopril Renogram

The glomerular filtration rate of a hypoperfused kidney is dependent on the contractile effects of AII on the efferent arterioles. Therefore, angiotensin-converting enzyme inhibitors produce marked falls in glomerular filtration rate without pronounced changes in renal blood flow. The diagnostic criterion for RVHTN is a decrease in the glomerular filtration rate as measured by [^{99m}Tc]-diethylenetriamine pentaacetic acid. After angiotensin-converting enzyme inhibitor, renal blood flow and, therefore, the delivery of Hippuran are maintained, yet their elimination is delayed because of the fall in glomerular filtration rate and enhanced tubular fluid reabsorption.

Diagnostic criteria for RVHTN from an [^{131}I]-Hippuran renogram include a delayed time to peak or, in extreme cases, progressive renal cortical accumulation of the tracer after angiotensin-converting enzyme inhibitor. The reported sensitivity and specificity of these tests are 80–96%. [^{99m}Tc]-mercaptoacetotriglycine$_3$ is handled by the kidney in a manner similar to Hippuran, but the ^{99m}Tc label provides superior imaging quality to the ^{131}I label of Hippuran.

Renal Arteriography

Anatomical information concerning renal artery stenosis may be obtained by angiography. To cause significant renal ischemia, a stenosis must usually occlude 75% of the arterial lumen; however, demonstration of an anatomical stenosis does not prove that it is the cause of the hypertension.

Treatment

The goal is to control or cure hypertension and, with atherosclerotic RVHTN, delay progression to impaired renal function.

Percutaneous transluminal renal angioplasty is successful in 80% of nonostial lesions; however, the long-term success rate in ostial lesions is <20%. Percutaneous transluminal renal angioplasty is an invasive procedure and occasionally leads to arterial rupture or dissection, atheroemboli to the kidney, acute renal failure, bleeding, or death.

Surgical revascularization is performed on some patients with ostial lesions, those who have failed percutaneous transluminal renal angioplasty, and those with concomitant disease of the abdominal aorta requiring surgery. Patients with a small, minimally functioning kidney may benefit from a nephrectomy.

PHEOCHROMOCYTOMA

Hypertension is caused by a tumor that secretes catecholamines.

Pathophysiology

Neural crest cells are found in the adrenal medulla, autonomic ganglia, organs of Zuckerkandl (lying anterior to the aortic bifurcation), and bladder. Pheochromocytomas may form at any of these sites, but 80–90% are found in or about a single adrenal gland. Tumors are bilateral in 10–20%, and less than 10% are malignant. Pheochromocytoma may be inherited as an autosomal dominant trait either alone or in combination with other endocrine diseases.

Clinical Features

Hypertension is the most common clinical manifestation. It is sustained in about 60% of patients. The paroxysm, which is caused by the sudden release of stored catecholamines, is often accompanied by severe hypertension, headache, sweating, and palpitations. Paroxysms may be precipitated by exercise, urination, defecation, sexual intercourse, anesthesia, contrast agents, or certain drugs, including vasodilators. Other clinical features include weight loss, fever, anxiety, sweating, and glucose intolerance. Orthostatic hypotension is common and may be secondary to diminished plasma volume and blunted sympathetic reflexes.

Screening Tests

The clinical features that suggest the need to screen for pheochromocytoma follow:

- Patients with hypertension and at least two of the characteristic triad of symptoms of headache, palpitations, or sweating;
- Patients with paroxysmal hypertension;
- Patients with sustained diastolic blood pressure of >120 mmHg.

The most accurate tests employ 24-hr urinary excretion of free catecholamines or their primary metabolites (metanephrines). Yield is increased if a collection is initiated after a hypertensive episode. The excretion of vanillylmandelic acid is less reliable.

Diagnostic Tests

With the clonidine suppression test, clonidine inhibits the sympathetic outflow from the brain by stimulating α-receptors in the vasomotor center. It reduces plasma catecholamine levels in normal subjects and those with anxiety but does not reduce levels in patients with an autonomously secreting pheochromocytoma. Details of the procedure for the clonidine suppression test follow; its sensitivity is approximately 97%.

- Withhold β–blockers and diuretics 2 weeks before the test;
- Patient is recumbent in a quiet room with an intravenous cannula in place 30 min before and during the test;
- Hold routine antihypertensives the morning of the test;
- Administer 0.3 mg oral clonidine;
- Obtain plasma for free catecholamines before and 3 hr after test;
- Test is positive if free catecholamines remain above 500 pg/mL or fail to fall by at least 50%.

Localization Tests

Abdominal computed tomography scan, magnetic resonance imaging, or selective venous sampling are common localization tests. Computed tomography and magnetic resonance imaging are accurate means of localizing tumors larger than 0.5–1 cm in diameter. Contrast agents occasionally induce a crisis; however, this can be prevented by prior α-blockade. Slices of 0.5 cm should be taken through the adrenal region, the anterior aspect of the aortic bifurcation, and the superior aspect of the bladder. Pheochromocytoma can often be differentiated from adrenal adenoma by its T_2-weighted image on magnetic resonance imaging. Occasionally, venous sampling for plasma catecholamines is required for localization.

Management

Surgical excision cures most patients. Preoperative stabilization with α-blockade and volume expansion is advised. After hypertension is controlled, a β-blocker can be administered to control tachycardia.

PRIMARY HYPERALDOSTERONISM

Hypertension is caused by autonomous secretion of aldosterone.

Pathophysiology

Aldosterone-producing adenomas (APA) of the zona glomerulosa cells, also called Conn's syndrome, account for 80–90% of cases. Bilateral glomerulosa cell hyperplasia, also called idiopathic hyperaldosteronism (IHA), accounts for most of the remainder. Multiple adenomas occur in 10%. The excessive production of aldosterone results in renal sodium retention causing extracellular fluid volume expansion, hypertension, and hypokalemic metabolic alkalosis.

Primary aldosteronism should be differentiated from secondary aldosteronism caused by excess renin secretion, as with RVHTN or edematous states, and from pseudohyperaldosteronism, a condition associated with excess intake of licorice and some types of chewing tobacco that contain glycyrrhizic acid.

Clinical Features

The hallmarks are hypertension with hypokalemic metabolic alkalosis and suppressed PRA but elevated aldosterone levels. Many of the other features relate to hypokalemia, which can cause

- Glucose intolerance secondary to insulin resistance;
- A urinary concentrating defect with polyuria and polydipsia;
- Muscular weakness;
- Cardiac arrhythmias and palpitations;
- Orthostatic hypotension from blunted postural reflexes.

Screening Tests

The clinical features that indicate the need to screen a hypertensive patient for primary hyperaldosteronism follow:

- Patients with unprovoked or severe diuretic-induced hypokalemia;
- Patients whose hypertension is resistant to therapy and who have suppressed PRA levels.

Screening should be undertaken after correction of potassium deficits, because hypokalemia suppresses aldosterone secretion even from adenomas. Primary hyperaldosteronism is suggested by

- 24-hr urine potassium > 30 mEq despite hypokalemia;
- Low basal or furosemide-stimulated PRA;
- Excessive 24-hr aldosterone excretion.

Diagnostic Tests

These tests are employed to confirm the diagnosis of primary hyperaldosteronism and to distinguish between APAs and IHAs.

Saline Suppression Test

This tests the sensitivity of the adrenal gland to AII. APAs exhibit autonomous secretion of aldosterone and will, therefore, show little to no response to this maneuver. The test is performed by infusing 1.25 L of 0.9% NaCl intravenously over 2 hr to suppress PRA and AII. Blood is drawn before and after the infusion for plasma cortisol and aldosterone. APAs should have a postsaline aldosterone level above 10 ng/dL and an aldosterone-to-cortisol ratio of >2.2, whereas those with normal adrenals and IHAs show a 50% reduction in aldosterone.

Postural Stimulation Test

This tests the regulation of aldosterone secretion by the renin-angiotensin system. Orthostasis stimulates PRA and AII. The test is performed during a time of day when adrenocorticotropic hormone and cortisol are normally undergoing a circadian decline. After 1 hr of recumbency, a blood sample is obtained at 8 AM for aldosterone, 18-hydroxycorticosterone (18-OHB), and cortisol, and the sample is repeated after 4 hr of upright ambulation. A decrease in cortisol confirms that adrenocorticotropic hormone has fallen over the test period. Results suggesting an APA include no increase in plasma aldosterone or 18-OHB and a basal 18-OHB above 50 ng/dL. Normals and those with IHA show an increase in plasma aldosterone and 18-OHB.

Computed Tomography Scan

A computed tomography scan may fail to detect adenomas smaller than 1 cm.

Adrenal Venous Sampling

This is required when no mass is seen on computed tomography scan; however, it is an invasive test and technically difficult. The adrenal venous effluent is assayed for plasma aldosterone and cortisol before and during adrenocorticotropic hormone infusion. A high aldosterone-to-cortisol ratio is found on the side of a tumor, whereas the contralateral side shows a low value. Patients with IHA have elevated levels in both adrenal veins.

Treatment

APAs are removed surgically. Blood pressure is normalized in 50–75%, and the biochemical abnormalities are corrected in all patients. IHA is best managed medically with amiloride or spironolactone.

Table 20.3
Additional Causes of Secondary Hypertension

Cause	Clinical Features
Preeclampsia	Pregnancy, proteinuria, edema
Cushing's syndrome	Central obesity, hirsutism, glucosuria
Coarctation of the aorta	Delayed pulses in legs
Hyperparathyroidism	Increased calcium
Congenital adrenal hyperplasia	
11-Hydroxylase deficiency	Virilization
17-Hydroxylase deficiency	Abnormal sexual development
Sleep apnea	Obesity, snoring, somnolence
Hypothyroidism	Bradycardia, hair loss
Acromegaly	Excessive growth
Carcinoid syndrome	Diarrhea, flushing
Baroreflex failure	Neck surgery, paroxysmal hypertension

DRUG-INDUCED HYPERTENSION

- Adrenergic agonists
    - Methylphenidate
    - Neosynephrine
    - Phenylephrine
    - Phenylpropanolamine
    - Pseudoephedrine
- Hypertension after abrupt withdrawal
    - Barbiturates
    - Clonidine
- Catecholamine-releasing drugs
    - Amphetamine
    - Cocaine
- Other agents
    - Cyclosporine
    - Disulfiram (plus alcohol)
    - Ergotamine
    - Estrogen and birth control pills
    - Ketamine
    - MAO inhibitors

OTHER CAUSES OF SECONDARY HYPERTENSION

Some other causes of secondary hypertension are presented in Table 20.3.

Suggested Readings

Arteaga E, Klein R, Biglieri EG. Use of the saline infusion test to diagnose the cause of primary aldosteronism. Am J Med 1985;79:722–728.

Davidson RA, Wilcox CS. Newer tests for the diagnosis of renovascular disease. JAMA 1992;268:3353–3358.

Davidson R, Wilcox CS. Diagnostic usefulness of renal scanning after angiotensin converting enzyme inhibitors. Hypertension 1991; 80: 299–303.

Grossman E, Goldstein DS, Hoffman A, et al. Glucagon and clonidine testing in the diagnosis of pheochromocytoma. Hypertension 1991; 17:733–741.

Klahr S, Levey AS, Beck JB, et al. The effects of protein restriction and blood-pressure control on the progression of chronic renal disease. N Engl J Med 1994;330:877–884.

Laragh JH, Brenner BM, eds. Hypertension: pathophysiology, diagnosis and management. New York: Raven, 1990.

Muller FB, Sealey JE, Case DB, et al. The captopril test for identifying renovascular disease in hypertensive patients. Am J Med 1986;80: 633–644.

Chapter 21

Treatment of Hypertension

Yousri M. H. Barri and Christopher S. Wilcox

The aim of controlling hypertension is to reduce the associated risk of stroke, myocardial infarction, and nephrosclerosis. Most physicians attempt to reduce blood pressure (BP) to 140/90 mmHg or less. Stricter reductions appear to be important in preventing progressive renal damage in patients with diabetic nephropathy or proteinuria above 1 g/day. More gradual reduction is required in patients with advanced renal failure, decompensated neurological deficits (evolving stroke, subarachnoid hemorrhage), severe fixed vascular obstruction (e.g., claudication with pain at rest), or evolving myocardial infarction.

NONPHARMACOLOGIC THERAPY

Restriction of Dietary Salt Intake

Approximately two-thirds of subjects (salt sensitive) derive a >10-mmHg fall in BP with dietary salt restriction. A "no added salt" diet, in which salt is not used in cooking or added directly to food, usually reduces daily sodium intake to 100–140 mEq. The dietary salt intake can be assessed from 24-hr sodium excretion provided the patient has not just started or stopped diuretic therapy. Salt sensitivity is common in patients with renal insufficiency.

Table 21.1
Stepwise Approach to Treatment

Step 1	Lifestyle modification: weight reduction, moderation of alcohol intake, regular physical activity, reduction of sodium intake, and smoking cessation
Step 2	Continue lifestyle modification. Initial pharmacologic selection: diuretics or β-blockers are preferred because reduction in morbidity and mortality has been demonstrated; ACE inhibitors, calcium antagonists, α-receptor blockers, and α- and β-blockers have not been tested nor shown to reduce morbidity and mortality
Step 3	Add a second drug of a different class, increase dose of first drug, or substitute another drug
Step 4	Add second and third agent and/or diuretic if not already prescribed
Step 5	Further evaluation at a specialist unit or a third or fourth drug can be added

Step down therapy
 For patients with mild hypertension with satisfactory control for at least 1 year, antihypertensive drugs may be reduced in a step-wise fashion while maintaining nonpharmacologic therapeutic recommendations

Other

Loss of body weight and increased daily exercise reduce BP. Increased dietary intake of calcium, potassium, or fish oils can lower BP. Consumption of more than 2 oz of alcohol per day increases BP. Stress management and biofeedback can lower BP, but the effect is often transient.

PRINCIPLES OF DRUG THERAPY

Step-Care Treatment

The 1993 Report of the Joint National Committee on Detection, Evaluation, and Treatment of High Blood Pressure recommends a stepwise approach to treatment as shown in Table 21.1.

Individualized Treatment

The patient's age and race should be considered in selection of antihypertensive therapy. β-Blockers and angiotensin-converting enzyme (ACE) inhibitors are more effective in young, white patients and those with high renin levels. In contrast, calcium antagonists, diuretics, and perhaps α-receptor blockers are more effective in elderly or African-American patients and those with lower renin values.

Use of more than one class of drug at low dose is preferable to a single drug at high dose. Antihypertensive drugs have widely divergent mechanisms of action and adverse effects. Therefore, addition of another drug from a different class may produce an additive fall in BP without precipitation of dose-dependent adverse effects. However, as the number of drugs prescribed increases so does the likelihood of noncompliance.

Anticipate adverse or unwanted effects. For example, unless there are compelling reasons, *do not use*

- β-Blockers in athletes (limits maximal levels of cardiac output), asthmatics (precipitates bronchospasm), or patients with bradyarrhythmias (reduces heart rate and atrioventricular nodal conduction);
- ACE inhibitors in patients with bilateral renal artery stenosis or stenosis of a single or dominant kidney (decreases renal function);
- Thiazide diuretics in patients with hypokalemia, gout, hyperglycemia, or hyperlipidemia;
- Centrally acting agents in depressed or lethargic patients;
- Vasodilators in patients with angina (reflex increase in cardiac work).

Consider cost and convenience of therapy. Drugs that are expensive and have to be given frequently are less likely to be taken.

Secondary Hypertension Requires Specific Therapy

Drugs are required during preparation for definitive therapy or in those unable to tolerate a curative procedure. The selection of therapy is important.

Renovascular Hypertension

Hypertension responds to β-blockers and ACE inhibitors. However, the latter can cause a reversible fall in glomerular filtration rate (GFR) in patients with stenosis of a single kidney (e.g., renal transplant recipients) or bilateral renal artery stenosis. The fall in GFR, which is usually reversible, is due to a fall in BP and a decrease in glomerular capillary pressure produced by relaxation of the efferent arteriole.

Chronic Renal Failure

Hypertension responds well to extracellular volume depletion. However, diuretics must be used carefully because they can reduce renal function further. Thiazides are ineffective when used alone in patients with a serum creatinine above 2–4 mg/dL. The following are significantly metabolized and relatively safe in renal failure:

- Short-acting β-blockers (metoprolol, propranolol, labetolol, timolol);
- Central-acting agents (clonidine, α-methyldopa);
- Prazosin;
- Vasodilators (minoxidil is preferable to hydralazine, whose metabolites may accumulate in renal failure);
- Calcium antagonists;
- ACE inhibitors (dose adjustment is required, except for fosinopril).

Pheochromocytoma

The following must be avoided, because they can precipitate a crisis:

- β-blockers (unopposed α-mediated vasoconstriction);
- Reserpine;
- Sympatholytic agents, e.g., guanethidine;
- Vasodilators.

Preoperative management requires blockade of α-receptors with phenoxybenzamine (irreversible antagonist of $α_1$- and $α_2$-receptors, long duration), prazosin, or terazosin (competitive antagonist of $α_1$-receptors). β-Blockers are used to control tachycardia only after effective α-blockade. The contracted plasma volume must be expanded (liberal salt intake, stop diuretics) to prevent a sharp fall in BP after removal of the tumor.

Hyperaldosteronism

Definitive therapy for adrenal adenoma is surgery, but for bilateral adrenal hyperplasia the therapy is spironolactone. Dose

Table 21.2
Selected Diuretics for Hypertension

Drug	Initial Dose	Usual Daily Dose	Site of Action	Duration of Action (hr)
Thiazide diuretics				
Hydrochlorothiazides (Hydrodiuril)	12.5 mg qd	25–50 mg	DCT	6–12
Chlorthalidone (Hygroton)	12.5 mg qd	25–50 mg	DCT	48–72
Metolazone (Zaroxolyn)	2.5 mg qd	2.5–5 mg	DCT	12–24
Loop diuretics				
Furosemide (Lasix)	20 mg bid	40–80 mg[a]	TAL	6–8
Bumetanide (Bumex)	0.5 mg bid	1–4 mg[a]	TAL	4–6
Ethacrynic acid (Edacrin)	25 mg bid	50–100 mg[a]	TAL	6–8
Potassium-sparing diuretics				
Spironolactone (Aldactone)	25 mg qd	25–100 mg	CD	48–72
Amiloride (Midamor)	5 mg qd	5–10 mg	CD	24
Triamterene (Dyrenium)	50 mg qd	100–200 mg	CD	7–9

DCT, distal convoluted tubule; TAL, thick ascending limb of the loop of Henle; CD, collecting duct.
[a]Higher doses are required in renal failure (see Chapter 9).

requirements increase in proportion to the plasma aldosterone level (i.e., up to 200–800 mg/day). Distal potassium-sparing diuretics (e.g., amiloride) are an effective alternative in some patients.

INDIVIDUAL DRUG CATEGORIES

The dose ranges given in Table 21.2 are generally those recommended in the Report of the Joint National Committee on Detection, Evaluation, and Treatment of High Blood Pressure.

Diuretics

Advantages

Diuretics with salt restriction are effective monotherapy for about two-thirds of hypertensives. They are inexpensive, convenient, and well tolerated by most subjects and are proven to reduce the risk of stroke in hypertension. They potentiate the antihypertensive actions of most other drugs. They need to be given only once daily.

Disadvantages

Diuretics may not reverse fully the increased risk of death from myocardial infarction. There is a small incidence of drug allergy (fever, rash, interstitial nephritis) and impotence. They produce unwanted biochemical changes including hypokalemia, metabolic alkalosis, hypomagnesemia, hyperlipidemia, prerenal azotemia, hypercalcemia (thiazides), glucose intolerance, and hyperuricemia. Loop diuretics, particularly ethacrynic acid in high doses, can cause deafness.

Combinations

Hydrochlorothiazide + triamterene (Dyazide, Maxzide); hydrochlorothiazide + amiloride (Moduretic); spironolactone + hydrochlorothiazide (Aldactazide).

b-**Blockers**

Because all β-blockers lower BP equivalently, the choice depends on cost, convenience, pharmacokinetics, and adverse effects (Table 21.3).

Advantages

β-Blockers are effective as monotherapy in approximately 50% of hypertensives or more if used with diuretics; they have proven efficacy in secondary prevention of myocardial infarction. They are well tolerated and have a relatively low cost. They are available as once or twice daily dosing regimens.

Disadvantages

They often require a diuretic for effective antihypertensive action. They are not universally effective in primary prevention of myocardial infarction. They cause a spectrum of mild adverse effects such as lethargy, malaise, sleep disturbance and vivid dreams, depression, impotence, and decreased capacity for prolonged exercise. Additional adverse effects occur in certain groups of patients.

Table 21.3
Characteristics of Selected b-Blockers in Specific Categories of Patients

β-Blocker	Cardioselective	ISA	Once Daily Dosing	Cumulative in Renal Failure	Dose Range (mg/day)
Propranolol (Inderal)					40–320
Nadolol (Corgard)			+	+	40–320
Metoprolol (Lopressor)	+		+		50–200
Atenolol (Tenormin)	+		+	+	50–100
Pindolol (Visken)		+			10–60
Acebutolol (Sectral)	+		+	+	200–1200
Labetalol (Normodyne, Trandate)	+				200–1800

Acebutolol has significant hepatic metabolism, but its active metabolites require renal excretion. Propranolol is available as a long-acting preparation that can be given once or twice daily. Labetalol has α-blockade effect. ISA, intrinsic sympathomimetic activity.

Cardioselective Drugs

These have less action on β-receptors in the bronchioles than in the heart. However, this selectivity is reduced at higher doses.

α-Blockade

This additional action increases efficacy.

Hepatic Metabolism

Shorter-acting drugs are safer in renal failure.

Bronchospasm

Cardioselective drugs (only at low dosage) or those with intrinsic sympathomimetic activity are preferable.

Peripheral Vascular Disease or Raynaud's Phenomenon

Nonselective and cardioselective β-blockers can reduce skin blood flow. Drugs with intrinsic sympathomimetic activity are safer.

Diabetes Mellitus

Epinephrine released during insulin-induced hypoglycemia causes many of the warning symptoms and also helps to counter prolonged hypoglycemia. Cardioselective agents are probably safer.

Hypercholesterolemia

Drugs with intrinsic sympathomimetic activity are preferable.

African-American and Elderly Subjects

Labetolol is more effective.

Angiotensin-Converting Enzyme Inhibitors

These drugs lower BP predominantly by preventing generation of angiotensin II from angiotensin I (Table 21.4).

Advantages

They are well tolerated. Usually these drugs do not impair exercise or sexual ability, lower cardiac output, or affect the central nervous system. They reduce proteinuria and slow the progression of renal disease in patients with diabetic nephropathy. They increase life expectancy in patients with severe congestive heart failure. They diminish diuretic-induced hypokalemia by reducing aldosterone secretion.

Disadvantages

They produce occasional drug allergy (rash, fever, eosinophilia), abnormal taste, and blood dyscrasias (agranulocytosis or pancytopenia). The most frequent adverse effect is nonproductive cough. Hyperkalemia is more common in patients with renal failure who, therefore, require careful monitoring. Most patients, especially those with mild renal parenchymal impairment (e.g., nephrosclerosis), actually have an *increase* in GFR and renal blood flow.

Table 21.4
Selected Angiotensin-Converting Enzyme Inhibitors for Hypertension

Drug	Initial Dose	Usual Daily Dose	Duration of Action (hr)
Captopril (Capoten)	12.5–25 mg bid/tid	12.5–50 mg bid/tid	6–12
Enalapril (Vasotec)	2.5–5 mg qd	5–10 mg qd/bid	12–24
Fosinopril (Monopril)	10 mg qd	20–40 mg qd	24
Lisinopril (Zestril, Prinivil)	5–10 mg qd	20–40 mg qd	24
Quinapril hydrochloride (Accupril)	10 mg qd	20–40 mg qd/bid	24
Ramipril (Altace)	2.5 mg qd	2.5–20 mg qd	24
Benzapril hydrochloride (Lotensin)	10 mg qd	20–40 mg qd/bid	24

Table 21.5
Selected Vasodilators for Hypertension

Agent	Initial Dose	Usual Daily Dose	Duration of Action (hr)
Hydralazine (Apresoline)	25 mg tid	25–50 mg tid/qid	10–12
Minoxidil (Loniten)	5 mg bid	10–20 mg qd/bid	75

Vasodilators

Advantages

These drugs are powerful antihypertensives. Minoxidil is effective in refractory renal hypertension due to renal disease. Selected vasodilators are listed in Table 21.5.

Disadvantages

Concurrent therapy is often required with diuretics and salt restriction to prevent fluid retention and β-blockers to prevent reflex cardiac stimulation. There is a high incidence of adverse

Table 21.6
Selected a_1 Receptor Antagonists

Agent	Initial Dose	Usual Daily Dose	Duration of Action (hr)
Prazosin (Minipress)	1 mg bid	2–5 mg tid/qid	6–12
Terazosin (Hytrin)	5 mg qd	10–20 mg qd	24
Doxazosin (Cardura)	1 mg qd	8–16 mg qd	24

effects including headaches, orthostatic hypotension, and impotence. Hydralazine in high dosage can cause a lupus-like syndrome, and minoxidil can cause hirsutism or pericardial effusion, particularly in patients with renal failure.

Special Precaution

These drugs are contraindicated in angina pectoris. The metabolites of hydralazine accumulate in renal failure.

a_1-Receptor Antagonists

Advantages

They cause little reflex cardiac stimulation, salt retention, or impotence. They are particularly effective in the elderly and African-American patients with low-renin hypertension. Selected drugs are listed in Table 21.6.

Disadvantages

Adverse effects include orthostatic hypotension, fatigue, malaise, and gastrointestinal upsets. Orthostatic hypotension after the first dose is sometimes severe with prazosin; therefore, the initial dose should be low and taken at bedtime and the patient warned appropriately.

Central Acting Agents

Advantages

These agents are effective in most hypertensives. They have little effect on renal hemodynamics. They have no reflex cardiac stimulation, salt retention, or increase in blood lipids. See Table 21.7 for a list of drugs.

Table 21.7
Selected Central Acting Agents

Agent	Initial Dose	Usual Daily Dose	Duration of Action (hr)
α-Methyldopa (Aldomet)	250 mg tid	250–500 mg bid/tid	24–48
Clonidine (Catapress)[a]	0.1 mg bid/tid	0.1–0.3 mg tid	4–8
Guanabenz (Wytensin)	4 mg bid	8–16 mg bid	12
Guanfacine (Tenex)	0.5 mg qd	1–3 mg qd	36

[a]Can also be prescribed as a skin patch once weekly, which is especially useful in noncompliant patients.

Disadvantages

They cause frequent, dose-related adverse effects, which include sedation, depression, headache, weight gain, sleep disturbance, impotence, nasal congestion, dry mouth, weakness, lethargy, constipation, diarrhea, and orthostatic hypotension. α-Methyldopa causes a positive Coombs' test in 20% of patients but hemolytic anemia in <1%; it can cause drug fever with rash and eosinophilia and occasionally hepatitis or cholestatic jaundice. A dangerous hypertensive crisis, associated with tachycardia, chest pain, nausea, and sweating, may occur on abrupt discontinuation of clonidine.

Calcium Antagonists

Calcium antagonists lower the basal arteriolar tone and the renal and aldosterone response to angiotensin II and increase NaCl excretion (Table 21.8).

Advantages

They are especially effective in the elderly or in those with severe hypertension. Efficacy is not improved by salt restriction. These agents are also useful in patients with angina and those with severe, low-renin hypertension (e.g., African-Americans).

Disadvantages

Verapamil often causes constipation, whereas nifedipine can cause edema.

Table 21.8
Selected Calcium Channel Blockers for Hypertension

Agent	Initial Dose	Usual Daily Dose	Duration of Action (hr)
Amlodipine (Norvasc)	2.5 mg qd	5–10 mg qd	24
Diltiazem CD (Cardizem CD)	180 mg qd	180–360 mg qd	24
Isradipine (DynaCirc)	2.5 mg bid	5–10 mg bid	12
Nifedipine GITS (Procardia XL)	30 mg qd	30–120 mg qd	24
Verapamil SR (Calan SR)	180 mg qd	240 mg qd/bid	12–24

Drug Interactions

Verapamil and diltiazem depress atrioventricular conduction and must be used cautiously with β-blockers. These two agents increase plasma digoxin levels by decreasing digoxin clearance. Dosage adjustments are required. Diltiazem and verapamil increase plasma levels of cyclosporin.

Other Drugs

Reserpine and adrenergic neuron antagonists (e.g., guanadrel, guanethidine, bretylium) are used only occasionally because of frequent adverse effects.

RESULTS OF CONTROLLED CLINICAL TRIALS IN HYPERTENSION

Treatment of malignant or severe hypertension undoubtedly prolongs life.

Results from placebo-controlled trials of treatment (for an average of 5 years) of mild hypertension (average diastolic BP 100 mmHg) have shown that death from stroke is reduced by 50%. Death from myocardial infarction is not reduced in most individual trials. However, meta-analysis of the largest trials shows that myocardial infarction is reduced overall by 15–20%. These trials mostly used diuretics as the primary treatment. The Medical Research Council trial compared a diuretic with propranolol; there was no overall benefit with the diuretic (see references in the 1993 Report of the Joint National Committee on Detection, Evaluation, and Treatment of High Blood Pressure for further information). Successful lowering of BP with a diuretic does not necessarily eliminate all excess risk of myocardial infarction. Use of a diuretic to treat hypertension or isolated systolic hypertension in the elderly reduces death from stroke or myocardial infarction.

Five trials have shown that β-blockers significantly reduce the risk of reinfarction in normotensive patients after a primary myocardial infarction. Therefore, β-blockers are strongly indicated in patients with a previous myocardial infarction. Recent studies have shown that an ACE inhibitor can slow or prevent the progression of type I diabetic nephropathy even in normotensive patients. Therefore, an ACE inhibitor is strongly indicated in patients with diabetes mellitus.

The Modification of Diet in Renal Disease study compared the effect of reducing the mean arterial pressure to 98 mmHg (equivalent to a BP of 130/80 mmHg) with that of 92 mmHg (equivalent to a BP of 125/75 mmHg). Patients with renal failure (GFR below 55 mL/min) and proteinuria above 1 g/day had a slower decline in GFR if randomized to the lower mean arterial blood pressure goal. Therefore, an attempt should be made to lower BP to 125/75 mmHg in such patients.

TREATMENT OF HYPERTENSIVE CRISIS

Severe hypertension requires immediate attention (Table 21.9). Two categories should be differentiated:

- Hypertensive emergencies: life-threatening situations with functional disturbance of the central nervous system, heart, or kidneys; BP must be lowered within 1 hr;
- Hypertensive urgencies: the immediate risk for end-organ damage is less, but prompt institution of therapy is required to control BP within 24 hr.

Hypertensive Emergencies

Hypertensive emergencies include the following:

- Hypertensive encephalopathy;
- Malignant hypertension (some cases);
- Severe hypertension accompanying myocardial infarction, acute aortic dissection, acute left ventricular failure or unstable angina;

Table 21.9
Choice of Agents in Patients with Special Categories of Hypertension

Clinical Condition	Agents of Choice[a]	Advantages
Hypertensive urgency	Nifedipine, po or bite and swallow	Fast acting, ↓ afterload, improves coronary flow
	Clonidine, po	Easy to administer, predictable action
Malignant hypertension	Nitroprusside, iv	Short half-life, fast action, little reflex tachycardia, ↓ afterload, dilates coronary arteries
	Labetalol, iv	Fast action, can be given as infusion, oral form available
Hypertension complicated by myocardial infarction	Nitroglycerin, iv	↓ Preload and afterload, dilates coronary vessels
	Nitroprusside, iv	As above
	Labetalol, iv	As above
Acute aortic dissection	Trimethaphan, iv	Short acting, smooth ↓ BP, ↓ left ventricular ejection rate
	β-Blocker + nitroprusside	β-Blocker must be given first to block any reflex effects on heart
	Labetalol	
Hypertensive encephalopathy or evolving stroke	Nitroprusside, iv	As above
	Labetalol, iv	As above
	Trimethaphan, iv	As above
Severe preeclampsia or eclampsia	Hydralazine, iv	Safe in pregnancy
	Methyldopa, po	Safe in pregnancy
Catecholamine excess	Phentolamine, iv	Effective α-blocker
	Prazosin, po	Effective α-blocker
	Clonidine, po	In cases of withdrawal

[a]For dosage and side effects, refer to Table 21.10.

- Severe hypertension accompanying intracranial hemorrhage;
- Catecholamine excess states;
- Eclampsia or severe hypertension in pregnancy;
- Hypertension in the immediate postoperative period.

General guidelines to therapy:

- Initiate treatment after a brief history and physical examination with emphasis on past history of hypertension, use of medications and drugs, presence of visual disturbances, funduscopic examination, and assessment of central nervous system;
- Patients should be monitored, preferably in an intensive care unit;
- A sharp drop in BP to normal or subnormal levels can lead to brain damage caused by a decrease in BP below the autoregulatory range of cerebral blood flow; diastolic BP should be maintained between 100 and 110 mmHg in the first 12–24 hr;
- An oral regimen should be initiated when tolerated by the patient to reduce the duration of parenteral therapy;
- Loop diuretics may be indicated in congestive heart failure or in patients with fluid overload.

Choice of Therapy

The choice of a parenteral agent in a patient with a hypertensive crisis should be guided by the clinical circumstance.

Neurologically Unstable Patient with Hypertension

Patients with hypertensive encephalopathy, intracranial or subarachnoid hemorrhage, or thrombotic or embolic stroke are at risk of further brain damage if their BP is reduced precipitously. Nitroprusside is the drug of choice because of a short half-life and easy achievement of goal BP. Labetalol is an acceptable alternative. Nimodipine is a calcium channel antagonist that reduces vasospasm and decreases mortality in patients with subarachnoid hemorrhage.

Malignant-Accelerated Hypertension

Malignant hypertension represents a true emergency when it is associated with rapid deterioration in critical organ function, which includes encephalopathy, rapidly failing vision, pulmonary edema, or rapid deterioration of renal function. Nitroprusside or labetalol parenterally are the agents of choice. Otherwise, malignant hypertension is considered a hypertensive urgency when nifedipine or other oral agents can be used to control BP within 24 hr.

Hypertension and Cardiac Instability

Patients with persistent hypertension complicating a myocardial infarction or unstable angina can be treated with intravenous nitroglycerin. This is also helpful in hypertension after cardiac bypass surgery, because it dilates coronary arteries and reduces the preload. Labetalol or propranolol plus nitroprusside are alternatives.

In patients with severe hypertension associated with pulmonary edema, nitroprusside is effective in reducing preload and controlling BP. Loop diuretics should be used with care, ideally with monitoring of pulmonary capillary wedge pressure.

Acute Aortic Dissection

The goal of initial therapy is to reduce BP and cardiac contractility. Vasodilators such as hydralazine or minoxidil, which lead to increased sympathetic activity, should be avoided. Trimethaphan (a short acting ganglionic blocker) is a logical choice, because it decreases the ventricular ejection rate. Intravenous labetalol provides α- and β-blockade and is hemodynamically adequate. Nitroprusside plus a β-blocker are also reasonable choices.

Catecholamine Excess States

Life-threatening hypertension caused by excessive catecholamine secretion occurs in association with (a) pheochromocytoma, (b) clonidine withdrawal syndrome, (c) administration of sympathomimetics, (d) ingestion of tyramine by a patient taking monoamine oxidase inhibitors, and (e) drug abuse with cocaine or amphetamine. Rapid intravenous injection of phentolamine is an effective initial therapy; prazosin is a useful alternative. β-Blockers are contraindicated initially, because unopposed α-activity increases vasoconstriction. More prolonged α-blockade can be produced later with phenoxybenzamine. The treatment of choice for clonidine withdrawal is to reinstitute the drug.

Severe Hypertension in Pregnancy

Management of a hypertensive crisis in pregnancy is complicated by concern about affecting uteroplacental blood flow. Intravenous hydralazine and methyldopa are the drugs of choice because there is extensive evidence of their safety. Preliminary evidence suggests that labetalol may be useful in the treatment of eclampsia, because it reduces BP without inducing fetal distress. Nifedipine has occasionally been used, but there is not yet sufficient evidence that it is safe. ACE inhibitors are contraindicated because of potential teratogenicity. Animal studies have suggested that sodium nitroprusside may entail risks to the fetus; therefore, it should be reserved for patients with hypertensive emergencies that are refractory to other agents.

Hypertensive Urgencies

These patients present with diastolic BP greater than 120 mmHg, without evidence of end-organ damage. They do not usually require parenteral therapy. However, they need close monitoring and aggressive management of BP, which can usually be achieved in the emergency room. Patients should be observed for 2–6 hr before discharge to ensure that the therapy has lowered BP without inducing untoward effects such as orthostatic hypotension. A follow-up visit should be arranged for the next day if admission is not indicated.

Common causes:

- Failure to comply with antihypertensive therapy;
- Accelerated hypertension;
- Scleroderma crisis;
- Perioperative hypertension;
- Hypertension associated with coronary artery disease;
- Severe hypertension in kidney transplant patients;
- Clonidine withdrawal syndrome.

Oral or sublingual medications are usually satisfactory for treating hypertensive urgencies. The oral agents include nifedipine, clonidine, captopril, labetalol, and minoxidil. Nifedipine is easy to use and acts within 20 min; sublingual captopril may be equally effective. It is important to institute an effective regimen for long-term control.

The details of the use of parenteral drugs to treat a patient with a hypertensive crisis are presented in Table 21.10.

Table 21.10
Selected Drugs for Management of Hypertensive Crisis

Parenteral Agents	Initial Dose	Onset of Action	Duration	Main Adverse Effects
Sodium nitroprusside	0.5–1.0 µg/kg/min titrate ↑ every 3–5 min	Immediate	2–3 min	Metabolized to cyanide and thiocyanate; accumulation after 3–5 days therapy (more rapidly in renal failure); maintain thiocyanate levels <10 mg/dL
Labetalol	20 mg iv bolus then repeated doses or infuse at 2 mg/min	<5 min	3–6 hr	May induce congestive heart failure, bronchospasm, or heart block
Hydralazine	5–10 mg im or iv	15–30 min	4–6 hr	Reflex sympathetic activation may cause cardiac ischemia
Trimethaphan	3–4 mg/min as an iv drip	5–10 min	5–10 min	Paralytic ileus, urinary retention, and tachyphylaxis
Phentolamine	5–10 mg iv	Immediate	15 min	Tachycardia, abdominal pain, cramps, diarrhea, and vomiting
Nitroglycerin	5–100 µg/min	2–5 min	5–10 min	Headache, tachycardia, nausea, vomiting, and methemoglobinemia
Nifedipine	10 mg bite and swallow	5–10 min	4 hr	Flushing, tachycardia and occasional hypotension, or coronary or central nervous system ischemia
Clonidine	0.2 mg po followed by 0.1 mg every hr	2–4 hr	6–8 hr	Induces somnolence and mental depression, can cause withdrawal syndrome
Enalaprilot	0.625–1.25 mg iv	15–60 min	6 hr	Deterioration in blood urea nitrogen with bilateral renal artery stenosis and hypotension

Suggested Readings

Bedoya LA, Vidt DG. Treatment of the hypertensive emergency. In: Jacobson HR, Striker GE, Klahr S, eds. The principles and practice of nephrology. Philadelphia: Decker, 1991:547–557.

Calhoun DA, Oparil S. Treatment of hypertensive crisis. N Engl J Med 1990;323:1177–1183.

Cunningham FG, Lindheimer MD. Current concepts: hypertension in pregnancy. N Engl J Med 1992;326:927–935.

Dequattro V. How to recognize hypertensive crises and their causes. J Crit Illness 1987;2:64–71.

Fifth Report of the Joint National Committee on Detection, Evaluation, and Treatment of High Blood Pressure. Arch Intern Med 1988;148:1023–1038.

Glassock RJ. Current therapy in nephrology and hypertension. Philadelphia: Decker, 1992.

Grokin JU. Managing the hypertensive crisis. Hosp Ther 1993;153:154–183.

Klahr S, Levey AS, Beck GJ, et al. The effects of dietary protein restriction and blood pressure control on the progression of chronic renal disease. N Engl J Med 1994;330:877–884.

Lewis EJ, Hunsicker LG, Bain RP, et al. The effects of angiotensin-converting-enzyme inhibition on diabetic nephropathy. N Engl J Med 1993;329:1456–1462.

Unwin RJ, Liguros M, Shakelton C, Wilcox CS. Diuretic treatment for hypertension. In: Laragh JH, Brenner BM, eds. Hypertension: pathophysiology diagnosis and management. New York: Raven, in press.

Chapter 22

Hemodialysis

Edward A. Ross and
Yousri M. H. Barri

Hemodialysis is defined as the movement of solute and water from the patient's blood across a semipermeable membrane (the dialyzer) into the dialysate. The dialyzer may also be used to remove large volumes of fluid. This is accomplished by ultrafiltration in which hydrostatic pressure causes the bulk flow of plasma water (with comparatively few solutes) through the membrane. With advances in vascular access, anticoagulation, and the production of reliable and efficient dialyzers, hemodialysis has become the predominant method of treatment for acute and chronic renal failure in the United States.

INDICATIONS FOR HEMODIALYSIS

Most patients with *acute renal insufficiency* are successfully managed without dialysis (see Chapter 8). Factors to be considered before initiating hemodialysis in patients with *chronic renal failure* should include comorbid conditions and patient preference. Timing of therapy is dictated by serum chemistries and symptoms. Hemodialysis is usually started when creatinine clearance decreases below 10 mL/min, which typically corresponds to a serum creatinine of 8–10 mg/dL. However, more important than the absolute laboratory values is the presence of uremic symptoms. At present most patients who are not terminal from another progressive illness, or who are so mentally incompetent as to present a danger to themselves or others, are offered dialysis therapy (Table 22.1).

Table 22.1
Indications and Contraindications for Hemodialysis

Indications

Relative
  Symptomatic azotemia including encephalopathy
  Dialyzable toxins (drug poisoning)
Absolute
  Uremic pericarditis
  Hyperkalemia, severe (see Chapter 11)
  Diuretic unresponsive fluid overload (pulmonary edema)
  Intractable acidosis

Contraindications

Relative
  Hypotension unresponsive to pressors
  Terminal illness
  Organic brain syndrome

VASCULAR ACCESS

Provision of dialysis requires reliable repeated access to the patient's circulation that can provide blood flow of 150–500 mL/min. Ideally the access should be created well before the need for chronic dialysis, typically when the creatinine clearance falls below approximately 15 mL/min.

Acute Vascular Access

Subclavian and internal jugular venous catheters have become the preferred temporary vascular access. Modern catheters provide dual lumens for bidirectional blood flow. Temporary catheters are placed for emergent dialysis and are useful until a more permanent access is ready. The flexible, silicone-based catheters, which are tunneled subcutaneously and sutured in place, may be left for extended periods. Possible complications include bleeding, infection, thrombosis or stenosis of the vessel, pneumothorax, and air embolus. Less commonly, femoral vein catheterization is used as a temporary access for up to 48 hr. It is not suitable for ambulatory patients and carries a significant risk of infection. Temporary dialysis catheters should not be used as routine intravenous lines, because breaks in sterile technique greatly increase the risk of infection and catheter thrombosis. Catheters obstructed by clot can often be successfully cleared using thrombolytic agents (streptokinase, urokinase).

In the presence of systemic bacteremia, temporary dialysis catheters should be removed, the appropriate cultures taken, including the catheter tip, and systemic antibiotics administered. The empiric antibiotic of choice is vancomycin, which covers the most common Gram-positive organisms. Effective blood levels may be maintained for up to 1 week with a single dose; however, close monitoring of blood levels is recommended, especially when high flux dialysis is used.

Chronic Vascular Access

Arteriovenous Fistula

The arteriovenous fistula is the preferred vascular access for chronic hemodialysis and may last for years. When progression to end-stage renal failure is imminent, an effort should be made to spare the nondominant arm from venipuncture and arterial puncture. Fistulae are created by the surgical anastomosis of an artery and vein, most commonly the radial artery to the cephalic vein. After approximately 1 month, the vein enlarges, matures ("arterializes"), and is then used for the two needle sites (to and from the dialyzer). Examination of the functioning arteriovenous fistula reveals a palpable pulsation and a bruit by auscultation.

Arteriovenous Grafts

When the patient's own vessels are inadequate to create an arteriovenous fistula, native, bovine, or preferably polytetrafluoroethylene grafts (i.e., Gore-Tex) can be used to form a conduit from artery to vein. Antibiotic prophylaxis to safeguard synthetic grafts should precede procedures for which bacteremia is anticipated.

Assessment of Vascular Access

Recirculation studies should be performed at regular intervals. If recirculation is >10–15%, further assessment of the access by a fistulogram is recommended. Fistulogram is helpful in studying the access and in the presence of stenosis angioplasty may correct the abnormality. In addition, it helps the surgeon to define the anatomy of the access in case surgical revision is necessary.

Complications of chronic vascular access follow:

- Stenosis leading to inadequate blood flow;
- Thrombosis requiring surgical intervention in 24–48 hr;
- Infection, skin erosion, or both;
- Failure to develop adequate venous outflow;
- Ischemic limb caused by vascular steal;
- Venous hypertension syndrome;
- High output cardiac failure;
- Pseudoaneurysms.

HEMODIALYSIS—THE PROCEDURE

The equipment used for hemodialysis prepares the dialysate, regulates dialysate and blood flow past a semipermeable membrane, and monitors functions involving the dialysate and extracorporeal blood circuit. Heparin administration provides systemic anticoagulation.

Blood and dialysate are perfused on opposite sides of the semipermeable membrane in a countercurrent direction for maximal efficiency of solute removal. Dialysate composition, the characteristics and size of the membrane in the dialyzer, and blood and solute flow rates all affect solute removal.

Dialysate Composition

The standard glucose concentration of dialysate is 200 mg/dL. Sodium, potassium, and calcium concentrations are prescribed as the clinical situation dictates. Low calcium baths may be used in the acute and chronic therapy of hypercalcemia.

The dialysate buffer base may be either acetate or bicarbonate. In the absence of liver dysfunction, acetate is converted mole per mole into bicarbonate. Acetate may cause hypotension, myocardial depression, nausea, vomiting, and headache. Bicarbonate dialysis, although more costly, usually prevents these symptoms. It is the therapy of choice in patients with respiratory compromise, hemodynamic instability, liver disease, and severe metabolic acidosis and in patients receiving high-flux dialysis.

Dialyzers

Dialyzers are manufactured in hollow fiber and parallel plate configurations. Hollow fiber dialyzers are composed of up to approximately 10,000 small diameter fibers through which blood circulates. Parallel plate dialyzers consist of a parallel arrangement of membrane sheets that form compartments for blood and dialysate. Commonly used membranes include cuprophane, cellulose acetate, and several high-porosity synthetic copolymer membranes (polyacrylonitrile, polymethyl-methacrylate, and polysulfone). The nonsynthetic membranes are relatively biocompatible in that they can activate the alternate complement pathway and lead to leukoagglutination and cytokine release. In comparison, the synthetic copolymer membranes exhibit better biocompatibility, improved ultrafiltration characteristics, and increased solute clearance, especially in the middle molecule (molecular mass 300–2000 daltons) range. These membranes are used in high-flux dialysis and hemofiltration. A disadvantage of the synthetic membranes is their high cost. Reprocessing or reuse of these dialyzers is commonly performed.

Allergic reactions, which may be due to the membrane plastic compounds or disinfectants, are manifested by pruritus and respiratory distress on initiation of dialysis. Reactions may be prevented by rinsing the dialyzer; however, once they occur, cessation of dialysis, treatment with antihistamines, and expectant management of respiratory difficulty are required.

High-Flux Dialysis

High-flux dialysis has gained rapid acceptance. Very permeable dialyzers and high flow rates are used to increase the efficiency of dialysis and shorten treatment time. Urea kinetic modeling is used to determine the adequacy of dialysis (see below).

AIMS OF DIALYTIC THERAPY

Incomplete understanding of the pathogenesis of uremic symptoms makes it difficult to define an optimum dialysis prescription. Although a predialysis blood urea nitrogen concentration of <80 mg/dL was once an aim of therapy, correlation of toxic manifestations of uremia with blood urea nitrogen is often poor. The National Cooperative Dialysis Study has shown low morbidity in chronic stable dialysis patients when time-averaged concentration urea levels are below 50 mg/dL. Time-averaged concentration urea is calculated from pre- and postdialysis blood urea nitrogen, dialysis time, and interdialytic time.

The prescription for dialysis therapy is increasingly guided by urea kinetic modeling as high-flux dialysis assumes greater prominence in chronic dialytic therapy. Key concepts in this model include the protein catabolic rate (a measure of the dietary protein intake), residual renal function, and the dimensionless parameter K_t/V urea. The latter term expresses the fractional urea clearance, where K is dialyzer urea clearance, t is dialysis treatment time, and V is body urea distribution volume. This ratio determines the magnitude of decline of blood urea nitrogen during a dialysis, and it serves as a measure of the dose of dialysis related to urea removal. This ratio should be at least 1.2 to minimize uremic symptoms.

COMPLICATIONS OF HEMODIALYSIS

Hypotension

Hypotension, which is the most frequent complication during hemodialysis, has been related to acetate dialysis, low sodium dialysate (130–135 mEq/L), atherosclerotic heart disease, autonomic neuropathy, and excessive fluid weight gain. Prevention of symptomatic hypotension can be achieved by accurate determinations of dry weight, precise ultrafiltration with newer technology dialysis machines, and reduction of antihypertensive medications immediately before dialysis.

Muscle Cramps

Muscle cramps occur commonly during rapid, high-volume ultrafiltration. Preventive measures include fluid restriction to gain no more than 2 kg between treatments, stretching exercises, and, if clinically disabling, quinine sulfate administration (i.e., 325 mg po before dialysis).

Dialysis Disequilibrium Syndrome

The dialysis disequilibrium syndrome is believed to result primarily from less rapid clearance of urea and other osmoles from the brain than from the blood, which results in an osmotic gradient between these compartments. This osmotic gradient leads to a net movement of water into the brain that results in cerebral edema. The syndrome is uncommon and is usually seen with the first dialytic treatments in severely azotemic patients. Symptoms, which can occur during or after the procedure, include headache, lethargy, nausea, muscular twitching, and malaise, with rare progression to mental status changes, seizures, and even cardiorespiratory arrest. After recognition of high-risk patients, the use of smaller surface area dialyzers and lower blood flow rates will lessen osmotic shifts. Intradialysis mannitol infusion (25–50 g) may lessen the frequency and severity of symptoms but carries a risk of pulmonary edema.

Hypoxemia

Hypoxemia during dialysis is important in patients with compromised cardiopulmonary function. Research implicates membrane incompatibility, acid-base changes induced by the dialysate base buffer, and hypoventilation. Predisposed patients should be given supplemental oxygen and dialyzed with synthetic copolymer membranes using bicarbonate baths.

Arrhythmias

Hypoxemia, hypotension, removal of antiarrhythmic agents during dialysis, and rapid changes in serum bicarbonate, calcium, magnesium, and potassium (especially in patients taking digoxin) all contribute to arrhythmias in predisposed patients. Continuous electrocardiogram monitoring during dialysis is necessary in high-risk patients.

Bleeding

Uremia causes platelet dysfunction, which is best assessed by measuring the bleeding time. Heparin is used to prevent clotting of the extracorporeal circuit, and the dose is adjusted according to the clotting time. The action of heparin may be reversed by protamine sulfate, but if protamine sulfate is administered in excess, it has an anticoagulant effect. Dialysis may be attempted without heparin if indicated. Cryoprecipitate, 1-deamino-8-arginine vasopressin (DDAVP) (0.3 μg/kg body weight), and conjugated estrogen may prove successful when uremic bleeding is unresponsive to adequate dialysis.

Transfusion-Related Diseases

The incidence of hepatitis B infection has decreased dramatically since the screening of donor blood and implementation of isolation techniques. Hepatitis B vaccine induces seroconversion in 40–70% of hemodialysis patients. The incidence of non-A, non-B (hepatitis C) infection is also declining as blood donors are screened for hepatitis C virus antibodies. Other possible infections include human immunodeficiency virus and cytomegalovirus. Generally, fewer blood transfusions are required with the introduction of erythropoietin therapy, and this decreases the risk of blood-borne disorders.

Metabolic Bone Disease

The causes of metabolic bone disease include secondary hyperparathyroidism, aluminum deposition (from aluminum-containing antacids used as phosphate binders), and a unique form of amyloid deposition (β_2-microglobulin). Clinical features common to dialysis bone disease include bone pain, arthralgias, fractures, bone cysts, and the carpal tunnel syndrome (for management, see Chapter 9).

Acquired Renal Cystic Disease

Multiple renal cysts develop in the kidneys in up to 80% of dialysis patients treated for more than 3 years. Screening of hemodialysis patients by ultrasonography or computed tomography after 3 years on dialysis is recommended to detect malignant changes.

Pericarditis

Two distinct patterns of pericarditis are encountered in patients with renal failure. Pericarditis can occur in uremic nondialyzed patients and in those already receiving dialysis therapy. Uremic pericarditis usually responds to intensive daily dialysis, and a correlation between resolution of pericarditis and improvement in the uremia has been shown. Conversely, pericarditis that occurs in patients already on hemodialysis may be related to inadequate dialysis or concurrent illnesses, such as systemic lupus erythematosus or viral pericarditis. Treatment is intensive dialysis without heparin anticoagulation. The patient should be monitored clinically and by echocardiography for features suggestive of pericardial tamponade. A pericardiocentesis tray should be kept at the bedside. Patients need to be intensively monitored to detect hemodynamic instability, changes in pericardial friction rub, and pulsus paradoxus. If pericardial tam-

Table 22.2
Indications for CAVH

Acute renal failure (with hemodynamic instability)
Need for parenteral nutrition in acute renal failure
Cardiogenic shock with pulmonary edema and inadequate urine output
Diuretic-unresponsive congestive heart failure

ponade develops, percutaneous pericardiocentesis, placement of a pericardial window, or pericardiectomy may be necessary.

Anemia and Recombinant Human Erythropoietin

The causes of anemia in dialysis patients include decreased red blood cell production and survival and blood loss in the extracorporeal circuit. Recombinant human erythropoietin is used routinely to correct the anemia. The recommended starting dose in hemodialysis patients is 50–100 IU/kg iv three times weekly. The dose is adjusted to keep the hematocrit between 30 and 36%. In addition to correction of anemia, recombinant human erythropoietin improves patient well-being, exercise tolerance, and cognitive function. Potential side effects include hypertension, seizures, thrombosis, iron deficiency, hyperkalemia, and flu-like symptoms. Resistance to recombinant human erythropoietin occurs in the presence of iron deficiency, aluminum toxicity, severe secondary hyperparathyroidism, infection, or other inflammatory diseases.

HEMOFILTRATION

Hemofiltration relies on ultrafiltration, rather than diffusion, to move solutes across a high-porosity, semipermeable membrane. In continuous arteriovenous hemofiltration, blood pressure alone provides the driving force for ultrafiltration. Large volumes of ultrafiltrate (up to 1200 mL/hr), with a composition similar to that of plasma water, can be generated (see Table 22.2 for indications). These losses are replaced by a balanced electrolyte solution (modified by the clinical situation and indicated in Table 22.3) in amounts determined by desired fluid losses or

Table 22.3
CAVH Replacement Solutions

Solution (connected by four-prong manifold)
  1 L 0.9% NaCl + 7.5 mL 10% $CaCl_2$
  1 L 0.9% NaCl + 1.6 mL 50% $MgSO_4$
  1 L 0.9% NaCl
  1 L D_5W + 150 mEq $NaHCO_3$

This yields (mEq/L)
Na	147
K	0
Cl	115
HCO_3	37.5
Ca	2.4
Mg	1.4
Glu	1250 mg/dL

gains. The quantity of solute removed is a function of the amount of ultrafiltrate generated. Variations of continuous arteriovenous hemofiltration exist using external pumps to augment blood flow. Solute removal may be enhanced by continuously passing dialysate solution across the hemofilter using an intravenous pump. This technique is known as continuous arteriovenous hemofiltration dialysis and is particularly useful in catabolic patients.

Arteriovenous access is obtained with large-bore catheters, most commonly in the femoral vessels. Systemic heparinization is usually required and necessitates regular monitoring.

A frequent problem in continuous arteriovenous hemofiltration is a sudden decrease in ultrafiltrate production caused by kinked blood lines, improper elevation of the ultrafiltrate collection bag, hypotension, blood leaks, or hemoconcentration. A 50- to 100-mL bolus of normal saline (with the arterial line momentarily clamped) can be used to check for a clotted hemofilter. Advantages and disadvantages of continuous arteriovenous hemofiltration are listed in Table 22.4.

Hemofiltration may also be performed using two venous catheters (continuous venovenous hemofiltration). This has the advantage of avoiding arterial access but the disadvantage of requiring a specialized pump.

Table 22.4
Advantages and Disadvantages of CAVH

Advantages
- Ease of initiation
- Gradual correction of uremia and electrolyte and acid-base abnormalities
- Precise fluid control
- Rare hypotension, less hemodynamic instability
- Large volumes of parenteral nutrition may be administered
- Technically less demanding

Disadvantages
- Intensive care unit setting only
- Poor emergent treatment for hyperkalemia and acidosis
- Systemic heparinization
- Possible inability to control nitrogen balance (intermittent hemodialysis needed)
- Requires adequate vascular (arterial) access
- Access site infection
- Requires strict fluid monitoring

Table 22.5
Common Drugs and Toxins Removed by Hemodialysis

Alcohols (methanol)	Mannitol
Aspirin	Radiocontrast dye
Ethylene glycol	Theophylline[a]
Lithium	

[a]Hemodialysis or hemoperfusion is effective.

DIALYTIC TECHNIQUES IN DRUG OVERDOSE

Hemodialysis and a related technique, hemoperfusion, are occasionally helpful in the management of overdose or toxins. Charcoal hemoperfusion utilizes coated or uncoated charcoal particles to adsorb toxins. Complications include thrombocytopenia.

In acute poisonings hemodialysis has the advantage of correcting any acid-base and electrolyte disturbances. Table 22.5 gives a brief listing of medications removed by hemodialysis or hemoperfusion. Antidepressants and benzodiazapines are poorly removed by dialytic techniques. Dialysis for poisoning should be considered only when supportive measures are ineffective or there is impending irreversible organ toxicity.

OTHER CONSIDERATIONS IN CARE OF DIALYSIS PATIENTS

The following are important practical aspects in the care of hemodialysis patients that must be emphasized.

- Fluid intake should be limited to 1–1.5 L/day to avoid fluid overload because these patients are usually oligo-anuric. For dietary therapy refer to Chapter 25.
- Phosphate binders, such as calcium carbonate, calcium acetate, and aluminum hydroxide, should be administered with meals.
- Many drugs, such as antibiotics and antiarrhythmics, are removed by hemodialysis. Therefore, alteration of dosage, supplemental doses, and monitoring of blood levels are frequently required. This may be especially problematic in patients undergoing hemofiltration.
- These patients are often on intravenous medications, such as recombinant human erythropoietin and vitamin D, as outpatients. These should be continued when the patients are admitted to the hospital.
- Magnesium-containing antacids and laxatives, or phosphorus-based (Fleets) enemas, should be avoided to prevent hypermagnesemia and hyperphosphatemia, respectively.
- If blood transfusions are required, they should be administered during hemodialysis to avoid fluid overload and hyperkalemia.
- Because these patients are immunosuppressed and frequently hypothermic, there should be a low threshold for an intensive work-up if they present with features suggestive of infection.
- Specific dialysis treatment goals, such as optimum fluid removal and target pulmonary capillary wedge pressure, should be discussed with the nephrologist.
- If invasive procedures are planned, the nephrologist should be informed in advance to modify the dialysis schedule, alter heparin dosage, and correct bleeding time abnormalities.

Suggested Readings

Blagg CR. The end-stage renal disease program: here are some of the data. JAMA 1987;257:662–663, 645.

Couch P, Stumpf JL. Management of uremic bleeding. Clin Pharm 1990;9:673–681.

Daugirdas JT, Ing TS, eds. Handbook of dialysis. Boston: Little, Brown, 1994.

Golper TA. Continuous arteriovenous hemofiltration in acute renal failure. Am J Kidney Dis 1985;6:373–386.

Henderson LW, Mion C, Man NK, eds. Contemporary management of renal failure. Kidney Int 1988;33(suppl 24):S1–S197.

Lazarus JM, Hakim RM. Medical aspects of hemodialysis. In: Brenner BM, Rector FJ, eds. The kidney, 4th ed. 1991:1791–1846.

Levin NW, Lazarus JM, Nissenson AR. National cooperative rHu erythropoietin study in patients with chronic renal failure—an interim report. The National Cooperative rHu Erythropoietin Study Group. Am J Kidney Dis 1993;22(2 suppl 1):3–12.

Chapter 23

Peritoneal Dialysis

Donald R. Mars and Edward A. Ross

Peritoneal dialysis has been used for treating acute renal failure since 1923, thus antedating hemodialysis by 20 years. Intermittent peritoneal dialysis was introduced in 1952 and the permanent indwelling Tenckhoff peritoneal dialysis catheter in 1968. Continuous ambulatory peritoneal dialysis evolved in 1978 for the treatment of end-stage kidney failure.

There are >170,000 patients on maintenance dialysis in the United States according to the United States Renal Data System directory; approximately 20,000 are on chronic peritoneal dialysis. In Canada, 21% of end-stage renal failure patients are being treated with chronic peritoneal dialysis, and in third world countries the figure approaches 85–90%.

TECHNIQUE

Warmed (37°C) dialysate, typically at least 2 L, is infused over 5–10 min into the peritoneal cavity through a permanent indwelling catheter. The volume is left to dwell for a variable period depending on the type of peritoneal dialysis being performed, the range being 20 min to 8 hr. Chemical and osmotic gradients permit solute removal and ultrafiltration. After the dwell period, the dialysate is drained by gravity over approximately 20 min, and the next 2-L exchange is repeated.

Urea Removal

The goal is to remove enough urea over 24 hr to maintain the blood urea nitrogen at approximately 70 mg/dL to prevent uremic symptoms, using the smallest intraperitoneal volume and the shortest dialysate dwell time possible. This is possible because urea is freely permeable across all tissue membranes, which allows it to equilibrate over time with the dialysate fluid in the abdomen so that urea in the drainage fluid approaches the same concentration as in the plasma. For a 70-kg man with a urea nitrogen generation rate of approximately 1.0 g/kg/day, approximately 10 L of *outflow* volume will be required to achieve the removal of the 70,000 mg being produced (70,000 mg/70 mg/dL = 10,000 mL or 10 L). Because most chronic maintenance dialysis patients remove approximately 2 L of excess fluid per day with ultrafiltration, dialyzing with approximately 8 L dialysate (four exchanges of 2 L each) will achieve the 10-L outflow volume needed for urea removal.

Creatinine Removal

Creatinine is better removed from the body with a longer intraperitoneal dwell time than urea because of its larger molecular size (112 daltons) and resultant delayed equilibration with the intraperitoneal dialysate. In general, different solutes will have variable dialysance based on their molecular sizes.

"Middle Molecule Removal"

As solutes increase in weight, they are more efficiently removed with *longer* intraperitoneal dialysate dwell times. For example, molecules the size of inulin (molecular mass 5200 daltons) diffuse from blood to dialysate fluid very slowly, and the blood-to-dialysate concentration gradient is maintained for a prolonged period. For this reason continuous ambulatory peritoneal dialysis is approximately six times better at removing this solute size than acute or intermittent peritoneal dialysis, both of which have much shorter dialysate dwell times.

Fluid Removal

Peritoneal dialysis maintains fluid balance by volume removal because of osmotic gradients between blood and dialysate. The gradients are generated with commercial dialysate solutions containing dextrose as the osmotic agent, in concentrations of 1.5, 2.5, and 4.25% (1500, 2500, and 4250 mg/dL) and an osmolality of 347, 400, and 486 mOsm/kg H_2O, respectively. Fluid removal (ultrafiltration) will typically range from 300 mL

Table 23.1
Comparative Clearances Using Different Dialysis Techniques

Technique	Treatment Time (hr/wk)	Dialysate Inflow		C_{urea}		C_{inulin}	
		L/hr	L/wk	mL/min	L/wk	mL/min	L/wk
Manual peritoneal	48	2	96	18	52	1	12
Continuous ambulatory and cyclic peritoneal	168	0.33	56	7	67	4	40
Hemodialysis	12	30	450	150	135	0.7	7

to 1 L per exchange, depending on the dextrose concentration and dialysate dwell time.

TYPES OF PERITONEAL DIALYSIS

- Manual peritoneal dialysis
- Intermittent peritoneal dialysis
- Continuous ambulatory peritoneal dialysis
- Continuous cyclic peritoneal dialysis
- Tidal peritoneal dialysis
- Nocturnal intermittent peritoneal dialysis

Continuous ambulatory peritoneal dialysis is the most common form of peritoneal dialysis in use today. A typical daily dialysis regimen consists of four exchanges. With each daytime exchange, 1.5–3.0 L warmed peritoneal dialysate are infused into the abdominal cavity through the peritoneal catheter and allowed to dwell for approximately 4–5 hr. The overnight exchange is the "long" dwell, with the dialysate remaining in the peritoneal cavity for approximately 8 hr. See Table 23.1 for comparison of different dialysis techniques.

Indications

Most patients who develop end-stage renal failure are potential candidates for peritoneal dialysis (Table 23.2). Continuous ambulatory peritoneal dialysis and continuous cyclic peritoneal dialysis are the most cost-effective forms of maintenance peritoneal dialysis and provide the best rehabilitative potential. Pa-

Table 23.2
Advantages and Disadvantages of Peritoneal Dialysis

Advantages
  Ease of performance
  High safety margin
  Portability
  Fewer dialysis-related symptoms
  No routine anticoagulation
  Better control of parathyroid hormone levels
  More liberal diet
  Fewer medications
Disadvantages
  Low efficiency
  Body image problem because of dialysis catheter
  Potential pulmonary compromise
  Potential protein loss and malnutrition
  Hypertriglyceridemia
  Potential for infection

tients with acute renal failure benefit particularly from the cardiovascular stability offered by peritoneal dialysis. Specific indications for peritoneal dialysis include the following:

- End-stage renal failure patients with cardiovascular or hemodynamic instability;
- Maintenance hemodialysis patients with vascular access failure (especially the diabetic patient);
- Patients for whom vascular access cannot be created (especially the diabetic patient);
- Living conditions making travel for in-center maintenance hemodialysis difficult;
- High risk of anticoagulation in a dialysis dependent patient.

Contraindications

Absolute

- Peritoneal fibrosis (>50%)
- Pleuroperitoneal leak (hydrothorax)

Relative Major

- Presence of a colostomy or nephrostomy
- Severe hypercatabolic state (e.g., the burn patient)

- Fresh aortic prosthesis
- Recent thoracic or abdominal surgery
- Extensive abdominal adhesions
- Inguinal or abdominal hernia

Relative Minor

- Polycystic kidney disease
- Diverticulosis
- Obesity
- Peripheral vascular disease
- Hyperlipidemia
- Lack of a telephone to communicate with dialysis staff

Relative Major for Self-Care

- Blindness
- Quadriplegia
- Mental retardation
- Poor motivation and compliance
- Crippling arthritis

TECHNICAL ASPECTS OF PERITONEAL DIALYSIS

Catheters

The most commonly used peritoneal dialysis catheter is a flexible, 25- to 30-cm piece of tubing with distal perforations at the tip end. It is anchored in position with either one or two Dacron cuffs, one near the skin surface and the other at the level of the peritoneum. Approximately 15 cm of catheter floats freely in the abdominal cavity, a 7- to 10-cm segment tunnels through the abdominal wall, and another 7- to 10-cm segment extends outside the abdomen to be connected to the dialysate tubing.

Composition of Standard Dialysate Solution

The composition of standard dialysate solution is listed in Table 23.3.

Dialysate is available in premixed flexible plastic bags ranging in size from 250 to 750 mL for pediatric patients and 1 to 3 L for adult patients. Most adults tolerate 2-L volumes without difficulty, whereas some can accommodate 3-L volumes. Preparations with low calcium and magnesium concentrations are

Table 23.3
Standard Dialysate Solution

Dialysate Component	Composition
Dextrose monohydrate	1.5%, 2.5%, 4.25%
Sodium	132 mEq/L
Potassium	0
Calcium	2.5 mEq/L
Magnesium	1.5 mEq/L
Phosphorus	0
Chloride	102 mEq/L
Lactate	35 mEq/L

useful for patients who are at risk for hypercalcemia or hypermagnesemia.

Appearance

The peritoneal dialysate effluent is normally clear or pale yellow. Whenever the outflow is cloudy, peritonitis must be suspected. If the outflow fluid contains precipitated material, consider the presence of fibrin and the possibility that the patient may be developing peritonitis.

Additives

Heparin

The usual dosage of 1000 U/2 L is indicated for the following situations:

- Fibrin in the dialysate outflow;
- Peritonitis;
- After placement of a dialysis catheter to maintain patency;
- Blood in the peritoneal dialysate.

Heparin is not absorbed in amounts sufficient to result in anticoagulation of the patient.

Insulin

Regular insulin is added to the dialysate solution in patients with known insulin-dependent diabetes mellitus, as well as in patients whose dialysate glucose absorption results in hyperglycemia. This is a particularly effective form of glucose control for intermittent peritoneal dialysis and continuous ambulatory peritoneal dialysis. Many methods of insulin administration are recommended, and none is universal. The following method is based on a goal to achieve a fasting glucose of 80–200 mg/dL and a 2-hr postprandial level of 144–244 mg/dL.

- Daytime (preprandial exchanges)
  1.5% dextrose: 0.175 units/L dialysate/kg body weight;
  4.25% dextrose: 0.25 units/L dialysate/kg body weight;
- Overnight exchange
  1.5% dextrose: 0.1 units/L dialysate/kg body weight;
  4.25% dextrose: 0.15 units/L dialysate/kg body weight.

Potassium

Potassium is not a routine additive in the dialysate because of the potential risk of hyperkalemia. However, during both acute peritoneal dialysis and long periods of continuous cyclic or manual peritoneal dialysis, hypokalemia may, in fact, occur. In such situations, potassium can be added to the dialysate at a concentration equal to the desired serum level (e.g., 3–4 mEq/L).

Antibiotics

Antibiotics are routinely added to the dialysate to treat peritonitis. The peritoneal route achieves therapeutic concentrations of the drug quickly at the site of infection, and dosing is often relatively easy (see "Peritonitis").

COMPLICATIONS

Mechanical

Mechanical complications include pain with dialysate inflow or outflow, dialysate leakage, poor outflow drainage (ball-valve effect), scrotal edema, intestinal perforation, catheter cuff extrusion, and lower back pain.

Cardiovascular

Cardiovascular complications include fluid overload, hypertension, hypotension, and dysrhythmias.

Pulmonary

Pulmonary complications include atelectasis, hydrothorax, aspiration pneumonia, and respiratory arrest.

Neurologic

Neurologic complications include seizures and the disequilibrium syndrome, which are rare.

Infectious and Inflammatory

Infectious and inflammatory complications include bacterial, fungal, and sclerosing peritonitis; catheter tunnel infections; catheter exit site infections; and pancreatitis.

Metabolic

Metabolic complications include hyperglycemia, postdialysis hypoglycemia (rare), hyperosmolar nonketotic coma, hyper- or hypokalemia, hyper- or hyponatremia, metabolic alkalosis, protein depletion, and hyperlipidemia.

PERITONITIS

Diagnostic signs and symptoms of peritonitis include the following:

- Cloudy outflow;
- Peritoneal fluid white blood cell count of >100/mL with >50% polymorphonuclear leukocytes;
- Abdominal pain and bowel symptoms (e.g., cramps, constipation, diarrhea) approximately 75% of the time;
- Gram stain that demonstrates organisms approximately 50% of the time.

Etiology

Gram-positive organisms account for 65–75% of the infections and include *Staphylococcus epidermidis*, *S. aureus*, and *Streptococcus* species. Gram-negative organisms make up 25–30% of the infections and include *Enterobacteriaceae*, *Proteus* species, *Escherichia coli*, *Klebsiella* species, *Enterobacter cloacae*, *Acinetobacter* species, and *Pseudomonas* species. Other organisms account for approximately 5% of the infections and include *Candida albicans*,

Table 23.4
Common Therapeutic Regimens for Peritonitis

Gram-positive organism
  Vancomycin alone
Gram-negative organism
  Aminoglycoside alone or a third generation cephalosporin
Mixed organisms (e.g., bowel perforation)
  Vancomycin (or ampicillin) + aminoglycoside + metronidazole (or clindamycin)
No organisms seen by Gram stain
  Vancomycin + aminoglycoside
Fungal forms
  Intravenous or intraperitoneal amphotericin
  Fluconazole intraperitoneal

Nocardia asteroides, *Aspergillus* species, *Fusarium* species, *Mycobacterium tuberculosis*, Nontuberculous mycobacteria, *Actinomyces* species, and *Pityrosporum ovale*.

Treatment

There are three steps in the management of patients with peritonitis. These are usually performed on an outpatient basis over 2–3 weeks:

- Immediate lavage of the abdomen with three rapid in-and-out flushes of dialysate fluid;
- Initiation of empiric antibiotic coverage (intraperitoneal) until dialysate cultures and sensitivities aid specific antibiotic selection (Table 23.4);
- Catheter removal if symptoms do not rapidly improve or dialysate cell counts fail to decline within a reasonable period.

Indications for hospitalization for peritonitis include the following:

- Infection that has not responded to routine therapy after 2–3 days;
- Unusually severe peritonitis with difficult to treat organisms, including *Pseudomonas*, fungus, and *S. aureus*;
- Persistent tunnel infection;
- Failure to respond to initial antibiotic therapy;
- Mycobacterial peritonitis; Fecal peritonitis.

Table 23.5 provides dosing information for several antibiotics that are used frequently in the treatment of peritonitis.

SPECIAL CONSIDERATIONS FOR HOSPITALIZED PATIENTS

Ordering Dialysis Supplies

Hospitalized patients who are not acutely ill can perform their own exchanges. The nephrologist should arrange for the correct brand and composition of solutions to match the patient's dialysis system.

Changing the Method of Peritoneal Dialysis

When hospitalized patients are too ill to perform their own exchanges, arrangements for assistance must be made either to continue a manual technique or to continue the peritoneal dialysis with an automated cycler.

Interrupting Dialysis for Procedures

Patients can continue their continuous ambulatory peritoneal dialysis treatments during most procedures; however, it may be advantageous to drain the abdomen and clamp or disconnect the external tubing. With the use of an automated cycler, it is often preferable to disconnect the patient in the morning and then reconnect the patient at night.

Serial Sampling of Dialysate

It is often necessary to analyze the peritoneal effluent serially (e.g., for cell counts, culture, amylase levels). To prevent contamination of the system, only members of the dialysis team should obtain the samples.

Managing Acute Changes in Fluid Volume

Physician orders specifying the dextrose concentration of the dialysate fluids are usually written in the morning and are selected to remove a specific volume of fluid. To adjust for acute or unanticipated changes in the volume status of the patient (e.g., after blood transfusions, hyperalimentation, radiocontrast dye), the nephrologist should be contacted to adjust the dialysate regime.

Table 23.5
Antibiotic Dosing with Common Agents

Antibiotic	Loading Dose/2L Bag[a]	Maintenance Dose[a]
Vancomycin	1000–2000	15–25
Vancomycin	3 mg/kg/wk (2–3 wk)	0
Cephalothin	1000	100–250
Cefazolin	500–1000	125–250
Tobramycin	1.7 mg/kg	4–8 mg
Gentamicin	1.7 mg/kg	4–8 mg
Netilmicin	2.5 mg/kg	4–8 mg
Amikacin	7.5 mg/kg	6–12 mg
Ampicillin	1000	50
Cloxacillin	1000	100
Ticarcillin	1000–2000	125–250
Azlocillin	500	250
Cefamandole	1000	125–250
Cefoperazone	2000	250–500
Ceftizoxime	1000	125–250
Cefuroxime	1000	125–250
Cefotaxime	2000	250
Ceftazidime	1000	125
Aztreonam	1000	250
TMP-SMX	320/1600 po	20–40/100–200 mg/L
Clindamycin	300	150
Fluconazole	200 mg po	100 mg/day po
5-Flucytosine	2000 mg po	1000 mg/day po
Ciprofloxacin	500 mg po	750 mg/12 hr po; 25 mg/L
Amphotericin	NR	1–4 mg/L, 30 mg/day iv
Miconazole	200	50–100
Imipenem	500–1000	50–100
Metronidazole	500 mg iv	500 mg iv every 8 hr
Isoniazid	300 mg po	300 mg po/day
Rifampin	600 mg po	600 mg po/day

[a]All doses are in mg/L administered intraperitoneally unless specified otherwise. NR, not recommended; TMP-SMX, trimethoprim-sulfamethoxazole.

Slow or Inadequate Drainage

Inadequate outflow can be corrected occasionally by repositioning the patient. Laxatives or enemas may help in a constipated patient. Catheter flow problems will usually require more aggressive evaluation including a dye study to determine the intraabdominal position of the catheter.

Physician Orders

Diet

Peritoneal dialysis patients require a higher protein intake than those on hemodialysis (see Chapter 25), usually 1.2–1.5 g/kg/day. The diet needs to be modified further with peritonitis because protein losses through the peritoneum may increase to >20–30 g/day.

Laxatives

Nonmagnesium containing laxatives should be used.

Erythropoietin

Erythropoietin may be given either intravenously or subcutaneously, the latter usually on a once to twice weekly basis.

Phosphate Binders

Optimal administration of these agents is with meals rather than on a three times a day schedule, because the latter often misses meal times.

Drug Levels

Because many drugs are removed by peritoneal dialysis, it is frequently necessary to monitor drug levels.

Suggested Readings

Keane WF, Everett ED, Fine RN, et al. Continuous ambulatory peritoneal dialysis (CAPD) peritonitis treatment recommendations: 1989 update. Perit Dial Int 1989;9:247–256.

Keane WF, Everett ED, Golper TA, et al. Peritoneal dialysis-related peritonitis treatment recommendations: 1993 update. Perit Dial Int 1993;13:14–28.

Nolph KD, ed. Peritoneal dialysis, 3rd ed. Boston: Kluwer, 1989.
Nolph KD. Peritoneal dialysis. In: Brenner BM, Rector FC, Jr., eds. The kidney, 4th ed. Philadelphia: Saunders, 1991:2299–2335.
Nolph KD, Kindblad AS, Novak JW. Current concepts: continuous ambulatory peritoneal dialysis. N Engl J Med 1988;318:1595–1600.
Schoenfeld P. Care of the patient on peritoneal dialysis. In: Cogan MG, Schoenfeld P, eds. Introduction to dialysis, 2nd ed. New York: Churchill Livingstone, 1991:181–240.

Chapter 24

Renal Transplant Patients

Eleanor L. Ramos

Renal transplantation has allowed remarkable rehabilitation and improved the quality of life in patients with end-stage renal failure. The transplant kidney can be obtained from cadaver or living-related or living-unrelated donors. In general, 1-year graft survival rates in recipients of living-related and cadaver transplants are approximately 90 and 80%, respectively.

RECIPIENT EVALUATION

The limited number of available organs requires comprehensive screening of potential candidates to ensure that resources are allocated to those with the best chance of a successful transplant. The following are accepted contraindications to renal transplantation: uncontrolled psychosis, ongoing substance abuse, medical noncompliance, age above 60–70 years, active infection, confirmed human immunodeficiency virus positivity, malignancy (life expectancy less than 1 year or less than 2–4 years after curative resection/therapy), severe secondary hyperparathyroidism, active peptic ulcer disease, and cardiovascular disease (severe coronary artery disease, severe left ventricular dysfunction).

Screening and evaluation for cardiovascular disease is particularly important in diabetic patients in whom there is a high incidence of silent coronary artery disease. Patients with hepatitis B antigenemia and possibly hepatitis C viremia with aggressive histologic changes on liver biopsy, such as chronic active hepatitis, are at high risk for progressive liver disease and hepatocellular cancer after transplantation. Thus, renal transplantation is a relative contraindication in these patients.

DONOR EVALUATION

Cadaver Donor

Individuals fulfilling the criteria for brain death are deemed potential organ donors. Organ donors should generally be younger than 65 years and should not suffer from any systemic or renal disease, severe hypertension, or malignancy.

Living Donor

Potential living-related donors also undergo a comprehensive screening procedure to exclude underlying conditions that may be exacerbated by donation. The following are relative contraindications to kidney donation: age >65 years, advanced medical illness, severe hypertension, diabetes mellitus, active infection, and preexisting renal disease.

There is concern that uninephrectomy places the kidney donor at risk for hyperfiltration injury and progressive renal disease. Many follow-up studies, however, have shown there is no apparent decline in function of the remaining kidney as long as 20 years after nephrectomy.

IMMUNOSUPPRESSIVE DRUGS

Maintenance immunosuppression is necessary to prevent immunologic rejection of the allograft, except in the situation of an identical twin transplant. Current immunosuppressive regimens usually consist of corticosteroids in combination with cyclosporin A (CsA), azathioprine, or both.

Azathioprine

The immunosuppressive effect of azathioprine (Imuran) is dependent on its conversion in the liver to 6-mercaptopurine, which is the active drug. It inhibits purine nucleotide metabolism, thereby interfering with DNA replication. The initial dose is usually 2–4 mg/kg/day. It is continued indefinitely at maintenance doses of 1.5–2.0 mg/kg/day. Oral and intravenous doses are equivalent.

The complications associated with the use of azathioprine include leukopenia, megaloblastic erythropoiesis, anemia and thrombocytopenia, hepatocellular injury, cholestatic jaundice, pancreatitis, arthritis, interstitial nephritis, hepatobiliary injury, pneumonitis, malignancy, and alopecia.

In the setting of leukopenia, azathioprine must be discontinued or the dose reduced. Concomitant administration with allopurinol should be avoided, because profound bone marrow suppression may occur. Allopurinol inhibits the enzyme xanthine oxidase, which is critical in the degradation of azathioprine. Because of the potential exacerbation of hepatocellular injury and an increased susceptibility to the myelosuppressive effects of azathioprine in patients with acute or chronic liver disease, the dose should be reduced or the drug discontinued altogether. It is unclear whether azathioprine alone can cause hepatocellular injury.

Corticosteroids

Corticosteroids are used as adjunctive therapy in combination with azathioprine or CsA for maintenance immunosuppression. In higher doses, they are also effective in the therapy of acute rejection episodes. They block the elaboration of critical cytokines including interleukin-1, interleukin-6, and tumor necrosis factor by activated macrophages, which is an important step in T cell activation. Prednisone is usually started at a dose of 0.5–2.0 mg/kg/day and is then gradually reduced to approximately 10 mg/day by 3–6 months after transplantation.

Complications of corticosteroid therapy include impaired glucose metabolism, hyperlipidemia, aseptic necrosis of bone, cataracts, myopathy, easy bruisability, acne, hypertension, and mood lability.

Cyclosporine

At present, CsA (Sandimmune) is the primary immunosuppressive agent used in solid organ transplantation. The drug inhibits the transcription of interleukin-2 mRNA, leading to decreased production of interleukin-2 and other cytokines critical to T cell activation and proliferation. The major route of elimination is via biliary excretion. Because of significant interpatient and intrapatient variability in the extent of absorption after oral administration, as well as enterohepatic recirculation, monitoring of CsA trough levels should be employed as a guide to dosing changes.

The usual oral starting dose is 8–15 mg/kg/day that is then tapered to a maintenance dose of 3–6 mg/kg/day approximately 6 months after transplantation. CsA is available in oral (liquid at 100 mg/mL and soft gelatin capsules at 25 and 100 mg/capsule) and intravenous forms, with the intravenous dose equivalent to one-third of the oral dose.

The most common complication seen with CsA is an acute decline in renal function. This is due to renal vasoconstriction, which leads to impaired glomerular hemodynamics but responds to dose reduction. Less commonly, CsA may cause a clinical picture resembling the hemolytic-uremic syndrome. This latter situation may respond to dose reduction or discontinuation of CsA. Additionally, chronic CsA nephrotoxicity manifested by small vessel obliteration resulting in glomerular ischemia and sclerosis, tubular atrophy, and interstitial fibrosis may be seen. The histologic changes associated with chronic CsA nephrotoxicity are difficult to distinguish from chronic rejection and may not respond to CsA dose reduction.

Other side effects associated with the use of CsA include hyperkalemia, hypomagnesemia, gingival hypertrophy, tremors, seizures, hypertension, and malignancies.

Many drug interactions that affect blood levels have been reported with CsA. This may precipitate or potentiate toxicity or place the patient at risk for underimmunosuppression and rejection. A partial listing of drugs that interact with CsA appears in Table 24.1.

ALLOGRAFT DYSFUNCTION

Etiology

A comprehensive evaluation is needed to eliminate prerenal, parenchymal, postrenal, and vascular etiologies. However, immunologic rejection and complications related to the surgical procedure are common problems that are unique to the transplant recipient.

Table 24.1
Drugs That Affect CsA Level

Increase	Decrease
Diltiazem	Carbamazepine
Erythromycin	Isoniazid
Fluconazole	Phenobarbital
Ketoconazole	Phenytoin
Metoclopramide	Rifampin
Nicardipine	
Verapamil	

Primary Nonfunction

Primary nonfunction is defined as the lack of function immediately after engraftment. Most of these grafts have sustained ischemic injury leading to acute tubular necrosis (ATN). Most will gain function in the 10–14 days after transplantation and are labeled as having delayed graft function. A minority of kidneys will never gain function and are thought to have primary allograft failure. This may be due to an immunologic process, a vascular catastrophe, or both.

Prerenal Disease

Prerenal azotemia immediately after transplantation may occur if excessive fluid losses caused by diuretic administration or osmotic diuresis as a result of hyperglycemia or clearance of uremic metabolites outpace fluid replacement. Primary cardiac disease, impaired vascular tone, and other causes of intravascular volume depletion must also be considered.

Parenchymal Disease

ATN

ATN caused by ischemia is the most common cause of delayed graft function. Generally, kidneys that have a long time interval from harvesting to engraftment have a high incidence of ATN. In addition to the unique factors surrounding organ harvesting and preservation, the transplanted kidney is subject to the same causes of ATN that lead to renal dysfunction in the native kidneys. Nephrotoxic insult (drugs, radiographic contrast, pigments, etc.) and acute hemodynamic insufficiency can contribute to ATN at any time.

Rejection

Immunologic rejection can be classified into four forms (hyperacute, accelerated, acute, and chronic) based on temporal, pathogenetic, and histologic distinctions.

Hyperacute rejection, which occurs within minutes to hours of engraftment, is the result of preexisting antibodies in the recipient directed against donor tissue. These antibodies may be directed against donor blood ABO or histocompatibility leukocyte antigens. The interaction of antibody with the transplant endothelium leads to activation of the complement pathway and inflammatory cell infiltration, resulting in microvascular thrombosis and cortical necrosis. The graft is almost invariably lost, necessitating nephrectomy.

Accelerated rejection, which generally occurs in the first 2–4 days after transplantation, can be mediated by either previously primed cellular (T cell) or humoral mechanisms (antibody). The histologic lesions are similar to those found in hyperacute rejection. Clinically, this form of rejection presents as primary nonfunction or early initial function with rapid deterioration manifested as minimal urine output and graft demise.

Acute rejection, which may occur as early as 5–7 days after transplantation, is generally encountered during the first 3 months after transplantation. It is due to the primary response of the immune system with participation of both the cellular and humoral components. The histologic changes include infiltration of the interstitium with mononuclear cells and invasion of the tubular basement membrane and vessels with lymphocytes. Clinically, the usual presentation is an elevation in the serum creatinine with or without diminished urine output. The classic signs of fever and graft tenderness, which may herald the onset of an acute rejection episode, are less pronounced in the CsA era.

Chronic rejection, which may occur as early as a few weeks after transplantation, is due to immunologic and nonimmunologic injuries. Immunologic injury is thought to be due to repetitive subclinical rejection, whereas nonimmunologic damage may be due to hyperfiltration injury resulting from reduced nephron mass. The histologic lesions include glomerulosclerosis, thickening and reduplication of the glomerular basement membrane (resembling membranoproliferative glomerulonephritis), tubular atrophy, interstitial fibrosis, and small vessel obliteration. The clinical presentation may include progressive azotemia, proteinuria, and hypertension.

Other

Renal syndromes associated with administration of antibiotics, nonsteroidal antiinflammatory agents, angiotensin-converting enzyme inhibitors, and other drugs are also encountered in the renal transplant patient. Pyelonephritis of the native kidneys generally does not cause renal dysfunction, but parenchymal bacterial infection of a single functioning allograft may lead to acute dysfunction. Although recurrence of native kidney disease in the allograft accounts for <4% of graft failures, it may cause renal insufficiency or recurrent proteinuria and hematuria. The most common recurrent primary glomerulopathies are type II membranoproliferative glomerulonephritis, IgA nephropathy, and focal segmental glomerulosclerosis. Recurrence of secondary glomerulopathies is seen in diabetic nephropathy, hemolytic-uremic syndrome, Schönlein-Henoch purpura, amyloidosis, and, rarely, systemic lupus erythematosus.

Postrenal Disease

Interruption of the flow of urine may be due to obstruction within, or extrinsic to, the collecting system. Fluid collections such as blood (hemorrhage), urine (urinoma), lymph (lymphocele), or pus (perinephric abscess) may compress the ureter and lead to hydronephrosis. Hemorrhage may be a postsurgical or postbiopsy complication or a result of fulminant rejection or blunt trauma to the allograft. A urinoma is usually the result of infarction of the renal pelvis or ureter. A lymphocele is caused by the interruption of lymphatic vessels around the surgical bed. These fluid collections, if large enough, may lead to leg edema and thrombosis of the transplant artery and vein. Blood clots (postsurgical or postbiopsy), calculi, and fungus balls may cause obstruction within the collecting system. Additionally, bladder outlet obstruction with prostatic enlargement, bladder stones, and neoplasms may cause obstructive uropathy.

Vascular Disease

Acute thrombosis of the graft artery or vein can lead to sudden oligoanuria. The incidence of graft artery and vein thromboses is low, but risk factors include difficulty with the surgical procedure and recipient hypotension. Most grafts with acute vascular thrombosis are not salvageable. Stenosis of the transplant renal artery, which is seen in 3–12% of patients is often due to atherosclerosis or fibrotic narrowing at the site of anastomosis. These patients usually present with hypertension with an allograft bruit or graft dysfunction or a rise in serum creatinine with angiotensin-converting enzyme inhibition.

Diagnosis of Graft Dysfunction

The approach to the diagnosis of graft dysfunction includes a thorough history, including drug intake, and a physical examination. Laboratory data that should be obtained include a complete blood count, electrolytes, blood urea nitrogen, serum creatinine, CsA trough level, urinalysis, and urine culture. In the setting of proteinuria, a 24-hr urine collection for protein should be obtained.

In the early posttransplant period, patency of the urinary catheter must be ensured. Thereafter, unless there is a contraindication to volume repletion, a trial of fluid replacement should be undertaken. If the CsA level is in the toxic range, the dose may be decreased and a serum creatinine should be repeated within the next 2–4 days. If there is no response to empiric volume challenge or CsA dose reduction and there is no evidence for a systemic or urinary tract infection, a Doppler ultrasound of the kidney transplant should be obtained.

The ultrasound may detect hydronephrosis with or without a fluid collection. Hydronephrosis without a fluid collection is due to obstruction within the collecting system. In the absence of bladder outlet obstruction, retrograde pyelography may be attempted; however, it may be technically difficult because of the surgically created ureterovesical anastomosis. Alternatively, a nephrostomy tube may be placed percutaneously to allow proximal drainage and resolution of acute graft insufficiency; an antegrade pyelogram may then be performed to locate the level of obstruction. In the setting of a fluid collection that may be causing obstruction, the nature of the collection must first be ascertained. Simultaneous determination of fluid, serum, and urine creatinine should be performed. If the fluid and serum creatinine are equivalent, this is suggestive of a lymphocele. If the fluid and urine creatinine are equivalent, this is suggestive of a urine leak.

In addition to detection of fluid collections and hydronephrosis, Doppler ultrasound can also assess blood flow to the graft. Lack of vascular pulsations is suggestive of vascular thrombosis. A renal nuclear scan or an angiogram can confirm the diagnosis of arterial thrombosis. If there is a suspicion for renal artery stenosis, an angiogram should be obtained.

In the absence of correctable prerenal, postrenal, and vascular causes, the next suggested diagnostic test is a kidney transplant biopsy. This may reveal ATN, rejection, CsA nephrotoxicity, or recurrent or de novo renal disease.

Management of Graft Dysfunction

In the setting of primary nonfunction caused by ischemic ATN, dialytic support is provided until graft function recovers. Diagnostic tests including urine culture, Doppler ultrasound, renal nuclear scan, or a transplant biopsy should be obtained every 10–14 days to eliminate correctable causes of persistent graft dysfunction.

Prerenal azotemia is treated with volume repletion and, if applicable, discontinuation of diuretics and optimization of cardiac function and vascular integrity.

ATN caused by nephrotoxic insult or hemodynamic insufficiency is managed with dialytic support if uremia supersedes, avoidance of nephrotoxins, and correction of hemodynamic instability. Bacterial pyelonephritis is treated with parenteral antibiotics.

In general, owing to severe parenchymal damage, grafts sustaining hyperacute or accelerated rejection are not salvageable. In the setting of an acute rejection episode, the therapeutic options include high-dose (pulse) corticosteroids and polyclonal or monoclonal antilymphocyte antibodies. High dose corticosteroids may be given intravenously (methylprednisolone 0.5–1.0

g every day for 3 days) or orally (prednisone 100–200 mg every day for 3–5 days). The usual dose of antithymocyte globulin is 10–15 mg/kg/day iv administered for approximately 14 days. OKT3 is given at 5 mg/day iv for 10–14 days. With the polyclonal and monoclonal antibodies, concomitant immunosuppression is lowered to prevent over-immunosuppression and infectious morbidity.

There is no specific therapy for chronic rejection. Baseline immunosuppression should be optimized, and hypertension should be aggressively controlled. Although there are no clinical data to suggest that protein restriction (0.6–0.8 g/kg/day) retards deterioration of graft function, this is recommended.

Fluid collections are drained acutely if they are causing obstructive nephropathy. Lymphoceles that recur despite percutaneous drainage may require creation of a peritoneal window to allow drainage into the intraperitoneal space. A urinoma resulting from infarction of the ureter is managed by reimplantation or anastomosis of the viable portion of the ureter or renal pelvis to the bladder. A blood collection should be drained to prevent infection, and surgical exploration may be necessary to ligate persistent bleeding vessels. Obstruction caused by stenosis of the distal ureter is repaired by reimplantation of the ureter.

Vascular thrombosis of graft vessels generally leads to graft demise. If detected within 30 min of acute thrombosis, surgical removal of the clot or antithrombolytic therapy may be attempted. Stenosis of the main renal transplant artery may be repaired by angioplasty or surgical revascularization, provided the renal parenchyma is viable.

LONG-TERM COMPLICATIONS

Infection

Chronic immunosuppression places the transplant recipient at risk for life-threatening infections. The length of time posttransplantation, the amount of immunosuppression, and the level of renal function are helpful in determining the etiology of infections. During the first 2–4 weeks after transplantation, infections are usually related to the surgical procedure (generally bacterial) and those that were acquired before transplantation (e.g., hepatitis B). Reactivation of herpes simplex virus with orolabial, esophageal, or genital involvement is also frequently seen.

Beyond the first month posttransplantation, opportunistic infections with cytomegalovirus (CMV), *Mycobacterium, Pneumocystis, Listeria, Aspergillus, Nocardia, Toxoplasma,* and *Cryptococcus* become evident. This is due to the peak immunosuppressive effect of drug therapy. Therefore, patients who receive excessive immunosuppression for severe or multiple rejection episodes are prone to develop an opportunistic infection. In contrast, patients on minimal immunosuppression with well-functioning grafts have essentially the same etiologic patterns of infectious disease as the general population.

CMV is one of the most serious infections encountered during the first 6 months after transplantation. The most common presentation is fever and leukopenia. Other clinical manifestations include chorioretinitis, pneumonitis, gastrointestinal involvement (esophageal, gastric, intestinal), hepatitis, and arthralgias. CMV seronegative recipients of CMV seropositive donor kidneys are at risk for developing primary infection and, consequently, more serious morbidity. Patients at risk for primary infection should receive prophylactic therapy with acyclovir or CMV hyperimmunoglobulin to attenuate the clinical manifestations. In patients with life-threatening (pneumonitis, gastrointestinal involvement) and sight-threatening (chorioretinitis) infections, immunosuppression should be reduced or discontinued, and therapy with a CMV antiviral agent should be initiated.

P. carinii pneumonia is also a life-threatening infection encountered in immunosuppressed patients. The prophylactic administration of trimethoprim-sulfamethoxazole (or dapsone and trimethoprim for sulfa allergic patients) during the first 6 months after transplantation may minimize the risk for developing pneumocystis infection.

Patients with central nervous system infections often present with unexplained fever with headache, photophobia, or mental status change. Because early clinical findings are often nonspecific and because mortality rates may be as high as 50%, cranial computed tomography or magnetic resonance imaging scanning, lumbar puncture, or both should not be delayed. Urinary tract infection is the most common infection encountered in renal transplant patients. During the first 3–4 months after transplantation, this may present as pyelonephritis and septicemia. In this situation, prolonged antibiotic therapy (total of 6 weeks) is indicated.

Cardiovascular Disease

Coronary artery disease is now becoming the most common cause of death in renal transplant recipients. It is likely that the same epidemiologic risk factors for coronary artery disease in the normal population are operational in renal transplant patients. Therefore, where appropriate, these risk factors should be minimized. Hypercholesterolemia is a common problem after transplantation that is often recalcitrant to dietary therapy. Pharmacologic treatment such as with a 3-hydroxy-3-methylglutaryl-coenzyme A (HMG-CoA) reductase inhibitor may be necessary. Because of the small risk of rhabdomyolysis associated with the use of HMG-CoA reductase inhibitors, creatine phosphokinase levels should be monitored along with liver function tests.

Hypertension is seen in approximately 40–60% of transplant patients. The etiology is multifactorial and may include preexisting essential hypertension, volume expansion, renin-producing native kidneys, acute and chronic rejection, renal artery stenosis, and drugs. Hypertension often responds to therapy with calcium-channel blockers, α- or β-blockers, angiotensin-converting enzyme inhibitors, diuretics, or a combination of these agents.

Malignancies

Immunosuppressive drugs induce alterations in the immune system and predispose transplant patients to develop certain types of tumors. Although there is no increased incidence of lung, breast, and colon cancer compared with the general population, transplant recipients are much more likely to develop skin cancer, most commonly squamous cell carcinoma. Other malignancies that occur at higher frequency in this patient population include non-Hodgkin's lymphoma; carcinomas of the cervix, uterus, vulva, perineum, and hepatobiliary system; and Kaposi's sarcoma.

Reduction or cessation of immunosuppressive therapy is indicated particularly in non-Hodgkin's lymphoma and Kaposi's sarcoma where tumor regression may be seen. Minimizing sun exposure and routine surveillance are of primary importance in preventing neoplastic complications.

Suggested Readings

Braun WE. Long-term complications of renal transplantation (Nephrology Forum). Kidney Int 1990;37:1363–1378.

Kirkman RL, Tilney NL. Surgical complications in the transplant recipient. In: Brenner BM, Stein JH, eds. Contemporary issues in nephrology. New York: Churchill Livingstone, 1989:231–245.

Ramos EL, Tilney NL, Ravenscraft MD. Clinical aspects of renal transplantation. In: Brenner BM, Rector FC, eds. The kidney. Philadelphia: Saunders, 1991:2361–2407.

Rubin RH. Infection in the renal and liver transplant patient. In: Rubin RH, Young LS, eds. Clinical approach to infection in the compromised host. New York: Plenum Medical, 1988:557–621.

Chapter 25

Nutrition in Renal Failure

Edward A. Ross

Patients with kidney disease have nutritional requirements that vary with the degree of renal insufficiency and proteinuria. The diet is restricted to reduce uremic symptoms from the accumulation of toxic metabolites, to facilitate electrolyte and water homeostasis, and to prevent renal osteodystrophy. Many patients with advanced chronic renal failure, however, ultimately develop protein-calorie malnutrition and require dietary supplementation.

GENERAL NUTRITIONAL CONCEPTS

Protein-Calorie Malnutrition

Patients with advanced renal insufficiency are at risk for malnutrition because uremic symptoms (anorexia, nausea, vomiting, and altered taste) are superimposed on the restricted diet, malabsorption, and urinary protein losses. This often results in hypoalbuminemia, abnormal profiles of blood amino acid levels, decreased protein and fat stores, and deranged white blood cell function. Merely the institution of an appropriate diet or initiation of dialysis therapy may not correct these deficits, however. It is frequently necessary to enlist the aid of a renal dietitian to assist in an aggressive program of enteral or parenteral nutrition. This includes the careful monitoring of nutritional parameters such as serum albumin and transferrin levels, total lymphocyte counts, and anthropometric measurements of fat and muscle bulk (triceps skinfold thickness and midarm muscle circumference).

Caloric Requirements

Patients with uncomplicated renal insufficiency have normal basal energy expenditure and caloric requirements. A diet containing at least 35 Kcal/kg body weight is usually prescribed. Individuals who are catabolic or have proteinuria have greater requirements; without additional carbohydrate intake, they deplete their fat and protein stores.

Macronutrients

Protein

Patients with renal disease have normal minimum daily protein requirements. Protein restriction will delay the need for dialysis by preventing the uremic symptoms caused by nitrogenous wastes. The quantity of protein necessary to avoid malnutrition depends on the food's biologic value (ratio of essential to nonessential amino acids). Fish, eggs, and milk are of higher biological value than poultry or beef, especially when compared with grains. Approximately 75% of the protein in renal diets should be of the high biologic value type.

The amount of protein prescribed is based on the patient's renal function, proteinuria, type of dialysis, and body weight. As described below, the protein recommendation ranges from 0.6 to 1.5 g/kg/day. For edematous patients, the calculation should be based on the usual or estimated "dry" weight. For obese patients, calculate the "adjusted" body weight from the ideal body weight plus 25% of the excess weight. Generally, diets are reasonably tolerated if they contain at least 40 g of high biologic value protein/day. Patients are usually in negative protein balance if their intake is restricted to 20 g/day unless they are provided with essential amino acid supplementation. α-Ketoanalogues (ketoacids) are experimental supplements that contain no nitrogen yet undergo liver transamination into the corresponding amino acid.

Intensive and repeated dietary counseling is helpful to improve compliance for protein restriction. A very useful monitor of dietary nitrogen intake (in grams) in a patient with stable renal function is to measure the 24-hr urine urea nitrogen ($U_{UN}V$):

$$I_N = U_{UN}V + NUN$$

where NUN is nonurea nitrogen excretion (in grams) and is estimated to be

$$NUN = 0.031 \times body\ weight$$

Daily nitrogen intake (I_N) is then converted to protein intake (in grams) as follows:

$$protein\ intake = 6.25 \times I_N$$

As an example, consider a lean, nonedematous 70-kg man whose 24-hr urine reveals 5 g of urea N:

$$I_N = 5\ g + (0.031 \times 70\ kg) = 7.17$$

Estimated protein intake (in grams per day) = $6.25 \times 7.17 = 48.8$, which is then compared with dietary protein prescription.

Lipids

Hyperlipidemia occurs in more than 50% of chronic renal failure patients and is of great concern because of the high mortality owing to atherosclerotic cardiovascular disease. Causes of the hypercholesterolemia and hypertriglyceridemia are multifactorial and include proteinuria in the nephrotic range, depressed lipoprotein lipase activity, decreased metabolism of remnant lipoproteins, and impaired cholesterol transport. Initiation of dialysis does not correct these disorders. Indeed, hypertriglyceridemia often worsens during peritoneal dialysis owing to the absorption of large quantities of dextrose from the dialysate.

Dietary lipid guidelines and goals for renal patients are the same as those for nonuremic individuals. These include performing routine lipoprotein analyses, restricting fats to 30% of calories, substituting polyunsaturated fats for saturated fats, and reducing cholesterol intake to <300 mg/day. However, it may be difficult to design a diet that provides adequate calories with concurrent fat and protein restrictions. Fruits (limited by their potassium content), sugars, and syrups are often useful.

Carbohydrates

Carbohydrates are a major source of calories in renal patients with multiple dietary restrictions and, thereby, are protein sparing. Sugars also permit the complete oxidation of fatty acids, which avoids ketone production. Grains, vegetables, and fruits are common sources of carbohydrate and have the added benefits of dietary fiber.

Micronutrients

Sodium and Chloride

Most patients with advancing renal insufficiency develop salt retention. This can be a management problem in patients with the nephrotic syndrome or oliguric renal failure. The dietary prescription is commonly expressed in either milliequivalents of NaCl or grams of sodium (100 mEq NaCl contain 2.3 g of sodium and 3.5 g of chloride).

Renal disease also may impair the patient's ability to conserve salt, which may lead to a superimposed prerenal azotemia. Many patients with acute renal failure have an initial oliguric phase when salt must be restricted and then a polyuric phase in which salt must be supplemented.

Potassium

The degree of dietary potassium restriction will depend on the amount of both renal and nonrenal losses. Foods high in potassium include citrus fruits, dairy products, and some vegetables and legumes. Because 40 g of protein contain 1 g (26 mEq) of potassium, a high-protein diet would preclude severe potassium restriction. In most patients, a diet limited to 1 mEq of potassium/kg body weight/day will prevent hyperkalemia. Additional potassium may need to be prescribed because of peritoneal dialysate or gastrointestinal losses.

Phosphorus

Hyperphosphatemia and secondary hyperparathyroidism develop with advancing renal insufficiency unless dietary phosphate is restricted concurrent with the use of phosphate binders. Patients on diets relatively high in protein will have an obligatory source of phosphorus and may require higher doses of binders. As noted in Chapter 9, calcium carbonate and calcium acetate are the preferred binders. However, these must be administered directly with the meals; a delay can lead to significant calcium absorption and cause hypercalcemia. Unless carefully specified in the physician orders, the proper timing of phosphate binders can be problematic in hospitalized patients because of variable meal schedules.

Vitamins and Minerals

Vitamin nutrition is complex in renal patients because some of these nutrients are deficient, whereas others can accumulate to the point of toxicity. The *fat-soluble* vitamins (A, E, and K) do not require supplementation, and excess vitamin A can be toxic in dialysis patients. The *water-soluble* vitamins, however, can become deficient because of losses into dialysate and decreased availability from the restricted diet, anorexia, or abnormal metabolism. Most patients require supplementation with folic acid, pyridoxine, thiamine, riboflavin, and pantothenic acid. Vitamin C is not supplemented beyond the normal recommended daily requirement because its metabolite (oxalate) accumulates and contributes to secondary oxalosis in dialysis patients. Because of the unique vitamin requirements of renal patients, routine multivitamin preparations are best avoided in preference for those formulated specifically for this population. Typical contents include folic acid 1 mg, pyridoxine 10 mg, thiamine 1.4–1.6 mg, riboflavin 1.6–2.0 mg, pantothenic acid 5–10 mg, and ascorbic acid 60 mg.

Iron

Iron deficiency is becoming increasingly common in renal patients because of the increased utilization during erythropoietin therapy. Repetitive, albeit small, blood losses during hemodialysis also contribute to the iron deficit. Oral repletion is difficult in renal patients because of poor dietary intake of iron and decreased absorption when administered with phosphate-binding antacids. Even when oral iron is administered in high dose (65–150 mg of elemental iron) between meals, parenteral repletion is often necessary.

Zinc

Zinc may become deficient in patients with advanced renal insufficiency because of decreased intake and absorption. This can be one of many causes of dysgeusia, alopecia, or impotence, and these may at least partially respond to zinc supplementation.

Magnesium

Because renal insufficiency decreases magnesium excretion, magnesium containing laxatives and antacids should be avoided.

SPECIFIC RECOMMENDATIONS

Acute Renal Failure Patients Managed without Dialysis

Macronutrients

The goal is to provide adequate nutrition without exceeding the patient's excretory capacity and inducing uremic symptoms. Caloric requirements typically increase with the stress of the acute illness to approximately 40–45 Kcal/kg, reflecting a rise in the metabolic rate by >20%. These extra calories are provided by a high carbohydrate diet, because protein must be limited to 0.6–0.8 g (of high biologic value)/kg/day. Patients who cannot tolerate oral feeding need parenteral nutrition with essential and nonessential amino acids, dextrose, and lipids.

Micronutrients

Oliguric patients at risk of volume overload need sodium to be restricted to 1–2 g/day and fluid intake decreased to 1.0–1.5 L/day. Depending on the degree of hyperkalemia, potassium may need to be limited to 50 mEq/day or less. Phosphate binders and a phosphorus intake of 0.6–1.0 g/day are necessary to prevent hyperphosphatemia. These restrictions must be liberalized in the setting of excessive nonrenal salt and water losses as well as after the onset of the diuretic phase of acute renal failure.

Chronic Renal Failure Patients (Predialysis)

Macronutrients

Because of the risk of malnutrition from chronically restricted diets, careful monitoring with the assistance of a dietitian is necessary. Clinical studies have suggested that low protein diets have a small benefit in slowing the decline of renal function in patients with moderate renal insufficiency. It is suggested that the daily protein intake be decreased to 0.6–0.8 g/kg with a diet containing approximately 35 Kcal/kg. Compliance with the diet can be assessed by periodically measuring the urine urea nitrogen appearance rate, as described above. The nonprotein calories are provided by fats (such as poly- or monounsaturated vegetable oils) and simple carbohydrates. However, diabetic patients benefit from the use of complex carbohydrates. Once the glomerular filtration rate has fallen below approximately 15 mL/min, a 0.6- to 0.8-g protein/kg/day diet will clearly minimize uremic symptoms and permit a brief delay in the initiation of dialysis to establish appropriate vascular or peritoneal access.

Micronutrients

The degree of salt and water restriction needs to be individualized based on the patient's residual renal function and associated electrolyte disorders (i.e., hyperkalemia, renal tubular acidosis). A daily 2- to 4-g sodium and 50- to 70-mEq potassium diet is often adequate in individuals retaining these salts. When the glomerular filtration rate declines below approximately 50 mL/min, patients benefit from a phosphate restriction of 0.8–1.2 g/day (later decreased to 0.6–0.8 g/day), phosphate binders, as well as monitoring of parathyroid hormone levels and 1,25-dihydroxyvitamin D therapy as necessary.

Patients with Nephrotic Syndrome

Macronutrients

Patients with the nephrotic syndrome present unique dietary problems because of the urinary protein losses, hypoalbuminemia, edema, and hyperlipidemia. Very high protein diets are generally ineffective in raising the serum albumin level and may exacerbate the proteinuria. There is recent evidence that dietary protein limited to 0.8 g/kg/day (supplemented with the amount lost in the urine) will provide adequate substrate for albumin synthesis and decreases proteinuria. Because of the associated lipid disorders, it is usually necessary to limit cholesterol intake to <300 mg/day with 30% of the dietary calories in fat (2:1 polyunsaturated-to-saturated fat ratio). The remainder of the 35 Kcal/kg/day preferably consists of complex carbohydrates.

Micronutrients

The degree of sodium restriction will depend on the magnitude of edema and typically ranges from 2–4 g/day. Potassium and phosphorus are limited as necessary if glomerular filtration rate declines.

Patients on Hemodialysis

Macronutrients

Once hemodialysis is initiated, there will be small protein and amino acid losses into the dialysate, and the dialysis prescription will be periodically adjusted to optimize clearance of nitrogenous waste products. The dietary protein should be liberalized to 1.0–1.2 g/kg/day with additional quantities added to compensate for any residual renal losses. Because a low serum albumin at the commencement of dialytic therapy is associated with high patient morbidity and mortality, it is hoped that these individuals will benefit from very aggressive feeding. Various palatable dietary supplements are now commercially available for patients unable to consume standard meals because of anorexia, nausea, or vomiting. Intradialytic parenteral nutrition with solutions of 10–20% dextrose, 10% amino acids, and 20% lipids is reserved for those who cannot achieve adequate oral intake. The diet generally contains 35 Kcal/kg/day of which 35–50% of the calories are from carbohydrates and 30% from fat (2:1 polyunsaturated-to-saturated fat ratio). Cholesterol intake should be guided by periodic lipoprotein analyses. For anabolic patients gaining weight, calories must be increased with the use of fats and simple carbohydrates.

Micronutrients

Sodium, potassium, and water restriction will depend on the residual renal function and urine output. Anuric patients typically require a daily restriction of 1.0–1.5 L fluid, 2–3 g sodium, and 70 mEq (1 mEq/kg) potassium. Phosphorus is limited to 0.8–1.0 g/day.

Patients on Chronic Peritoneal Dialysis

Macronutrients

Malnutrition is a very common problem in peritoneal dialysis patients. Diminished appetite is mainly due to the dialysate, which distends the abdomen, causes intermittent discomfort, and leads to dextrose absorption. The calories from dextrose are significant and can be estimated based on a 70–80% peritoneal absorption rate and 3.4 Kcal/g. For example, 2 L of 4.25% dextrose will yield a total of 85 g, of which an estimated 80% (or 68 g) can be absorbed after a long dwell time. This would provide 68 × 3.4 or approximately 231 Kcal. Protein nutrition is, however, much more of a problem because as much as 2–3 g can be lost with each dialysate exchange. During episodes of peritonitis, the losses can exceed 15 g protein/day. For this reason patients are placed on a 1.2- to 1.5-g protein/kg/day diet, which is increased during peritonitis. Balancing the types of nutrients to provide a total of 35 Kcal/kg/day is further complicated when fat intake is limited because of hyperlipidemia. Dietary fat is usually reduced to 30% of the prescribed calories, with a 2:1 polyunsaturated-to-saturated fat ratio. Malnutrition is so common that it has led to the development of aggressive strategies for enteral food supplementation as well as the use of experimental dialysate solutions containing amino acids.

Micronutrients

Salt and water balance is less problematic than in hemodialysis because patients can compensate for their diet by adjusting the type and frequency of peritoneal dialysate exchanges. However, the chronic use of high dextrose concentrations to increase ultrafiltration may worsen the hyperlipidemia. Thus, sodium intake occasionally needs to be limited to 2–4 g/day in 1.0–1.5 L of fluid. Hyperkalemic patients should limit their potassium intake to 70 mEq/day; however, hypokalemia frequently occurs because of significant peritoneal potassium losses, and this permits the diet to be liberalized. The high protein prescription makes it difficult to decrease phosphorus to less than approximately 1.0 g/day.

Kidney Transplant Patients

Postoperative kidney transplant patients receiving glucocorticoids require close attention to assure they are receiving increased nutrients. Even if the allograft has initial nonfunction, these patients should receive 1.5 g protein/kg/day. The increased protein and caloric intake commonly demands more intensive dialytic therapy. Subsequent dietary guidelines depend on the degree of allograft function. Steroid-induced hyperglycemia may limit the permissible simple carbohydrate intake. Calcium intake should be monitored to achieve approximately 1 g/day. Particular attention should be focused on dietary modification for control of hyperlipidemia. In addition, potassium intake may need to be reduced because of the hyperkalemia associated with cyclosporine therapy.

Suggested Readings

Anderson S. Low protein diets and diabetic nephropathy. Semin Nephrol 1990;10:287–293.

Hoy WE, Sargent JA, Freeman RB, et al. The influence of glucocorticoid dose on protein catabolism after renal transplantation. Am J Med Sci 1986;291:241–247.

Kaysen GA. Effect of dietary protein intake on albumin homeostasis in nephrotic patients. Kidney Int 1986;29:572–577.

Klahr S, Levey AS, Beck GJ, et al. The effects of dietary protein restriction and blood-pressure control on the progression of chronic renal disease. N Engl J Med 1994;330:877–884.

Kopple JO, Blumenkrantz MJ. Nutritional requirements for patients undergoing continuous ambulatory peritoneal dialysis. Kidney Int 1983;24(suppl 16):S295–S302.

Mitch WE. Dietary protein restriction in chronic renal failure: nutritional efficacy, compliance and progression of renal insufficiency. J Am Soc Nephrol 1991;2(suppl 4):823–831.

Mitch WE, Klahr S. Nutrition and the kidney, 2nd ed. Boston: Little, Brown, 1993.

Chapter 26

Use of Drugs in Renal Failure

Nicolas J. Guzman

The activity of any drug is related to the concentration of free drug in the tissue compartment where the effect occurs (Fig. 26.1). The kidney is a major route of drug elimination through both excretion and metabolism; therefore, patients with renal disease and also the elderly who have reduced renal function because of aging are more susceptible to drug toxicity. Drug interactions are also more common in patients with renal insufficiency because they are frequently receiving many drugs. Uremia alters gastrointestinal absorption, hepatic metabolism, protein affinity, and tissue responses to various pharmacological agents. Protein binding of drugs is also diminished by hypoalbuminemia. Active metabolites may accumulate in renal insufficiency and produce undesired effects. Finally, some drugs may trigger or exacerbate metabolic disorders that occur as a result of renal disease, whereas others may accelerate the progression of renal failure by causing acute or chronic injury to the kidney. The nephrotoxicity of commonly used therapeutic agents is discussed in detail in Chapter 8.

GASTROINTESTINAL ABSORPTION AND BIOAVAILABILITY

Any change in the extent or rate of absorption of a drug will lead to variations in blood drug levels that may result in therapeutic failure or toxicity. Gastrointestinal absorption of drugs is unchanged by mild or moderate renal insufficiency. With severe

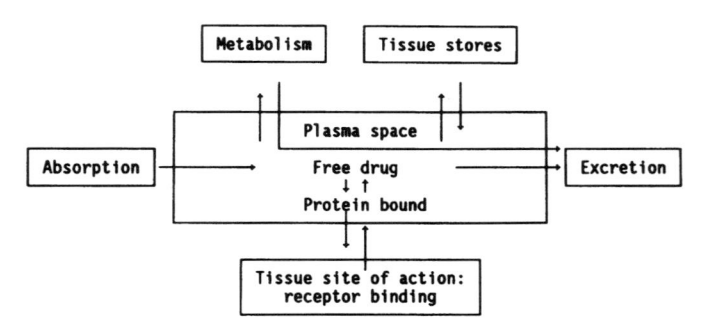

```
┌──────────────┐  ┌──────────────┐
│  Metabolism  │  │ Tissue stores│
└──────┬───────┘  └──────┬───────┘
       │ ↑↓              │ ↑↓
┌──────────────┐  ┌─────────────────────┐
│              │  │   Plasma space      │
│  Absorption  │──→│   Free drug        │──→  Excretion
│              │  │   ↓ ↑               │
└──────────────┘  │   Protein bound     │
                  └──────────┬──────────┘
                             │ ↑↓
                  ┌─────────────────────┐
                  │ Tissue site of action:│
                  │   receptor binding  │
                  └─────────────────────┘
```

Figure 26.1. Relationship among absorption, distribution, protein binding, and excretion of a drug and its concentration at locus of action.

renal insufficiency, however, several situations can impair drug absorption.

Uremia

Uremia commonly causes gastritis, which leads to nausea and vomiting. Uremia may also cause gastroparesis, and because most drugs are absorbed in the proximal small intestine, delayed gastric emptying (particularly when associated with vomiting) will diminish peak drug plasma concentrations and total drug absorption. This is especially important for drugs that require rapid onset of action.

Association of Renal Failure with Other Conditions That Impair Gastrointestinal Motility

Diabetes mellitus causes autonomic neuropathy and gastroparesis, which may delay drug absorption, or, if diarrhea is present, decrease contact time for intestinal absorption. Patients on peritoneal dialysis occasionally develop peritonitis, which slows intestinal peristalsis and may interfere with drug absorption.

Renal Failure and Adverse Drug Effects and Drug Interactions

This is the most important mechanism by which renal failure affects drug absorption. Phosphate-binding antacids, at the doses used in renal failure, produce a marked rise in gastric pH that delays gastric emptying and impairs drug absorption. Antacids may also decrease the absorption of some drugs (e.g., cimetidine) and reduce the activity of others (e.g., sucralfate). Aluminum-based antacids may cause constipation and increase drug bioavailability by increasing contact time for intestinal absorption. On occasion, drugs may accelerate gastric emptying and intestinal transit. This will also impair drug absorption. Peak plasma concentrations will be increased and occur earlier with more rapid gastric emptying. This situation is common in patients with diabetic gastroparesis after initiation of metoclopramide.

DRUG DISTRIBUTION

Uremia causes changes in albumin binding that frequently result in a higher free fraction of drug in the plasma. Three mechanisms have been implicated in the decrease of albumin-bound plasma drug levels observed in these patients.

Decreased Serum Albumin

This is a problem in patients with nephrotic syndrome or protein malnutrition and in those receiving peritoneal dialysis.

Accumulation of Substances in Uremic Plasma That Displace Acidic Drugs from Albumin Binding Sites

Processes that displace drugs from albumin do not have a therapeutic impact if binding to albumin is <90%. These considerations are important mainly for acidic drugs. Basic drugs, such as propranolol and lidocaine, bind to glycoproteins and do not seem to be affected by protein displacement.

Alterations in Capacity of Albumin to Bind Drugs

This can result from uremia or acidosis. Reductions in the amount of albumin-bound drug lead to a decrease in *total* plasma drug concentrations. Therefore, in situations where a highly albumin-bound drug has been displaced from its protein binding sites, total plasma drug concentrations do not accurately reflect actual *free* drug levels and *therapeutic* response. In most cases, when a highly albumin-bound drug is displaced from its protein binding site, there is a transient rise in free drug levels. However, free drug levels will usually return to steady state at the same level that existed before displacement occurred, i.e., therapeutic levels. Because the fraction of drug bound to albumin is now decreased, total plasma drug levels will also be decreased. Lack of awareness of this fact will prompt the physician to increase drug dosages to reestablish "therapeutic" total plasma drug levels, and, not infrequently, this will result in drug toxicity. This phenomenon is particularly common with phenytoin. In these circumstances, measurement of free plasma drug concentrations is indicated to avoid drug toxicity.

CLEARANCE

The total plasma clearance of a drug is equal to the sum of renal elimination, hepatic metabolism and conjugation, and other metabolic and excretory pathways in other tissues. Renal elimination of drugs is determined by glomerular filtration, active secretion primarily in the proximal tubule, and reabsorption. Protein-bound drugs are poorly filtered, but they may be efficiently cleared by proximal secretion. Unbound drugs are usually freely filtered at the glomerulus; their renal elimination depends on volume of distribution, glomerular filtration rate, and drug reabsorption. Drugs with large volumes of distribution and large tissue reservoirs are not available for glomerular filtration. For dose adjustment of drugs that are cleared primarily by the kidney, glomerular filtration rate can be estimated using the Cockcroft and Gault formula (see Chapter 2).

Hepatic metabolism gains importance in patients with renal insufficiency. Whenever possible, drugs with significant hepatic elimination should be used. However, patients with chronic renal insufficiency exhibit decreased hepatic metabolism of some drugs, e.g., the reduction of drugs such as hydrocortisone and the acetylation of drugs such as isoniazid. In addition, drugs that are avidly cleared by the liver or have high first pass effect tend to achieve higher peak levels after oral administration in uremic patients. For example, propranolol typically shows increased bioavailability after standard oral doses in patients with renal insufficiency. This has been attributed to decreased first pass effect. In renal failure, previously minor hepatic metabolic pathways may become the major mechanism for elimination of a drug. Therefore, concomitant hepatic failure can result in severe overdosage and toxicity.

HEMODIALYSIS OF DRUGS

The degree to which a drug is removed by hemodialysis is directly proportional to the plasma concentration of free drug (not bound to plasma proteins) and to the clearance characteristics of the dialysis membrane. Hemodialysis clearance is inversely proportional to the amount of tissue binding or volume of distribution. Many drugs, particularly antibiotics, are removed by hemodialysis, and it is important to supplement the dose after a treatment. Occasionally symptoms will occur because of an inadequate drug level toward the end of a treatment. Arrhythmias may break through because N-acetyl procainamide, the acetylated active metabolite of procainamide, is dialysable. Opiates and ethanol are dialysable, and their removal can precipitate withdrawal or inadequate analgesia.

PERITONEAL DIALYSIS OF DRUGS

Most drugs are poorly removed by peritoneal dialysis. Drug administration in the dialysate fluid is similarly a difficult way to obtain a systemic drug level. Antibiotics are frequently used intraperitoneally to treat dialysis-related peritonitis, and removal of systemic antibiotics can be avoided by placing therapeutic drug levels into the dialysate.

TABLES

Tables 26.1–26.3 provide specific information about commonly used drugs that require dose adjustments in patients with renal disease. Included is information on the major route of elimination, percentage of protein binding, percentage of a normal dose removed by dialysis, and dosing recommendations in patients with renal insufficiency relative to the normal dose. This information is a guideline and should be used to start therapy with the understanding that individual adjustments will be the rule rather than the exception. With the few exceptions described in Tables 26.1–26.3, most psychotrophic, analgesic, anti-inflammatory, and antineoplastic drugs undergo extensive hepatic metabolism, and therefore dose adjustments are not necessary in patients with renal insufficiency. These agents have been omitted from the tables. The tables have been adapted from Brater (1991), listed under "Suggested Readings."

Table 26.1
Antimicrobial Agents

Drug	Major Route of Elimination	Protein Binding (%)	% Removed by		Dosing When C_{cr} (mL/min)		
			Hemodialysis	CAPD	>50	20–50	<20
Antibiotics							
Aminoglycosides	Renal	0	50	20–25	1/3	1/2	1/4
Carbapenes							
Imipenem	Renal	20	80–90			1/2	1/4
Cephalosporins							
Cefaclor	Renal	25	33			1/2	1/4
Cefamandole	Renal	74	>50	5	1/2	1/3	1/4
Cefazolin	Renal	85	50	20	1/2	1/4	1/6
Cefotaxime	Renal	30	60	Negligible		1/2	1/4
Cefotetan	Renal	85	Negligible	Negligible	1/2	1/4	1/10
Cefoxitin	Renal	74	>50	Negligible	1/2	1/4	1/6
Ceftazidime	Renal	17	50	Negligible	1/2	1/5	1/10
Ceftriaxone	Renal	90		Negligible			
Cefuroxime	Renal	40		20		1/2	1/4
Cephalexin	Renal	15	>50	Negligible		1/3	1/10
Cephalothin	Renal	65	50		2/3	1/2	1/6
Macrolides							
Clindamycin	Hepatic	60–90	Negligible	Negligible			
Erythromycin	Hepatic	85	Negligible	Negligible			

Drug	Route					
Monobactams						
Aztreonam	Renal	50-60	40	Negligible	1/2	1/3	1/4
Penicillins						
Amoxicillin	Renal	17	30			1/2	1/6
Ampicillin	Renal	18	40		1/2	1/4	1/10
Carbenicillin	Renal	50	50		1/3	1/5	1/10
Cloxacillin	Hepatic	95	Negligible				
Dicloxacillin	Hepatic	96	Negligible				
Methicillin	Renal	40	Negligible			1/2	1/4
Mezlocillin	Renal	30	20–25	Negligible	1/2	1/4	1/8
Nafcillin	Hepatic	90	Negligible				
Oxacillin	Hepatic	92	Negligible				
Penicillin	Renal	60	>50			1/5	1/8
Piperacillin	Renal	21	50			1/2	1/3
Ticarcillin	Renal	50	50		1/2	1/3	1/4
Quinolones						
Ciprofloxacin	Renal	20	Negligible	Negligible			1/2
Norfloxacin	Hepatic	14	Negligible				1/2
Ofloxacin	Renal	32					1/2
Sulfonamides						
Sulfamethoxazole	Renal	65	50	Negligible			1/2
Sulfisoxazole	Renal	90			3/4	1/2	1/4
Tetracyclines[a]						
Doxycycline	Renal	90	Negligible			Avoid	Avoid
Minocycline	Hepatic	70				Avoid	Avoid
Tetracycline	Renal	65				Avoid	Avoid

Table 26.1. Continued

Drug	Major Route of Elimination	Protein Binding (%)	% Removed by Hemodialysis	% Removed by CAPD	Dosing When C_cr (mL/min) >50	20-50	<20
Others							
Chloramphenicol	Hepatic	25-50			1/2	1/3	1/10
Vancomycin	Renal		Negligible	Negligible	2/3	1/2	1/10
Trimethoprim	Renal	70	50				1/2
Antifungals							
Amphotericin B	Hepatic	95	Negligible				
Flucytosine	Renal	3-4	50	Negligible	1/2	1/3	1/4
Ketoconazole	Hepatic	99	Negligible	Negligible			
Miconazole	Hepatic	98	Negligible				1/3
Fluconazole	Renal	12	>50			1/2	1/4
Antimalarials							
Chloroquine	Renal	55	Negligible				
Quinine	Hepatic	90	Negligible				
Antiparasitics							
Metronidazole	Hepatic	10	25-50	Negligible			
Antituberculous agents							
Ethambutol	Renal	20-30	33-50			1/2	1/3
Isoniazid	Hepatic	0	75				1/2
Aminosalicyclic acid	Renal	60	>50				
Rifampin	Hepatic	90					

Antivirals

Acyclovir	Renal	9–22	60	1/2	1/5
Amantadine	Renal	0	Negligible	1/2	1/10
Ganciclovir	Renal	0	50	1/2	1/10
Foscarnet	Renal	14–17	50	1/2[b]	1/3[c]	Avoid

[a]These drugs have an antianabolic effect that raises blood urea nitrogen independent of renal function. In addition, they are nephrotoxic, and most compounds have renal elimination. CAPD, continuous ambulatory peritoneal dialysis; C_{cr}, creatinine clearance.

[b]Dosing recommendations are for induction therapy only.

[c]Discontinue therapy if creatinine clearance falls below 30 mL/min.

Table 26.2
Cardiovascular Drugs, Antihypertensives, Diuretics, Bronchodilators, Antianginals, and Antiarrhythmics

Drug	Major Route of Elimination	Protein Binding (%)	% Removed by Hemodialysis	% Removed by CAPD	Dosing When C_{cr} (mL/min) >50	Dosing When C_{cr} (mL/min) 20–50	Dosing When C_{cr} (mL/min) <20
Antiarrhythmics							
Amiodarone	Hepatic	96	Negligible				
Bertylium	Hepatic	8–10	Negligible				1/5
Disopyramide	Renal	50–70	Negligible			1/2	1/5
Lidocaine	Hepatic	50	Negligible				
Mexiletine	Hepatic-renal	50	Negligible				
Procainamide	Renal	15	Negligible	Negligible			
N-acetylprocainamide	Renal	10	50	Negligible		1/2	1/4
Quinidine	Hepatic	70–95	Negligible				
Antihypertensives							
Angiotensin-converting enzyme inhibitors							
Captopril	Renal	30	40		1/2	1/6	1/12
Enalapril	Hepatic	50	50			1/3	1/5
Lisinopril	Renal	0					
β-Blockers							
Acebutolol	Hepatic	15	Negligible			1/2	1/3
Atenolol	Renal	5	50			1/2	1/4
Labetolol	Hepatic	50	Negligible	Negligible			
Metoprolol	Hepatic	12	Negligible				1/2

Drug	Route	Col3	Col4	Col5	Col6	Col7	Col8
Nadolol	Renal	25			3/4	1/2	1/4
Pindolol	Hepatic	57	Negligible				
Propranolol	Hepatic	99	Negligible				
Timolol	Hepatic	10	Negligible				
Calcium channel antagonists							
Diltiazem	Hepatic	80	Negligible	Negligible			
Nifedipine	Hepatic	95	Negligible	Negligible			
Nitrendipine	Hepatic	98	Negligible	Negligible			
Verapamil	Hepatic	90	Negligible	Negligible			
Central agents, α_2-agonists							
Clonidine	Renal	25	Negligible			1/2	1/3
Guanabenz	Hepatic	90					
Guanfacine	Hepatic	65	Negligible				1/2
Methyldopa	Hepatic	10					
Diuretics							
Amiloride	Renal	0–10				Avoid	Avoid
Bumetanide[a]	Renal	96					
Chlorthalidone	Renal	98				Avoid	Avoid
Ethacrynic acid[a]	Hepatic	95					
Furosemide[a]	Renal	95					Avoid
Mannitol	Renal	0	>90				
Metolazone[a]	Renal	95					
Spironolactone	Hepatic	98				Avoid	Avoid
Thiazides	Renal	95				Avoid	Avoid
Triamterene	Renal	50					Avoid

Table 26.2. Continued

Drug	Major Route of Elimination	Protein Binding (%)	% Removed by Hemodialysis	% Removed by CAPD	Dosing When C_{cr} (mL/min) >50	Dosing When C_{cr} (mL/min) 20–50	Dosing When C_{cr} (mL/min) <20
Vasodilators							
Hydralazine	Hepatic	90					
Minoxidil	Hepatic	0	24–34				
Prazosin	Hepatic	90					
Terazosin	Hepatic	90					
Inotropes							
Amrinone	Hepatic	40					
Digitoxin	Hepatic	90					
Digoxin	Renal	25	Negligible	Negligible	1/2	1/3	1/5

[a]Decreased drug effect in renal failure. Dose must be increased to obtain same effect. CAPD, continuous ambulatory peritoneal dialysis; C_{cr}, creatinine clearance.

Table 26.3
Drugs Used in Psychiatry and Neurology

Drug	Major Route of Elimination	Protein Binding (%)	% Removed by Hemodialysis	% Removed by CAPD	Dosing When C_{cr} (mL/min) >50	Dosing When C_{cr} (mL/min) 20–50	Dosing When C_{cr} (mL/min) <20
Antimaniacal agents							
Lithium	Renal	0	Considerable	Considerable			
Antihistamine drugs							
Cimetidine	Renal	19	10–20	Negligible		1/2	1/6
Famotidine	Renal	17	Negligible				1/3
Ranitidine	Renal	15	50–60		1/2	1/3	1/4
Nizatidine	Renal	15	>50			1/2	1/4
Hypouricemic drugs							
Allopurinol	Renal	5	40		2/3	1/3	1/6
Colchicine	Hepatic	31					1/2
Antidopaminergic agents							
Metoclopramide	Hepatic	40	Negligible			1/2	1/4
Lipid-lowering agents							
Clofibrate	Hepatic	96			1/2	1/4	1/10

CAPD, continuous ambulatory peritoneal dialysis; C_{cr}, creatinine clearance.

Suggested Readings

Brater DC. Drug use in clinical medicine, 3rd ed. Toronto: Decker, 1987.

Brater DC. Use of drugs in uremia and dialysis. In: Suki WN, Massry SG, eds. Therapy of renal diseases and related disorders. Boston: Kluwer, 1991:853–865.

Gilman AG, Rall TW, Nies AS, Taylor P. Goodman and Gilman's: the pharmacological basis of therapeutics, 8th ed. New York: Pergamon, 1990.

Perucca E, Grimaldi R, Cieme A. Interpretation of drug levels in acute and chronic disease states. Clin Pharm 1985;10:498–513.

Reed WE, Sabatini S. The use of drugs in renal failure. Semin Nephrol 1986;6:259–295.

Reidenberg MM, Drayer DE. Alteration of drug-protein binding in renal disease. Clin Pharm 1984;9(suppl 1):18–26.

Index

Page numbers followed by "t" denote tables; those followed by "f" denote figures.

Abortion, septic, acute tubular necrosis in, 75–76
Abruptio placentae, acute tubular necrosis in, 75–76
Abscess, renal, 164t, 166
Absorption, drug, in renal failure, 277–279, 278f
Accelerated hypertension, 191
Accelerated rejection, in renal transplantation, 259
Acebutolol, in hypertension, 215t
Acetaminophen, tubulointerstitial nephritis from, 174
Acetate, in hemodialysis, 231
Acid-base disorders (*see also* Acidosis; Alkalosis)
  classification, 121
  compensatory response in, 122t, 123–124, 132
  etiology, 122t
  evaluation, 123–124
  mixed, 134–135, 136t, 137
  pathophysiology, 123–124
  terminology, 121
  triple, 135, 137
Acidemia, 121
Acidosis
  definition, 121
  metabolic, 124–130 (*see also* Renal tubular acidosis)
    causes, 127–129, 127t
    in chronic renal failure, 90
    clinical presentation, 124–125, 126t
    compensatory response to, 122t, 123–124
    definition, 121, 124
    differential diagnosis, 126t–127t
    elevated anion gap, 125, 126t
    in HIV infection, 185
    hypokalemia and, 113
    mechanisms, 122t, 124
    in mixed acid-base disorders, 135, 136t
    normal anion gap, 125, 127t
    potassium metabolism and, 108
    treatment, 125, 127–129
    uremic, 125
  renal tubular (*see* Renal tubular acidosis)
  respiratory, 121, 122t, 130–131, 131t
    in mixed acid-base disorders, 135, 136t
  types, 121
ACNAs (antineutrophilic cytoplasmic antibodies), 50–52
Acquired immunodeficiency syndrome (*see* Human immunodeficiency virus infection)
Acute diseases (*see under specific disease*)
Acute fatty liver syndrome, in pregnancy, acute tubular necrosis in, 76
Acute renal failure
  clinical presentation, 70–71
  in cyclosporine therapy, 257
  definition, 69
  differential diagnosis, 77–79, 77t–79t
  etiology, 70

Acute renal failure — *continued*
  in glomerulonephritis
    postinfectious proliferative, 40
    rapidly progressive, 41
  in HIV infection, 183–184
  hypercalcemia in, 141
  nutrition in, 272
  parenchymal (*see* Acute tubular necrosis)
  pathophysiology, 69
  peritoneal dialysis in, 244
  prerenal, 69–72
    in renal transplantation, 258
  renal biopsy in, 22
  reversible, 79
  in Schönlein-Henoch purpura, 54
  treatment, 71–72
  in tubulointerstitial nephritis, 168, 171–172
Acute tubular necrosis, 72–77
  in aminoglycoside therapy, 72–73
  in amphotericin B therapy, 73
  in cisplatin therapy, 74
  clinical features, 76–77, 79–80
  in contrast agent use, 73–74
  course, 79–80
  in crystal deposition, 75
  definition, 72
  differential diagnosis, 77–79, 77t–79t
  in ethylene glycol poisoning, 74
  etiology, 72–76, 73t
  in hepatorenal syndrome, 76
  in hypoperfusion, 72
  incidence, 72
  laboratory findings, 76–77
  mortality in, 81
  in multiple myeloma, 75
  nonoliguric, conversion to, 80
  pathophysiology, 76
  phases, 79–80
  in pregnancy, 75–76
  prognosis for, 81
  recovery from, 80
  in renal transplantation, 258–259, 262–263
  in rhabdomyolysis, 74–75
  from toxins
    endogenous, 73t, 74–76
    exogenous, 72–74, 73t
  treatment, 80–81, 81t
    in renal transplantation, 262–263
Acute urethral syndrome, 163
Addison's disease, hyperkalemia in, 117
Adenoma, adrenal gland, hyperaldosteronism in, 204–206
Adrenal gland
  adenoma, hyperaldosteronism in, 204–206
  insufficiency, hyperkalemia in, 117
  pheochromocytoma, 202–204
Adrenal vein, blood sampling from
  in hyperaldosteronism, 206
  in pheochromocytoma, 204
AIDS (*see* Human immunodeficiency virus infection)
AIDS-related complex, dialysis in, 185
Albumin
  vs. calcium concentration, 138
  deficiency (*see* Hypoalbuminemia)
  drug binding to, 279–280
  glomerular filtration, 31
Alcoholism, hypomagnesemia in, 150
Aldosterone
  deficiency, acidosis in, 129–130
  hypersecretion (*see* Hyperaldosteronism)
  in potassium uptake, 108
Alkalemia, 121
Alkalosis
  definition, 121
  metabolic, 121, 122t, 131–133, 133t
    causes, 131–132

clinical presentation, 132–133, 133t
compensatory response to, 132
definition, 121
in hyperaldosteronism, 205
in mixed acid-base disorders, 135, 136t
treatment, 133
potassium metabolism and, 108–109
respiratory, 121, 122t, 134, 134t
hypocalcemia in, 145
in mixed acid-base disorders, 135, 136t
types, 121
Allergy
drug, nephritis in (*see* Tubulointerstitial nephritis)
to hemodialysis components, 232
Allograft, renal (*see* Transplantation, renal)
Allopurinol
in hyperuricosuria, 160
interactions with azathioprine, 256
$Alpha_2$-agonists, pharmacokinetics, 287t
$Alpha_1$-receptor antagonists, in hypertension, 218, 218t
Alport's syndrome, hematuria in, 27
Aluminum toxicity, in hemodialysis, 235
Amikacin, acute tubular necrosis from, 72–73
Amiloride
in hyperaldosteronism, 206
in hypertension, 213t
in hypokalemia, 114
Aminoglycosides, acute tubular necrosis from, 72–73
Aminopyrine, tubulointerstitial nephritis from, 174
Amiodipine, in hypertension, 220t
Amniotic fluid embolism, acute tubular necrosis in, 75–76

Amoxicillin, in urinary tract infection, 165t
Amphotericin B, acute tubular necrosis from, 73
Amyloidosis, 59–60
in hemodialysis, 235
in multiple myeloma, 59
Analgesic nephropathy, 173–175
Anasarca, in nephrotic syndrome, 32, 34
Anemia
in chronic renal failure, treatment, 92
in hemodialysis, 236
hemolytic, in thrombotic microangiopathy, 55
in systemic lupus erythematosus, 46
in tubulointerstitial nephritis, 174
Aneurysm, cerebral, in polycystic kidney disease, 179
Angiography, in polyarteritis nodosa, 51
Angioplasty, renal artery, in hypertension, 202
Angiotensin-converting enzyme inhibitors
advantages, 216
in chronic renal failure, 91
disadvantages, 216
in hypertension, 216, 217t
in diabetic nephropathy, 66–67
in nephrotic syndrome, 34
pharmacokinetics, 286t
in progressive systemic sclerosis, 57–58
Anion gap, normal, 125
Anorexia, in chronic renal failure, 92
Antibiotics
acute tubular necrosis from, 72–73
clearance, 282t–284t
dosage alterations in, in renal failure, 282t–284t
in peritoneal dialysis, 247
with peritonitis, 249, 251t

Antibiotics — *continued*
  pharmacokinetics, in renal failure, 282t–284t
  in polycystic kidney disease, 179
  protein binding, 282t–284t
  tubulointerstitial nephritis from, 170, 171t
Antibodies
  antilymphocyte, in renal graft rejection, 262
  antineutrophilic cytoplasmic, 50–52
  antinuclear, 46, 56
  to donor tissue, in renal allograft rejection, 259
  glomerular basement membrane (Goodpasture's syndrome), 27, 42–43
  in glomerulonephritis, 42
Anticentromere antibodies, in progressive systemic sclerosis, 56
Anticoagulants, in renal vein thrombosis, 35
Antidiuretic hormone
  action/release, drugs affecting, 100
  deficiency, hypernatremia in, 104
  inappropriate secretion, 99
  in water regulation, 95
Antiglomerular basement membrane disease (Goodpasture's syndrome), 27, 42–43
Antihypertensive agents (*see also* Hypertension, treatment)
  pharmacokinetics, 286t–288t
Antilymphocyte antibodies, in renal graft rejection, 262
Antineutrophilic cytoplasmic antibodies
  in polyarteritis nodosa, 51–52
  in Wegener's granulomatosis, 50
Antinuclear antibodies
  in progressive systemic sclerosis, 56
  in systemic lupus erythematosus, 46

Antistreptolysin O titer, in glomerulonephritis, 41
Antithymocyte globulin, in renal graft rejection, 263
Anuria, in acute tubular necrosis, 76
Aortic dissection, hypertension in, treatment, 222t, 224
Arcuate arteries, anatomy, 2f, 11
Arrhythmias, cardiac, in hemodialysis, 234
Arterial blood gas, in acid-base disorders, 124
Arteriography, 21
  in hypertension, 196, 303
Arteriovenous fistula, in hemodialysis, 230
Arteriovenous graft, in hemodialysis, 230
Arteriovenous malformation, hematuria in, 28
Ascites
  in nephrotic syndrome, 32, 34
  treatment, 34–35
Aspirin
  in thrombotic microangiopathy, 55–56
  tubulointerstitial nephritis from, 174
Atenolol, in hypertension, 215t
ATN (*see* Acute tubular necrosis)
Autoregulation, glomerular filtration rate, 69
Autosomal polycystic kidney disease (*see* Polycystic kidney disease)
Azathioprine, in renal transplantation, 255–256
Azotemia
  acute prerenal (*see* Prerenal acute renal failure)
  in acute tubular necrosis, 72, 77

Bacteremia, in hemodialysis, 230
Bacteriuria
  asymptomatic, in diabetes mellitus, 67
  in cystitis, 165
  significant, definition, 163
Base deficit, calculation, 125

Basement membrane,
  glomerular, 4, 5f
  antibodies against
    (Goodpasture's syndrome),
    27, 42–43
  thin, hematuria in, 27
Bence Jones protein, detection,
  15
Benzapril, in hypertension, 217t
Berger's disease (IgA
  nephropathy), 27, 44
β-Blockers
  advantages, 214
  bronchospasm from, 215
  cardioselective, 215
  in diabetes mellitus, 216
  disadvantages, 214
  hepatic metabolism, 215
  hypercholesterolemia and, 216
  in hypertension, 214–216,
    215t, 221, 222t, 224
    in diabetic nephropathy, 67
  in peripheral vascular disease,
    216
  pharmacokinetics, 286t–287t
  in pheochromocytoma, 204
Bicarbonate (*see also* Sodium
    bicarbonate)
  deficit, calculation, 125
  fractional excretion, 129
  in hemodialysis, 231
  in metabolic acidosis, 125,
    128–129
  monitoring, in acute tubular
    necrosis, 80
  reabsorption, in renal tubular
    acidosis, 128–129
  in renal tubular acidosis, 128–
    129
  secretion, alkalosis and, 131–
    132
Bicarbonate buffer system, in
  acid-base homeostasis, 123
Bicarbonaturia
  hyponatremia in, 99
  in renal tubular acidosis, 128
Bilirubinuria, 13
Biopsy, renal, 22–24
  complications, 24
  contraindications for, 23
  in diabetic nephropathy, 66
  in glomerulonephritis
    membranous, 39
    postinfectious, 41
  in graft rejection, 262
  in immunoglobulin A
    nephropathy, 44
  indications for, 22–23
  in nephrotic syndrome, 34
  patient preparation for, 23–24
  in progressive systemic
    sclerosis, 57
  in Wegener's granulomatosis,
    50
Bladder infection (cystitis), 162,
  165
Bleeding
  in hemodialysis, 234
  in renal biopsy, 24
  in renal graft rejection, 260,
    263
Blood, urine (*see* Hematuria)
Blood chemistries, in nephrotic
  syndrome, 33
Blood gas, arterial, in acid-base
  disorders, 124
Blood pressure
  abnormalities (*see*
    Hypertension; Hypotension)
  measurement, 193
Blood transfusion, complications,
  in hemodialysis, 234–235
Blood urea nitrogen
  in glomerular filtration
    assessment, 16
  goals for
    in hemodialysis, 232–233
    in peritoneal dialysis, 241–
      242
  in hyponatremia, 96
  as osmole, 95
  retention, in chronic renal
    failure, 85
Body water balance (*see* Water
  balance)
Bone disease, metabolic
  in chronic renal failure, 84–85
  in hemodialysis, 235
Brain
  aneurysm, in polycystic kidney
    disease, 179

Brain — *continued*
  edema
    in hemodialysis, 233–234
    in hyponatremia, 100–101
Bretylium, in hypertension, 220
Broad casts, in urine, 16t
Buffers, in acid-base homeostasis, 123
Bumetanide
  in chronic renal failure, 89
  in hypertension, 213t
BUN (*see* Blood urea nitrogen)

Cadaver donor, for renal transplantation, 255
Calcitonin
  in calcium homeostasis, 139
  in hypercalcemia, 144
Calcium
  abnormalities (*see* Hypercalcemia; Hypocalcemia)
  balance
    in chronic renal failure, 90–91
    factors affecting, 138–139
  forms of, 138
  in hypermagnesemia, 150
  ionized, 138
  monitoring, in acute tubular necrosis, 81
  normal levels, 138
  urinary, 155, 155t–156t, 158–159
Calcium acetate, in chronic renal failure, 90
Calcium carbonate, in chronic renal failure, 90
Calcium channel blockers
  in diabetic nephropathy, 67
  in hypertension, 219–220, 220t
  pharmacokinetics, 287t
Calcium chloride
  in hyperkalemia, 118t
  in hypocalcemia, 146–147
Calcium gluconate
  in chronic renal failure, 90
  in hyperkalemia, 118, 118t
  in hypocalcemia, 146–147
Calcium lactate, in hypocalcemia, 147
Calcium oxalate
  deposition, in ethylene glycol poisoning, 74
  stones, 153f, 155t, 156, 157t
Calcium stones, 155, 155t–156t, 158–159
Calculi, renal (*see* Renal stone disease)
Caloric requirements, in renal failure, 268
Cancer, in renal transplantation, 265–266
Candiduria, catheter-related, 166
Captopril, in hypertension, 217t, 225
Captopril test, in hypertension, 200–201
Carbohydrate requirements, in renal failure, 270
Carbon dioxide
  partial pressure, definition, 121
  total, definition, 121
Cardiac arrhythmias, in hemodialysis, 234
Cardiac output, reduced, acute renal failure in, 70
Cardioselective β-blockers, 215
Cardiovascular complications
  in peritoneal dialysis, 247
  in renal transplantation, 265
Casts, urine, 16, 16t
  in acute tubular necrosis, 77
  "dirty-brown," in hyperkalemia, 117
  erythrocyte, in Wegener's granulomatosis, 50
  in glomerulonephritis, 36
  in hematuria, 26t
  in multiple myeloma, 58
  in urinary tract infection, 163
Catecholamines
  excessive, hypertension in, 202–203, 222t, 224
  potassium metabolism and, 108
Catheter
  peritoneal, for dialysis, 241, 245
  urinary, infection from, 166

vascular
  for hemodialysis, 229–230
  for hemofiltration, 237
Cellulose sodium phosphate, in hypercalciuria, 159
Central acting agents, in hypertension, 218, 219t
Central diabetes insipidus
  clinical presentation, 105–106
  diagnosis, 105–106, 105t
  pathogenesis, 104
  treatment, 106
Central nervous system (*see also* Brain)
  infections, in renal transplantation, 264
Centromeres, antibodies to, in progressive systemic sclerosis, 56
Cerebral aneurysm, in polycystic kidney disease, 179
Cerebral demyelination syndrome, in hyponatremia correction, 101–102
Cerebral edema
  in hemodialysis, 233–234
  in hyponatremia, 100–101
Charcoal hemoperfusion, in drug overdose, 238
Chlorambucil, in minimal change disease, 38
Chloride loss, metabolic alkalosis in, 132–133, 133t
Chlorthalidone, in hypertension, 213t
Cholesterol, excessive (*see* Hypercholesterolemia)
Chronic renal failure, 83–93
  vs. acute renal failure, 77, 77t
  causes, 87t
  clinical features, 85–86
  definition, 83
  etiology, 83
  evaluation, 86, 87t
  fluid and electrolyte changes in, 84–85, 85t
  in HIV infection, 184–185
  hormonal changes in, 85, 85t
  hypertension in, treatment, 212
  incidence, 83
  monitoring in, 86–87
  nutrition in (*see* Nutrition, in renal failure)
  pathophysiology, 83–84
  in pregnancy, 88
  reversible factors in, 86, 87t
  treatment, 87–92
    acid-base balance in, 90
    anemia, 92
    calcium balance in, 90–91
    diuretics in, 89–90
    drugs in, 88
    electrolyte abnormalities, 88–91
    gastrointestinal symptoms, 92
    goals, 88t
    hemodialysis in, 228
    hypertension control in, 91
    phosphorus balance in, 90–91
    potassium balance in, 90
    protein restriction in, 91
    pruritus, 91
    reversible factors, 87–88
    sodium balance in, 88–89
    uremic symptoms, 91–92
    water balance in, 89
  uremia in, 84–85
  waste product retention in, 85
Chvostek's sign, in hypocalcemia, 146
Cirrhosis, acute tubular necrosis in, 76
Cisplatin, acute tubular necrosis from, 74
Citrate, urinary, renal stone disease and, 155t, 156, 159
Clearance
  creatinine (*see* Creatinine clearance)
  drug
    in hemodialysis, 281, 282t–289t
    in peritoneal dialysis, 281, 282t–289t
    in renal failure, 278f, 280
  inulin, in peritoneal dialysis, 242, 243t
Clonidine, in hypertension, 219t, 222t, 224–225, 226t

Clonidine suppression test, in pheochromocytoma, 203
Clots
 formation, in hematuria, 26t
 removal, 29
Coagulation disorders
 in hemodialysis, 234
 in nephrotic syndrome, 32, 35
Cockcroft-Gault formula, in glomerular filtration rate estimation, 17
Colic, renal, in tubulointerstitial nephritis, 174
Collagen-vascular diseases, hematuria in, 27
Collecting duct
 anatomy, 2, 3f, 9–10, 10f–11f
 potassium excretion in, 109
Color, urine, 13
Complement
 deficiency, in systemic lupus erythematosus, 46
 deposition, in Schönlein-Henoch purpura, 54
 in glomerulonephritis, 43
Computed tomography, 20, 21t
 in hyperaldosteronism, 206
 in hypertension, 196
 in pheochromocytoma, 204
 in polycystic kidney disease, 178
 in renal cystic disease, 181
 in urinary tract infection, 164t
Connecting segment, anatomy, 3f, 8–9
Conn's syndrome, 204–206
Continuous ambulatory peritoneal dialysis, 243, 243t
Continuous arteriovenous hemofiltration, 236–237
 advantages, 238t
 disadvantages, 238t
 replacement solutions for, 236, 237t
Continuous venovenous hemofiltration, 237
Contrast agents, nephrotoxicity, 73–74, 88
Coronary artery disease, in renal transplantation, 265

Corticosteroids
 in Addison's disease, 117
 deficiency, hyponatremia in, 98
 in glomerulonephritis
  membranous, 40
  rapidly progressive, 42
 in Goodpasture's syndrome, 42
 in hyporeninemic hypoaldosteronism, 117
 in immunoglobulin A nephropathy, 44
 in lupus nephritis, 47
 in minimal change disease, 38
 in multiple myeloma, 59
 in polyarteritis nodosa, 52
 in renal graft rejection, 262–263
 in renal transplantation, 256
 in Schönlein-Henoch purpura, 54
 in thrombotic microangiopathy, 55
 in tubulointerstitial nephritis, 172
 in Wegener's granulomatosis, 51
Cramps, muscle, in hemodialysis, 233
Creatinine, increased
 in acute tubular necrosis, 76–77
 in chronic renal failure, 83
 in glomerular filtration assessment, 16–17
Creatinine clearance
 in chronic renal failure, 86
 drug dosage alterations based on, 282t–289t
 in glomerular filtration rate estimation, 17
 vs. hemodialysis initiation, 228
 in nephrotic syndrome, 33
 in peritoneal dialysis, 242, 243t
Crescents, in glomerulonephritis, 42
Cryoglobulinemia, hematuria in, 27

INDEX

Cryoprecipitate, in bleeding, in hemodialysis, 234
Crystallography, in renal stone disease, 154
Crystalluria
 in renal stone disease, 153, 153f
 urine color in, 13
Crystals, deposition, acute tubular necrosis in, 75
Culture, urine, in urinary tract infection, 162
Cyclophosphamide
 in glomerulonephritis, rapidly progressive, 42
 in Goodpasture's syndrome, 42
 in lupus nephritis, 47
 in minimal change disease, 38
 in polyarteritis nodosa, 52
 in Schönlein-Henoch purpura, 54
 in Wegener's granulomatosis, 51
Cyclosporine
 drug interactions with, 257, 258t
 in renal transplantation, 256–257, 258t, 261
 in thrombotic microangiopathy, 56
Cystine stones, 153f, 157, 160
Cystitis
 clinical features, 165
 pathophysiology, 162
 treatment, 165
Cytomegalovirus infection
 in renal transplantation, from immunosuppressive therapy, 264
 in transfusion, 235

1-Deamino-8-arginine vasopressin
 in bleeding, in hemodialysis, 234
 in hypernatremia, 106
Demeclocycline, in hyponatremia, 102
Dense-deposit disease, 43

Desmopressin, in bleeding, in hemodialysis, 234
Dextran 70, in thrombotic microangiopathy, 55–56
Dextrose (*see* Glucose)
Diabetes insipidus
 in amyloidosis, 60
 clinical presentation, 105–106
 diagnosis, 105–106, 105t
 pathogenesis, 104
 treatment, 106
Diabetes mellitus
 β-blockers in, 216
 drug absorption in, 278
 incidence, 62
 ketoacidosis in, 124
  hypokalemia and, 113
 retinopathy in, 66
Diabetic nephropathy, 62–68
 clinical presentation, 62–64
 dialysis in, 68
 differential diagnosis, 66
 end-stage renal failure in, 64
 evaluation, 66
 hyperfiltration in, 63
 hyperglycemia in, 67
 hypertension in, 66–67
 hypertrophy in, 63
 incidence, 62
 incipient, 63
 overt, 63–64
 pathogenesis, 65
 pathology, 64, 65t
 pathophysiology, 62–64
 renal insufficiency in, 67
 renal tubular acidosis in, 130
 silent, 63
 stages, 62–64
 transplantation in, 68
 treatment, 66–68
 urinary tract infection in, 67
Dialysate
 for hemodialysis, 231
 for peritoneal dialysis, 245–246, 246t
Dialysis (*see also* Hemodialysis; Peritoneal dialysis)
 in acute tubular necrosis, 81, 81t
 in AIDS-related complex, 185

Dialysis — *continued*
  in amyloidosis, 60
  in diabetic nephropathy, 68
  in glomerulonephritis, 40
  in HIV infection, 184–187, 187t
  in hyperkalemia, 118–119
  in multiple myeloma, 59
  in progressive systemic sclerosis, 58
  renal cystic disease in, 181
  in tubulointerstitial nephritis, 172
  urinary tract infection in, 167
Dialysis disequilibrium syndrome, in hemodialysis, 233–234
Dialyzers, 231–232
Diet (*see* Nutrition)
1,25-Dihydroxyvitamin D_3
  in calcium homeostasis, 139
  in chronic renal failure, 91
Diltiazem, in hypertension, 220t
Diphenhydramine, in pruritus, 91
Dipstick tests, urine (*see under* Urine)
Disseminated intravascular coagulation, in pregnancy, acute tubular necrosis in, 75–76
Distribution, drug, in renal failure, 278f, 279–280
Diuresis, osmotic, hyponatremia in, 99
Diuretics
  advantages, 213
  in amyloidosis, 60
  in chronic renal failure, 89–90
  combinations of, 214
  disadvantages, 214
  hypercalcemia from, 142
  in hypercalciuria, 159
  in hyperkalemia, 119
  in hyperkalemic renal tubular acidosis, 117
  in hypernatremia, 106
  hypernatremia from, 103
  in hypertension, 213–214, 213t
  in hypokalemia, 114
  hypokalemia from, 111, 113

  in hyponatremia, 101
  hyponatremia from, 98
  in nephrotic syndrome, 34–35
  pharmacokinetics, 287t
  in renal tubular acidosis, 130
  tubulointerstitial nephritis from, 171t
Doxazosin, in hypertension, 218t
Doxorubicin, in multiple myeloma, 59
Drugs
  antidiuretic hormone release/action and, 100
  diabetes insipidus from, 104
  dosage alterations
    in hemodialysis, 239
    in peritoneal dialysis, 252
  hyperkalemia from, 116, 116t
  hypertension from, 207
  interactions, in renal failure, 278–279
  nephrotoxicity, in HIV infection, 184
  overdose, hemodialysis in, 238, 238t
  pharmacokinetics, in renal failure, 277–290, 282t–289t
    absorption, 277–279, 278f
    clearance, 278f, 280
    distribution, 278f, 279–280
    dosage alterations in, 282t–289t
    in hemodialysis, 281, 282t–289t
    in peritoneal dialysis, 281, 282t–289t
    protein binding, 277, 278f, 279–280, 282t–289t
  tubulointerstitial nephritis from (*see* Tubulointerstitial nephritis)
Dyspnea, in nephrotic syndrome, 32–33
Dysuria, in cystitis, 165

Echocardiography, in hypertension, 196
Eclampsia
  acute tubular necrosis in, 75–76

treatment, 222t, 225
Edema
  cerebral
    in hemodialysis, 233–234
    in hyponatremia, 100–101
  in glomerulonephritis
    membranoproliferative, 43
    postinfectious proliferative, 40
  in hyperkalemic renal tubular acidosis, 117
  in hyponatremia, 96
  hyponatremia in, 100
  in minimal change disease, 38
  in nephrotic syndrome, 32, 34
  in renal tubular acidosis, 130
  treatment, 34–35
Effective osmoles, 95
Electrocardiography, in hyperkalemia, 114, 115t
Electrolyte abnormalities, in chronic renal failure, 84–85
Electrophoresis, in proteinuria, in glomerulonephritis, 37
Embolism
  amniotic fluid, acute tubular necrosis in, 75–76
  renal artery, hematuria in, 28
Enalapril, in hypertension, 217t
Enalaprilot, in hypertension, 226t
Encephalopathy, hypertensive, treatment, 222t, 223
Endocarditis
  glomerulonephritis after, 40
  hematuria in, 27
Endothelium, glomerular, 4, 5f
  damage, in thrombotic microangiopathy, 55
End-stage renal failure
  in diabetic nephropathy, 64
  in drug-induced tubulointerstitial nephritis, 173
  in HIV infection, 184–185
  hypercalcemia in, 141
  hypertension in, 198
  in medullary cystic kidney disease, 181
  peritoneal dialysis in, 243
  progression to, 83
  in systemic lupus erythematosus, 47, 49t
Eosinophilia and eosinophiluria, in tubulointerstitial nephritis, 169–171
Epithelial cells, tubular, in urinary sediment, 15–16, 16t
Epithelium, glomerular, 4, 5f, 6
Erythrocytes, in urine, 15, 25 (see also Hematuria)
  in casts, 16t, 50
Erythropoietin, in anemia
  in chronic renal failure, 92
  in hemodialysis, 236
  in peritoneal dialysis, 252
Escherichia coli, in urinary tract infection, 161
Estrogens, in bleeding, in hemodialysis, 234
Ethacrynic acid, in hypertension, 213t
Ethylene glycol, acute tubular necrosis from, 74
Etidronate, in hypercalcemia, 144
Euvolemic hyponatremia, 97f, 99–100, 102
Extracellular fluid, distribution, 94
Extracorporeal shock-wave lithotripsy, in renal stone disease, 158

Fanconi's syndrome
  hematuria in, 28
  in tubulointerstitial nephritis, 170
Femoral vein, for hemodialysis access, 229
Fenoprofen, tubulointerstitial nephritis from, 170
Fetal death, acute tubular necrosis in, 75–76
Fibrillary glomerulonephritis, 44–45
Fistula, arteriovenous, in hemodialysis, 230
Fludrocortisone
  in hyperkalemia, 119
  in renal tubular acidosis, 130

Fluid(s)
    removal, in peritoneal dialysis, 242–243
    restriction
        in acute tubular necrosis, 80
        in glomerulonephritis, 41
        in hemodialysis, 239
Fluid deprivation test, in hypernatremia, 105, 105t
Fluid therapy
    in acute renal failure, 71–72
    in hypernatremia, 106
    in renal graft rejection, 261
    in rhabdomyolysis, 75
Focal segmental glomerulonephritis, 39
Folic acid requirements, in renal failure, 271
Foot processes, epithelial cell, 4, 5f
Fosinopril, in hypertension, 217t
Fractional excretion
    bicarbonate, 129
    sodium, in acute renal failure, 70
Free water deficit, calculation, 106
Furosemide
    in acute tubular necrosis, 80
    in chronic renal failure, 89–90
    in hypercalcemia, 142, 144
    in hypertension, 213t
    in hyponatremia, 101
    in renal tubular acidosis, 130
    in rhabdomyolysis, 75

Gastrointestinal absorption, drugs, in renal failure, 277–279, 278f
Gastrointestinal symptoms, in chronic renal failure, 92
Genetic counseling, in polycystic kidney disease, 180
Genetic factors, in hypertension, 192
Gentamicin, acute tubular necrosis from, 72–73
Glomerular filtration
    assessment, 16–17
    in drug clearance, 280
Glomerular filtration rate
    autoregulation, 69
    decreased
        in acute renal failure, 69
        in acute tubular necrosis, 72
    estimation, 17
        renography in, 18
    increased
        in diabetic nephropathy, 63–65, 67
        in tubulointerstitial nephritis, 169
Glomerulonephritis, 36–45
    acute, vs. acute renal failure, 78–79
    clinical presentation, 36–37
    fibrillary, 44–45
    focal segmental glomerulosclerosis, 39
    in Goodpasture's syndrome, 42–43
    immunoglobulin A nephropathy, 27, 44
    laboratory evaluation, 37
    membranoproliferative, 43–44
    membranous, 39–40
    in microscopic polyarteritis, 52–53
    minimal change disease, 38
    necrotizing, in Wegener's granulomatosis, 50–51
    pathogenesis, 37
    in polyarteritis nodosa, 52
    postinfectious proliferative, 40–41
    poststreptococcal, hematuria in, 27
    primary, 36
    rapidly progressive, 41–42
    recurrent, in renal graft rejection, 260
    in Schönlein-Henoch purpura, 54
    secondary, 36
    treatment (*see specific type*)
Glomerulopathy

in diabetic nephropathy, 65t
hematuria in, 26–27
proteinuria in, 30–31
Glomerulosclerosis
in diabetic nephropathy, 64
in HIV infection, 184
nodular intercapillary, 64
Glomerulus, anatomy, 2, 4, 5f, 6
Glucose (*see also* Hyperglycemia)
control, in peritoneal dialysis, 246–247
in dialysate, 242
in hemodialysis, 231
in hyperkalemia, 118t
hypokalemia and, 113
as osmole, 95
urine, 14
Glucose tolerance test, in nephrotic syndrome, 34
Goodpasture's syndrome, 42–43
hematuria in, 27
Graft
arteriovenous, in hemodialysis, 230
renal (*see* Transplantation, renal)
Granular waxy casts, in urine, 16t
Granulomatosis, Wegener's (*see* Wegener's granulomatosis)
Granulomatous disease, hypercalcemia in, 140
Guanabenz, in hypertension, 219t
Guanadrel, in hypertension, 220
Guanethidine, in hypertension, 220
Guanfacine, in hypertension, 219t

Hematuria, 25–29
benign essential, 27
clinical features, 26t
in cystitis, 165
definition, 25
detection, 25
differential diagnosis, 27–28
evaluation, 26–27
glomerular causes, 26–27
in glomerulonephritis, 36
membranoproliferative, 43
postinfectious proliferative, 40
in immunoglobulin A nephropathy, 44
in infection, 26
in medullary sponge kidney, 180–181
microscopic, 25
in minimal change disease, 38
in polyarteritis nodosa, 52
in polycystic kidney disease, 177–178
in progressive systemic sclerosis, 57
renal biopsy in, 22
in renal cystic disease, 28
in renal stone disease, 153
in rhabdomyolysis, 74
in Schönlein-Henoch purpura, 53–54
in systemic lupus erythematosus, 47, 49t
in thrombotic microangiopathy, 55
treatment, 28–29
in tubulointerstitial disease, 28, 170, 174
unknown etiology, 27
vascular causes, 27–28
in Wegener's granulomatosis, 50
Hemoconcentration, in hyponatremia, 96
Hemodialysis, 228–240
in acute tubular necrosis, 75
allergy in, 232
anemia in, 236
anticoagulation in, 231
bacteremia in, 230
bleeding in, 234
cardiac arrhythmias in, 234
clearances, vs. peritoneal dialysis, 243t
complications, 233–236
contraindications to, 229t
definition, 228
in diabetic nephropathy, 68
dialysate composition, 231
dialysis disequilibrium syndrome in, 233–234

Hemodialysis — *continued*
  dialyzers, 231–232
  drug clearance in, 281, 282t–289t
  in drug overdose, 238, 238t
  equipment for, 231–232
  erythropoietin in, 236
  goals, 232–233
  guidelines, 239
  high-flux, 232
  in HIV infection, 184–185, 187
  in hyperkalemia, 119
  hypotension in, 233
  hypoxemia in, 234
  indications for, 228, 229t
  membranes for, 232
  metabolic bone disease in, 235
  muscle cramps in, 233
  nutrition in, 274–275
  pericarditis in, 235–236
  precautions in, 239
  prescription for, 232–233
  principles, 228
  procedure for, 231–232
  renal cystic kidney disease in, 235
  transfusion-related diseases in, 234–235
  ultrafiltration (hemofiltration) in, 236–237, 236t–238t
  vascular access for, 229–231
    acute, 229–230
    assessment, 231
    chronic, 230–231
    complications, 231
    failure, 244
Hemodilution, in hyponatremia, 96
Hemofiltration, 236–237
  advantages, 238t
  disadvantages, 238t
  replacement solutions for, 236, 237t
Hemoglobinuria, 13–14
Hemolytic anemia, in thrombotic microangiopathy, 55
Hemolytic-uremic syndrome, 54–56
  clinical features, 54–55
  management, 55–56
  prognosis for, 55–56
  renal involvement in, 55
Hemorrhage, pulmonary, in Goodpasture's syndrome, 42
Henderson-Hasselbalch equation, 123
Heparin
  in hemodialysis, 231, 234
  in peritoneal dialysis, 246
  reversal, 234
Hepatitis B, in transfusion, 234–235
Hepatitis C, in transfusion, 235
Hepatorenal syndrome, acute tubular necrosis in, 76
Hereditary nephritis, hematuria in, 27
High-flux dialysis, 232
Hippuran
  in hypertension, 196, 201
  in renography, 18
Histocompatibility antigens, antibodies to, in renal allograft rejection, 259
HIV infection (*see* Human immunodeficiency virus infection)
Hollow fiber dialyzers, 231–232
Human immunodeficiency virus infection, 183–188
  dialysis in, 184–187, 187t
  epidemiology, 183
  fluid and electrolyte disorders in, 185
  renal failure in
    acute, 183–184
    chronic, 184–185
  renal transplantation and, 185–186
  in transfusion, 235
  universal precautions in, 186–187, 187t
Hyaline casts, in urine, 16t
Hydralazine, in hypertension, 217t, 222t, 224–225, 226t
Hydrochlorothiazide
  in hypercalciuria, 159
  in hypertension, 213t
  in nephrotic syndrome, 35

Hydronephrosis
  in renal graft rejection, 260
  in renal transplantation, 261
  ultrasonography, 19
3-Hydroxy-3-methylglutaryl-coenzyme A reductase inhibitor, in renal transplantation, 265
Hyperacute rejection, in renal transplantation, 259
Hyperaldosteronism, 204–206
  clinical features, 205
  diagnosis, 205–206
  hypertension in, 192, 199
    treatment, 212–213
  idiopathic, 204
  pathophysiology, 204
  screening tests for, 205
  secondary, 204
  treatment, 206
Hyperalimentation
  in acute tubular necrosis, 80
  phosphorus in, 147–148
Hypercalcemia, 139–144
  clinical features, 140t, 142
  definition, 139
  diagnosis, 142, 143f
  differential diagnosis, 142, 143f
  etiology, 140–142
  pathogenesis, 140–142
  pathophysiology, 139
  treatment, 142, 144
Hypercalciuria
  etiology, 155
  renal stone disease in, 155, 155t–156t, 158–159
Hypercholesterolemia
  beta-blockers and, 216
  in nephrotic syndrome, treatment, 35
  in renal failure, dietary guidelines in, 269–270
  in renal transplantation, 265
Hypercoagulability, in nephrotic syndrome, 32, 35
Hyperfiltration, glomerular, in diabetic nephropathy, 63, 65
Hyperglycemia, control, in diabetic nephropathy, 65, 67
Hyperkalemia, 114–119
  in acute tubular necrosis, treatment, 80
  asymptomatic, 114
  chronic, treatment, 119
  in chronic renal failure, 84, 90
  definition, 108
  diagnosis, 114, 116–117, 116t, 118t
  drug-induced, 116, 116t
  electrocardiography in, 114, 115t
  etiology, 115t
  evaluation in, 114, 115t
  in HIV infection, 185
  in hypokalemia treatment, 113
  "overshoot," 113
  pathogenesis, 108–109
  vs. pseudohyperkalemia, 116
  in renal tubular acidosis, 129–130
  renal tubular acidosis in, 116–117
  spurious, 114, 115t
  treatment, 90, 117–119, 118t
Hyperkalemic hypertensive syndrome, 117
Hyperlipidemia
  hyponatremia in, 96, 98
  in nephrotic syndrome, 32, 35
  in renal failure, dietary guidelines in, 269–270
Hypermagnesemia, 149–150
  prevention, in hemodialysis, 239
Hypernatremia, 103–106
  in chronic renal failure, 84
  clinical features, 105–106, 105t
  definition, 103
  etiology, 103–105
  incidence, 103
  pathophysiology, 103
  treatment, 106
Hyperosmolar hyponatremia, 97f, 102–103
Hyperoxaluria, renal stone disease in, 153f, 155t, 156, 157t
Hyperparathyroidism
  calcium concentration and, 139

Hyperparathyroidism — *continued*
  in chronic renal failure, 84–85
  in hemodialysis, 235
  hypercalcemia in, 140
  renal stone disease in, 155t
Hyperphosphatemia
  acute, treatment, 149
  in acute tubular necrosis, treatment, 80
  clinical presentation, 148
  definition, 148
  etiology, 148
  hypocalcemia in, 146
  prevention
    in hemodialysis, 239
    in renal failure, 270–271
  treatment, 148–149
Hypersensitivity, to drugs, tubulointerstitial nephritis in (*see* Tubulointerstitial nephritis)
Hypertension
  accelerated, 191
  in aldosteronism, 204–206, 212–213
  with aortic dissection, treatment, 222t, 224
  benign, 190
  blood pressure measurement in, 193
  captopril test in, 200–201
  in catecholamine excess, treatment, 222t
  in chronic renal failure, 83–84, 91, 212
  classification, 190–191
  clinical presentation, 193–194
  definition, 189
  in diabetic nephropathy, 65–67
  diagnosis, 194, 196
  dietary causes, 192
  drug-induced, 207
  essential, 191
    clinical presentation, 193–194
    etiology, 191–193
  etiology, 191–193, 199t
  genetic factors in, 192
  in glomerulonephritis
    fibrillary, 44
    postinfectious proliferative, 40
  in hyperkalemic renal tubular acidosis, 117
  hypokalemia in, 111, 113
  incidence, 189–190
  isolated systolic, 189
  laboratory tests for, 194, 196
  malignant, 191, 222t, 223–224
  in minimal change disease, 38
  in myocardial infarction, treatment, 222t, 224
  nutrition in, 221
  in pheochromocytoma, 202–204, 212
  in polyarteritis nodosa, 51
  in polycystic kidney disease, 177, 179–180
  in pregnancy, treatment, 222t, 225
  prevalence, secondary, 198, 199t
  in progressive systemic sclerosis, 57
  renal function and, 192
  in renal parenchymal disease, 198
  in renal transplantation, 265
  in renal tubular acidosis, 130
  renin-angiotensin-aldosterone axis dysfunction in, 192
  renovascular (*see* Renovascular hypertension)
  retinopathy in, 193, 195t
  risk factors for, 190
  in Schönlein-Henoch purpura, 53
  secondary, 191, 198–208
    in aldosteronism, 204–206, 212–213
    drug-induced, 207
    etiology, 199t, 207t
    in pheochromocytoma, 202–204, 212
    prevalence, 198, 199t
    in renal parenchymal disease, 198

renovascular (*see*
　Renovascular
　hypertension)
treatment, 211–213
severity, 189
in stroke, treatment, 222t, 223
sympathetic nervous system
　and, 192
in systemic lupus
　erythematosus, 47, 49t
systolic, 189
treatment, 209–227
　α_1-receptor antagonists in,
　　218, 218t
　angiotensin-converting
　　enzyme inhibitors in, 216,
　　217t
　with aortic dissection, 222t,
　　224
　β-blockers in, 214–216,
　　215t
　calcium antagonists in, 219–
　　220, 220t
　in catecholamine excess,
　　222t, 224
　central acting agents in,
　　218–219, 219t
　in chronic renal failure, 91,
　　212
　clinical trials, 220–221
　cost considerations in, 211
　in diabetic nephropathy,
　　65–67
　diuretics in, 213–214, 213t
　in encephalopathy, 222t,
　　223
　goals, 209
　in hyperaldosteronism,
　　212–213
　hypertensive crisis, 221–226,
　　222t
　individualized, 210–211
　malignant, 222t, 223–224
　multiple drugs in, 211
　in myocardial infarction,
　　222t, 224
　nonpharmacologic, 209–
　　210, 221
　in pheochromocytoma, 212
　in polycystic kidney disease,
　　179–180
　precautions in, 211
　in pregnancy, 222t, 225
　in renal graft rejection, 263
　in renal parenchymal
　　disease, 198
　renovascular, 211–212
　salt restriction, 209
　secondary, 211–213
　step-care approach, 210,
　　210t
　in stroke, 222t, 223
　vasodilators in, 217–218,
　　217t
in tubulointerstitial nephritis,
　170, 174
Hypertensive crisis, 221–226
　categories, 221
　hypertensive emergency, 221,
　　222t, 223–225
　hypertensive urgency, 222t,
　　225
　treatment, 221, 222t, 223–225,
　　226t
Hypertensive emergency, 221,
　222t, 223–225
Hypertensive encephalopathy,
　treatment, 222t, 223
Hypertensive urgency, treatment,
　222t, 225
Hypertriglyceridemia
　hyponatremia in, 96, 98
　in nephrotic syndrome,
　　treatment, 35
　in renal failure, dietary
　　guidelines in, 269–270
Hypertrophy, kidney, in diabetic
　nephropathy, 63, 65
Hyperuricosuria, renal stone
　disease in, 155t, 156–157
Hyperventilation, respiratory
　alkalosis in, 134
Hyperviscosity syndromes, acute
　renal failure in, 70
Hypervolemia, clinical features,
　96, 97f
Hypervolemic hyponatremia
　clinical presentation, 97f, 100–
　　101

Hypervolemic hyponatremia — *continued*
  treatment, 102
Hypoalbuminemia
  drug distribution in, 279–280
  in nephrotic syndrome, 32, 34
  treatment, 34
Hypoaldosteronism, hyporeninemic, potassium secretion in, 117
Hypocalcemia, 144–146
  in chronic renal failure, 84–85
  clinical presentation, 145
  definition, 144
  differential diagnosis, 145
  etiology, 144–145
  in hypomagnesemia, 150
  treatment, 145–146
  true, 146
Hypocitraturia, renal stone disease in, 155t, 156, 159
Hypocomplementemia, hematuria in, 27
Hypokalemia, 109–114
  artifactual, 111
  chronic, treatment, 114
  clinical manifestations, 109, 111t
  definition, 108
  differential diagnosis, 109, 110t
  evaluation in, 109, 110t–111t, 111, 112f
  in HIV infection, 185
  in hyperaldosteronism, 205
  in hypomagnesemia, 150
  pathogenesis, 108–109
  treatment, 113–114
Hypomagnesemia, 150–151
  hypocalcemia in, 145
Hyponatremia
  acute
    clinical features, 100
    treatment, 101–102
  in Addison's disease, 117
  chronic
    clinical features, 101
    treatment, 101–102
  in chronic renal failure, 84, 89
  classification, 96, 97f
  in HIV infection, 185
  hyperosmolar, 97f, 102–103
  hypoosmolar, 97f, 98–102
    euvolemic, 97f, 99–100, 102
    hypervolemic, 97f, 100–102
    hypovolemic, 97f, 98–99, 102
  isoosmolar, 96, 97f, 98
  pathophysiology, 96
  treatment, 101–102
Hypoosmolar hyponatremia
  euvolemic, 97f, 99–100, 102
  hypervolemic, 97f, 100–102
  hypovolemic, 97f, 98–99, 102
Hypoperfusion, renal
  acute tubular necrosis in, 72
  hypertension in, 199
Hypophosphatemia
  clinical presentation, 146, 147t
  definition, 146
  differential diagnosis, 146–147, 147t
  etiology, 147t
  treatment, 147–148
Hyporeninemic hypoaldosteronism, potassium secretion in, 117
Hypotension
  acute renal failure in, 69
  in hemodialysis, 233
Hypothalamus, in water regulation, 95
Hypouricemia, in inappropriate antidiuretic hormone secretion, 99
Hypovolemia, clinical features, 96, 97f
Hypovolemic hyponatremia, 97f, 98–99, 102
Hypoxemia, in hemodialysis, 234

Ibuprofen, tubulointerstitial nephritis from, 170
IgA (*see* Immunoglobulin A)
Immobilization, hypercalcemia in, 141

Immune complexes
  in glomerulonephritis, 43
  in polyarteritis nodosa, 52
  in Schönlein-Henoch purpura, 53
Immunoglobulin A, deposits, in Schönlein-Henoch purpura, 53
Immunoglobulin A nephropathy, 44
  hematuria in, 27
Immunosuppressive therapy
  in renal transplantation, 255–257, 258t
    infection in, 263–265
  in thrombotic microangiopathy, 56
  in Wegener's granulomatosis, 51
Ineffective osmoles, 95
Infection
  glomerulonephritis after, 40–41
  in hemodialysis, 239
  hemolytic-uremic syndrome in, 55
  in peritoneal dialysis, 248
  in polycystic kidney disease, 178–179
  in renal cystic disease, 167
  in renal graft rejection, 260
  in renal stone disease, 153
  in renal transplantation, from immunosuppressive therapy, 263–265
  urinary tract (*see* Urinary tract infection)
Infective endocarditis, hematuria in, 27
Inotropic agents, pharmacokinetics, 288t
Insulin
  in diabetic nephropathy, 67
  in hyperkalemia, 118t
  in peritoneal dialysis, 246–247
  in potassium uptake, 108
Intercalated cells, in collecting duct, 9–10, 11f
Interstitium, anatomy, 10–11
Intracellular fluid, 94

Intravenous pyelography, 19–20, 20t
  in hypertension, 196
  in urinary tract infection, 164t
Inulin clearance, in peritoneal dialysis, 242, 243t
Iron supplementation, in renal failure, 271–272
Isradipine, in hypertension, 220t

Jugular vein, for hemodialysis access, 229
Juxtaglomerular apparatus, anatomy, 6

Kayexalate
  in chronic renal failure, 90
  in hyperkalemia, 118t, 119
Ketoacidosis, diabetic, 124
  hypokalemia and, 113
Ketonuria, hyponatremia in, 99
Kidney
  anatomy, 1–12
    collecting duct, 9–10, 10f–11f
    distal tubule, 8–9, 9f
    glomerulus, 2, 4, 5f, 6
    gross, 1–2, 2f–3f
    Henle's loop, 2f, 7–8
    innervation, 23
    interstitium, 10–11
    juxtaglomerular apparatus, 6
    proximal tubule, 6–7, 7f
    vasculature, 2f, 11
  evaluation
    biopsy in, 22–24
    glomerular filtration in, 16–17
    radiologic, 18–22, 18t–21t
    urinalysis in, 13–16, 16t
  hypertrophy, in diabetic nephropathy, 63, 65
  solitary, in living transplant donor, 255
  transplantation (*see* Transplantation)
K_t/V parameter, in hemodialysis, 233

Labetalol, in hypertension, 215t, 222t, 223–225, 226t
Laxatives, in peritoneal dialysis, 252
Leukocytes, in urine, 14–15
  in casts, 16t
Light chain disease, proteinuria in, 31–32
Lipids
  alterations, in nephrotic syndrome, 32, 35
  dietary, in renal failure, 269–270
Lipoid nephrosis (minimal change disease), 38
Lisinopril, in hypertension, 217t
Lithiasis, renal (see Renal stone disease)
Lithium carbonate, in hyponatremia, 102
Liver
  disease, acute tubular necrosis in, 76
  drug clearance in, 280, 282t–289t
  fatty, in pregnancy, acute tubular necrosis in, 76
Loop of Henle
  anatomy, 2, 3f, 7–8
  function, 8
Lupus nephritis
  clinical features, 47, 48t–49t
  management, 47–49
  prognosis for, 47–49
  World Health Organization classification, 47–49, 48t–49t
Lymphatics, renal, 11
Lymphocele, in renal graft rejection, 260, 262–263

M protein, in amyloidosis, 60
Macula densa, anatomy, 6
Magnesium
  abnormalities, 145, 149–151, 239
    in chronic renal failure, 84
  excretion, 149
    in renal failure, 272
  normal levels, 149
  reabsorption, 149

Magnesium oxide, in hypomagnesemia, 151
Magnesium sulfate
  in hypercalcemia, 144
  in hypomagnesemia, 151
Magnetic resonance imaging, 20, 21t
  in pheochromocytoma, 204
Malignancy
  hypercalcemia in, 140
  in renal transplantation, 265–266
Malignant hypertension, 191
  treatment, 222t, 223–224
Malnutrition, protein-calorie, in renal failure, 267–268
Mannitol, in rhabdomyolysis, 75
Medulla, anatomy, 1, 2f–3f
Medullary cystic kidney disease, 177t, 181
Medullary sponge kidney, 177t, 180–181
Melphalan
  in amyloidosis, 60
  in multiple myeloma, 59
Membranes, for hemodialysis, 232
Membranoproliferative glomerulonephritis, 43–44
Membranous glomerulonephritis, 39–40
Mesangium, glomerular, 4, 5f, 6
Metabolic acidosis (see under Acidosis)
Metabolic alkalosis, 122t
  in hyperaldosteronism, 205
  in mixed acid-base disorders, 135, 136t
Metabolic bone disease
  in chronic renal failure, 84–85
  in hemodialysis, 235
Metabolic disorders, in peritoneal dialysis, 248
Methicillin, tubulointerstitial nephritis from, 170
Methyldopa, in hypertension, 219t, 222t, 225
Methylprednisolone
  in lupus nephritis, 47
  in renal graft rejection, 262–263

in Schönlein-Henoch purpura, 54
in Wegener's granulomatosis, 51
Metolazone
in chronic renal failure, 90
in hypertension, 213t
in nephrotic syndrome, 35
Metoprolol, in hypertension, 215t
Microalbuminuria, 15
in diabetic nephropathy, 63–64
Microangiopathy, thrombotic, 54–56
Microscopic polyarteritis, 52–53
Microscopy, urine
in hematuria detection, 25
in nephrotic syndrome, 33
"Middle molecule" removal, in peritoneal dialysis, 242
Milk-alkali syndrome, hypercalcemia in, 141
Minimal change disease, 38
Minoxidil, in hypertension, 217t, 224–225
Mithramycin, in hypercalcemia, 144
Mononeuritis multiplex, in polyarteritis nodosa, 51
Multiple myeloma
acute tubular necrosis in, 75
clinical features, 58
management, 59
proteinuria in, 31–32
renal involvement in, 58–59
Muscle cramps, in hemodialysis, 233
Myeloma, multiple (see Multiple myeloma)
Myocardial infarction, hypertension in, treatment, 222t, 224
Myoglobinuria, 13

Nadolol, in hypertension, 215t
Naproxen, tubulointerstitial nephritis from, 170
Nausea and vomiting, in chronic renal failure, 92
Necrosis
papillary
drug-induced, 174–175
hematuria in, 28
tubular, acute (see Acute tubular necrosis)
Necrotizing vasculitis (see also specific disease)
renal involvement in, 49–54
Nephrectomy, in living transplant donor, kidney function after, 255
"Nephritic urinary sediment," 36
Nephritis
acute
in Schönlein-Henoch purpura, 53
in systemic lupus erythematosus, 47
in glomerulonephritis, 43
in Goodpasture's syndrome, 42
hereditary, hematuria in, 27
hypersensitivity interstitial, hematuria in, 28
lupus, 47–49, 48t–49t
salt-losing, hyponatremia in, 98
tubulointerstitial (see Tubulointerstitial nephritis)
Nephrogenic diabetes insipidus
clinical presentation, 105–106
diagnosis, 105–106, 105t
pathogenesis, 104
treatment, 106
Nephrolithiasis (see Renal stone disease)
Nephrons, anatomy, 1–2, 3f
Nephropathy
analgesic, 173–175
diabetic (see Diabetic nephropathy)
HIV-associated, 184–185
immunoglobulin A, 27, 44
Nephrosis, lipoid (minimal change disease), 38
Nephrostomy tube, in renal graft rejection, 261–262
Nephrotic syndrome, 30–35
in amyloidosis, 60
ascites in, 34–35
blood chemistries in, 33

Nephrotic syndrome — *continued*
cardinal features, 30, 30t
causes, 30, 31t
childhood, 38
clinical presentation, 32–33
definition, 30
in diabetes mellitus, vs.
 diabetic nephropathy, 66
edema in, 34–35
in glomerulonephritis, 36
 focal segmental, 39
 membranous, 39–40
glucose tolerance test in, 34
hypercoagulability in, 32, 35
hypoalbuminemia in, 32, 34
idiopathic, 30
in immunoglobulin A
 nephropathy, 44
investigations, 33
lipid alterations in, 32, 35
in minimal change disease, 38
nutrition in, 273–274
pathophysiology, 30–32
renal biopsy in, 22
from rifampin, 173
in Schönlein-Henoch purpura, 54
serologic tests in, 33–34
special studies, 33–34
Starling forces in, 32
in systemic lupus
 erythematosus, 47, 49t
treatment, 34–35
twenty-four-hour urine
 collection in, 33
ultrasonography in, 33
urinalysis in, 33
Nephrotoxicity
acute tubular necrosis in, 72–74, 73t
contrast agents, 73–74, 88
drugs, in HIV infection, 184
in immunosuppressive therapy, 257
in renal graft rejection, 260
Neurologic disorders, in
 peritoneal dialysis, 248
Nifedipine, in hypertension, 220t, 222t, 224–225, 226t
Nil (minimal change) disease, 38
Nimodipine, in hypertension, 223

Nitrites, urine, 14
Nitrogen, retention, in chronic
 renal failure, 85
Nitroglycerin, in hypertension, 222t, 224, 226t
Nitroprusside, in hypertension, 222t, 223–224, 226t
Nocturia, in tubulointerstitial
 nephritis, 174
Nodular intercapillary
 glomerulosclerosis, in diabetic
 nephropathy, 64
Nonsteroidal antiinflammatory
 drugs
in nephrotic syndrome, 34
tubulointerstitial nephritis
 from, 170, 172–173
Nonurea nitrogen excretion, 269
Nutrition
in acute tubular necrosis, 80, 81
in hemodialysis, 274–275
in hypercystinuria, 160
in hypertension, 192, 221
in hyperuricosuria, 160
in nephrotic syndrome, 34, 273–274
in peritoneal dialysis, 252, 275–276
in renal failure, 267–276
 acute, without dialysis, 272
 caloric requirements in, 268
 carbohydrates in, 270
 lipids in, 269–270
 micronutrients in, 270–272
 predialysis, 273
 protein in, 268–269
 protein-calorie malnutrition
  and, 267–268
in renal stone disease,
 hypercalciuric, 158
in renal transplantation, 276

Obstructive uropathy
vs. acute renal failure, 78, 78t
clinical features, 78t
infection in, imaging in, 164t
in renal graft rejection, 260–262
in renal stone disease, 153
renal tubular acidosis in, 130

OKT3 monoclonal antibody, in renal graft rejection, 263
Oliguria
  in acute tubular necrosis, 76
  in obstructive uropathy, 78
Opportunistic infections, in renal transplantation, from immunosuppressive therapy, 264
Orthoiodohippurate, radioiodinated, in renography, 18
Osmolality
  body fluids, 94–95
  urine, 95
Osmolar gap, 95
Osmostat, reset, hyponatremia in, 99
Osmotic diuresis, hyponatremia in, 99
Osteodystrophy, renal, 84–85
Osteomyelitis, glomerulonephritis after, 40
Oxalate stones, 153f, 155t, 156, 157t

Pain
  in cystitis, 165
  in hematuria, 26t
  in peritoneal dialysis, 247
  in polycystic kidney disease, 177–178
  in renal stone disease, 153, 157–158
Pancreatitis, hypocalcemia in, 146
Papillary necrosis
  drug-induced, 174–175
  hematuria in, 28
Parallel plate dialyzers, 232
Paraproteins, in urine, 31–32
Parathyroid hormone
  in calcium homeostasis, 139
  deficiency, hypocalcemia in, 145–146
  excessive (*see* Hyperparathyroidism)
Parathyroid intact hormone assay, in hypercalcemia, 142, 143f
Parietal epithelium, 6
Pediatric patients
  hemolytic-uremic syndrome in, 54–56
  minimal change disease in, 38
  renal tubular acidosis in, 127, 129
D-Penicillamine, in hypercystinuria, 160
Pericarditis, in hemodialysis, 235–236
Perinephric abscess, 164t, 166
Peripheral vascular disease, beta-blockers in, 216
Peritoneal dialysis, 241–253
  in acute tubular necrosis, 81
  additives in, 246–247
  advantages, 244t
  antibiotics in, 247, 251t
  catheters for, 245
  changing method, 250
  complications, 247–250, 249t, 251t
  continuous ambulatory, 243, 243t
    in diabetic nephropathy, 68
  contraindications, 244–245
  creatinine removal in, 242, 243t
  dialysate sampling in, 250
  dialysate solution for, 245–246, 246t
  disadvantages, 244t
  drainage problems in, 252
  drug clearance in, 281, 282t–289t
  drug dosage alterations in, 252
  effluent in, 246
  erythropoietin in, 252
  fluid removal in, 242–243
  fluid volume changes in, management, 250
  heparin in, 246
  historical aspects, 241
  in HIV infection, 185–186
  in hospitalized patients, 250, 252
  in hyperkalemia, 119
  incidence, 241
  indications for, 243–244, 244t
  insulin in, 246–247
  interruption, 250
  inulin clearance in, 243t

Peritoneal dialysis — *continued*
  laxatives with, 252
  manual technique for, 243, 243t
  "middle molecule" removal in, 242
  nutrition in, 252, 275–276
  ordering supplies for, 250
  peritonitis in, 248–250, 249t, 251t
  phosphate binders in, 252
  physician orders in, 252
  potassium in, 247
  technical aspects, 245–247, 246t
  technique for, 241–243
  types, 243–245, 243t–244t
  urea removal in, 241–242
Peritonitis
  drug absorption in, 278
  in peritoneal dialysis, 248–250
    clinical features, 248
    etiology, 248–249
    treatment, 249–250, 249t, 251t
pH
  blood
    calcium concentration and, 138
    normal, 123
  definition, 121
  urine, 14
Phenacetin, tubulointerstitial nephritis from, 173–175
Phenazone, tubulointerstitial nephritis from, 174
Phentolamine, in hypertension, 222t, 224, 226t
Pheochromocytoma, 202–204
  clinical features, 202–203
  diagnostic tests, 203
  hypertension in, treatment, 212
  localization, 204
  pathophysiology, 202
  screening test, 203
  treatment, 204
Phosphate binders
  in hemodialysis, 239
  in hyperphosphatemia, 148–149
  in peritoneal dialysis, 252
  in renal failure, 271
Phosphorus and phosphate abnormalities (*see also* Hyperphosphatemia)
    in chronic renal failure, 84
    hypophosphatemia, 146–148, 147t
  balance, in chronic renal failure, 90–91
  calcium concentration and, 139
  monitoring, in acute tubular necrosis, 80
  normal levels, 146
  reabsorption, 146
  restriction
    in chronic renal failure, 90
    in renal failure, 270–271
Pindolol, in hypertension, 215t
Plasmapheresis
  in glomerulonephritis, 42
  in multiple myeloma, 59
  in Schönlein-Henoch purpura, 54
  in thrombotic microangiopathy, 56
  in Wegener's granulomatosis, 51
Pneumocystis carinii pneumonia, in renal transplantation, from immunosuppressive therapy, 264
Podocytes, 4, 5f
Poisoning, hemodialysis in, 238
Polyarteritis, microscopic, 52–53
Polyarteritis nodosa, 51–52
Polycitra, in metabolic acidosis, 128
Polycystic kidney disease
  clinical features, 177–178, 177t
  diagnostic criteria for, 178, 178t
  genetic counseling in, 180
  hematuria in, 28
  in hemodialysis, 235
  prognosis for, 180

treatment, 178–180
Polydipsia
  in diabetes insipidus, 105–106
  psychogenic, hyponatremia in, 99
Polyneuropathy, in polyarteritis nodosa, 51
Polyuria
  in diabetes insipidus, 105–106
  hypotonic, 103
Porphyria, urine color in, 13
Postinfectious proliferative glomerulonephritis, 40–41
Postrenal disease, in renal graft rejection, 260–261
Poststreptococcal glomerulonephritis, hematuria in, 27
Postural stimulation test, in hyperaldosteronism, 206
Potassium
  abnormalities (*see* Hyperkalemia; Hypokalemia)
  balance, in chronic renal failure, 90
  excretion, 108–109
    reduced, 116–117
  intracellular, 94
  loss
    in hypomagnesemia, 150
    metabolic alkalosis in, 131
  monitoring, in acute tubular necrosis, 80
  in peritoneal dialysis, 247
  physiology, 108–109
  reabsorption, 109
  regulation, 109
  replacement with, in hypokalemia, 113–114
  restriction
    in chronic renal failure, 90
    in hyperkalemia, 119
    in renal failure, 270
  secretion, 109
  uptake, 108
Potassium citrate
  in hyperuricosuria, 159
  in metabolic acidosis, 128

Prazosin, in hypertension, 67, 218t, 222t
Prednisone
  in amyloidosis, 60
  in glomerulonephritis, 39
  in minimal change disease, 38
  in renal graft rejection, 263
  in renal transplantation, 256
  in Wegener's granulomatosis, 51
Preeclampsia, treatment, 222t, 225
Pregnancy
  acute tubular necrosis in, 75–76
  chronic renal failure in, 88
  hypertension in, treatment, 222t, 225
  hyponatremia in, 99
  urinary tract infection in, 162
Prerenal acute renal failure, 69–72
  clinical features, 70–71
  definition, 69
  etiology, 70
  pathophysiology, 69
  in renal transplantation, 258
  treatment, 71–72
Principle cells, in collecting duct, 9, 10f
Progressive systemic sclerosis
  clinical features, 56
  management, 57–58
  prognosis for, 57–58
  renal involvement in, 57
Propranolol, in hypertension, 215t
Prostacyclins, in thrombotic microangiopathy, 56
Prostatitis, 166–167
Protamine sulfate, in heparin reversal, 234
Protein
  biologic value, 268
  reabsorption, 31
  requirements, in renal failure, 268–269
  restriction
    in acute tubular necrosis, 80

Protein — *continued*
  restriction — *continued*
    in chronic renal failure, 91
    in glomerulonephritis, postinfectious, 41
    in renal graft rejection, 263
  requirements, 268–269
Protein binding, drugs, in renal failure, 277, 278f, 279–280, 282t–289t
Protein catabolic rate, in hemodialysis, 233
Protein-calorie malnutrition, in renal failure, 267–268
Proteinuria, 30–35
  in amyloidosis, 59–60
  ascites in, 34–35
  blood chemistries in, 33
  causes, 30, 31t
  clinical presentation, 32–33
  definition, 30
  in diabetic nephropathy, 63–64, 66
  edema in, 34–35
  in glomerulonephritis, 36
    electrophoresis in, 37
    fibrillary, 44
    focal segmental, 39
    membranoproliferative, 43
    membranous, 39
    postinfectious proliferative, 40
  glucose tolerance test in, 34
  in hematuria, 26t
  in HIV infection, 184
  hypercoagulability in, 32, 35
  hypoalbuminemia in, 32, 34
  idiopathic, 30
  in immunoglobulin A nephropathy, 44
  investigations, 33
  lipid alterations in, 32, 35
  in multiple myeloma, 58
  vs. normal protein values, 30
  pathophysiology, 30–32
  in polycystic kidney disease, 178
  renal biopsy in, 22
  in Schönlein-Henoch purpura, 53
  serologic tests in, 33–34
  special studies, 33–34
  Starling forces in, 32
  in systemic lupus erythematosus, 47, 49t
  testing for, 14
  in thrombotic microangiopathy, 55
  treatment, 34–35
  tubular, 31
  in tubulointerstitial nephritis, 169–170, 174
  twenty-four-hour urine collection in, 33
  ultrasonography in, 33
  urinalysis in, 33
  in Wegener's granulomatosis, 50
Pruritus, in chronic renal failure, 91
Pseudohyperaldosteronism, 204
Pseudohyperkalemia, 116
Pseudohyponatremia (isoosmolar hyponatremia), 96, 97f, 98
Psychogenic polydipsia, hyponatremia in, 99
Pulmonary hemorrhage, in Goodpasture's syndrome, 42
Purpura
  Schönlein-Henoch (*see* Schönlein-Henoch purpura)
  thrombotic thrombocytopenic, 54–56
Pyelography, intravenous, 19–20, 20t
  in hypertension, 196
  in urinary tract infection, 164t
Pyelonephritis
  acute, 162
    imaging in, 164t
  bacterial, hematuria in, 28
  chronic, 162
    imaging in, 164t
  clinical features, 165
  in diabetes mellitus, 67
  pathophysiology, 162

in renal transplantation, from
  immunosuppressive therapy,
  264–265
 treatment, 165–166
 in tubulointerstitial nephritis,
  174
Pyuria
 in glomerulonephritis, 36
 with hematuria, 26
 urine color in, 13

Quinapril, in hypertension, 217t

Radial artery, for hemodialysis
  access, 230
Radiology, 28–33 (*see also specific
  technique*)
 arteriography, 21
 computed tomography, 20, 21t
 contrast agents for, acute
  tubular necrosis from, 73–74
 intravenous pyelography, 19–
  20, 20t
 magnetic resonance imaging,
  20, 21t
 in renal stone disease, 153–
  154
 renography, 18, 18t
 ultrasonography, 18–19, 19t
 venography, 21
Radionuclide scan
 in hypertension, 196
 in tubulointerstitial nephritis,
  172
Ramipril, in hypertension, 217t
Rapidly progressive
  glomerulonephritis, 41–42
Rash, in Schönlein-Henoch
  purpura, 53
Raynaud's phenomenon,
  β-blockers in, 216
Rejection, in transplantation (*see
  under* Transplantation)
Renal artery
 anatomy, 2f, 11
 angioplasty, in hypertension,
  202
 embolism, hematuria in, 28

revascularization, in
  hypertension, 202
 stenosis (*see also* Renovascular
  disease; Renovascular
  hypertension)
  arteriography in, 196
  in graft, 261
  hypertension in, 199
  in renal transplantation,
   263
 thrombosis, in graft, 261
Renal cystic disease (*see also*
  Polycystic kidney disease)
 acquired, 181
 clinical features, 177t
 complex, 19
 computed tomography, 176
 etiology, 176
 infection in, 167
 medullary, 177t, 181
 medullary sponge kidney,
  177t, 180–181
 simple, 18
 treatment, 181
 types, 176, 177t
 ultrasonography, 18–19, 176
Renal failure
 acute (*see* Acute renal failure)
 chronic (*see* Chronic renal
  failure)
 end-stage (*see* End-stage renal
  failure)
 pharmacokinetics in, 277–290,
  282t–289t
  absorption, 277–279, 278f
  clearance, 278f, 280
  distribution, 278f, 279–280
  dosage alterations in, 282t–
   289t
  in hemodialysis, 281, 282t–
   289t
  in peritoneal dialysis, 281,
   282t–289t
  protein binding, 277, 278f,
   279–280, 282t–289t
 in polyarteritis nodosa, 52
 rapidly progressive, in systemic
  lupus erythematosus, 47, 49t

Renal insufficiency
  in amyloidosis, 60
  in diabetes mellitus, vs. diabetic nephropathy, 66
  in diabetic nephropathy, 66–67
  in hyperkalemic renal tubular acidosis, 117, 129–130
  in polycystic kidney disease, 179–180
  in tubulointerstitial nephritis, 170
Renal osteodystrophy, 84–85
Renal stone disease, 152–160
  asymptomatic, 153
  brushite stones in, 153f
  clinical presentation, 152–153
  cystine stones in, 153f, 157, 160
  diagnosis, 153–154, 153f
  etiology, 154–157, 154t–157t
  in hypercalciuria, 155, 155t–156t, 158–159
  in hyperoxaluria, 153f, 155t, 156, 157t
  in hyperuricosuria, 155t, 156
  in hypocitraturia, 155t, 156, 159
  incidence, 152
  in medullary sponge kidney, 180–181
  pathophysiology, 152
  in polycystic kidney disease, 179
  spontaneous stone passage in, 158
  struvite stones in, 153f, 155t, 156–157, 159
  treatment
    acute, 157–158
    chronic, 158–160
    follow-up in, 160
  uric acid stones in, 153f, 157, 159–160
Renal transplantation (*see* Transplantation)
Renal tubular acidosis, 125–130
  in amyloidosis, 60
  causes, 125, 127
  differential diagnosis, 126t–127t
  in hyperkalemia, 116–117
  in medullary sponge kidney, 180–181
  treatment, 181
  in tubulointerstitial nephritis, 170, 174
  type I (classic distal), 127–128
  type II (proximal), 128–129
  type III, 127
  type IV (hyperkalemic), 129–130
Renal vein
  anatomy, 2f, 11
  thrombosis
    in graft, 261
    hematuria in, 27–28
    in nephrotic syndrome, 35
Renin-angiotensin-aldosterone axis, hypertension and, 192, 199
Renography, 18, 18t
  in hypertension, 201
Renomedullary cells, 10–11
Renovascular disease, acute
  vs. acute renal failure, 78, 79t
  clinical features, 79t
  etiology, 79t
Renovascular hypertension, 199–202
  clinical features, 200
  definition, 199
  diagnosis, 201–202
  pathophysiology, 199–200
  screening tests for, 200–201
  treatment, 202, 211–212
Reserpine, in hypertension, 220
Respiratory acidosis, 121, 122t, 130–131, 131t
  in mixed acid-base disorders, 135, 136t
Respiratory alkalosis, 121, 122t, 134, 134t
  hypocalcemia in, 145
  in mixed acid-base disorders, 135, 136t

Respiratory system
  peritoneal dialysis effects on, 248
  Wegener's granulomatosis manifestations in, 50
Retinopathy
  diabetic, 66
  hypertensive, 193, 195t
Revascularization, in hypertension, 202
Rhabdomyolysis, acute tubular necrosis in, 74–75
Rifampin, nephrotoxicity, 173

Salicylamide, tubulointerstitial nephritis from, 174
Saline solution
  in acute renal failure, 71–72
  excessive use, hypernatremia from, 104–105
  in hypercalcemia, 142, 144
  in hypernatremia, 106
  in hyperphosphatemia, 149
  in hyponatremia, 101–102
  in metabolic alkalosis, 133
Saline suppression test, in hyperaldosteronism, 205–206
Salt (*see also* Saline solution)
  restriction
    in amyloidosis, 60
    in hypertension, 209
    in nephrotic syndrome, 34
Salt wasting, hyponatremia in, 98
Schönlein-Henoch purpura
  clinical features, 53
  hematuria in, 27
  management, 54
  prognosis for, 54
  renal involvement in, 53–54
Scleroderma
  clinical features, 56
  management, 57–58
  prognosis for, 57–58
  renal involvement in, 57
Scleroderma renal crisis, 57
Sediment, urinary (*see* Urine, sediment)

Septicemia, in renal transplantation, from immunosuppressive therapy, 264–265
Serologic tests, in nephrotic syndrome, 33–34
Shohl's solution, in metabolic acidosis, 128
SLE (*see* Systemic lupus erythematosus)
Slit pores, glomerular, 4, 5f
Sodium (*see also* Saline solution; Salt)
  abnormalities (*see* Hypernatremia; Hyponatremia)
  balance, in chronic renal failure, 88–89
  deficit, calculation, 102
  dietary, in renal failure, 270
  in extracellular fluid, 94–95
  loss, 98–99
  monitoring, in acute tubular necrosis, 80
  in potassium regulation, 109
  restriction, in glomerulonephritis, 41
Sodium bicarbonate
  in chronic renal failure, 90
  in hyperkalemia, 118–119, 118t
  in hyperuricosuria, 159
  in rhabdomyolysis, 75
Sodium phosphate, neutral, in hypercalciuria, 159
Sodium polystyrene sulfonate
  in chronic renal failure, 90
  in hyperkalemia, 118t, 119
Specific gravity, urine, 14
Spironolactone
  in hyperaldosteronism, 206
  in hypertension, 212–213, 213t
  in metabolic alkalosis, 133
Splenectomy, in thrombotic microangiopathy, 56
Starling forces, in nephrotic syndrome, 32

Stones, renal (*see* Renal stone disease)
Streptococcal infections, glomerulonephritis after, 27, 40–41
Stroke, hypertension in, treatment, 222t, 223
Struvite stones, 153f, 155t, 156–157, 159
Subclavian vein, for hemodialysis access, 229
Sympathetic nervous system, hypertension and, 192
Syndrome of inappropriate antidiuretic hormone secretion, 99
Systemic disease (*see also specific disease*)
  renal involvement in, 46–61
    amyloidosis, 59–60
    microscopic polyarteritis, 52–53
    multiple myeloma, 58–59
    polyarteritis nodosa, 51–52
    progressive systemic sclerosis, 56–58
    Schönlein-Henoch purpura, 53–54
    systemic lupus erythematosus, 46–49, 48t–49t
    thrombotic microangiopathy, 54–56
    vasculitis, 49–54
    Wegener's granulomatosis, 50–51
Systemic lupus erythematosus
  clinical features, 46
  hematuria in, 27
  management, 47–49
  prognosis for, 47–49
  renal involvement in, 47, 48t–49t

Tamm-Horsfall protein, in multiple myeloma, 58
Tamponade, pericardial, in hemodialysis, 235–236
Taste disorders, in chronic renal failure, 92
Technetium compounds
  in radionuclide scan, in hypertension, 196, 201
  in renography, 18
Terazosin, in hypertension, 218t
Tetany, in hypocalcemia, 146
Thirst, in water regulation, 95
Thrombosis
  in renal graft rejection, 260–261
  renal vein
    hematuria in, 27–28
    in nephrotic syndrome, 35
Thrombotic microangiopathy, 54–56
  clinical features, 54–55
  management, 55–56
  prognosis for, 55–56
  renal involvement in, 55
Thrombotic thrombocytopenic purpura, 54–56
  clinical features, 54–55
  management, 55–56
  prognosis for, 55–56
  renal involvement in, 55
Thyroid disease, hypercalcemia in, 141
Tobramycin, acute tubular necrosis from, 72–73
Topoisomerase, antibodies to, in progressive systemic sclerosis, 56
Tourniquet, calcium concentration and, 138
Toxicity, renal (*see* Nephrotoxicity)
Transfusion, complications, in hemodialysis, 234–235
Transplantation, renal, 254–266
  in amyloidosis, recurrence after, 60
  azathioprine in, 255–256
  cardiovascular disease in, 265
  complications, 263–266
  contraindications to, 254–255
  corticosteroids in, 256

cyclosporine in, 256–257, 258t
in diabetic nephropathy, 68
donor evaluation in, 255
graft dysfunction in, 257–263
    acute tubular necrosis, 258–259
    diagnosis, 261–262
    etiology, 257
    management, 262–263
    parenchymal disease, 258–260
    postrenal disease, 260–261
    prerenal disease, 258
    primary nonfunction, 258
    vascular disease, 261
HIV infection and, 185–186
hypercalcemia in, 141
immunosuppressive drugs in, 255–257, 258t
infection in, 263–265
malignancies in, 265–266
nutrition in, 276–277
in progressive systemic sclerosis, recurrence after, 58
recipient evaluation in, 254–255
rejection in
    accelerated, 259
    acute, 259
    chronic, 259–260
    hyperacute, 259
    monitoring, biopsy in, 23
    treatment, 262–263
renal tubular acidosis in, 130

Triamterene
  in hypertension, 213t
  in hypokalemia, 114

Trimethaphan, in hypertension, 222t, 224, 226t

Trimethoprim-sulfamethoxazole
  prophylactic, in renal transplantation, 264
  in urinary tract infection, 165t, 167

Trousseau's sign, in hypocalcemia, 146

Tuberculosis, renal, imaging in, 164t

Tubules
  atrophy, in progressive systemic sclerosis, 57
  distal
    anatomy, 2, 3f, 8–9, 9f
    defect in, renal tubular acidosis in, 127–128
    dysfunction, in tubulointerstitial nephritis, 170
  epithelial cells from, in urinary sediment, 15–16, 16t
  necrosis, acute (see Acute tubular necrosis)
  obstruction, in multiple myeloma, 58
  proximal
    anatomy, 1, 3f, 6–7, 7f
    defect in, renal tubular acidosis in, 128–129
    dysfunction, in tubulointerstitial nephritis, 170
    protein reabsorption in, 31
    reabsorption in, 7

Tubulointerstitial disease
  in diabetic nephropathy, 65t
  hematuria in, 28
  renal tubular acidosis in, 130
  in systemic lupus erythematosus, 47

Tubulointerstitial nephritis, 168–175
  acute drug-induced hypersensitivity, 170–173
    clinical manifestations, 171–172, 172t
    etiology, 170, 171t, 172–173
    hematuria in, 28
    histology, 171
    investigations in, 172
    pathophysiology, 170–171
    prognosis for, 172
    treatment, 172

Tubulointerstitial nephritis — *continued*
  chronic drug-induced, 173–175
    clinical manifestations, 174
    incidence, 173
    investigations, 175
    pathophysiology, 174
    treatment, 175
  clinical manifestations, 169–170
    acute, 171–172, 172t
    chronic, 174
  definition, 168
  etiology, 168–170
    acute, 170, 171t, 172–173
Tumors
  adrenal gland, hyperaldosteronism in, 204–206
  hematuria in, 28
  hypercalcemia in, 140
  pheochromocytoma, 202–204
  in renal transplantation, 265–266
  ultrasonography, 19

Ultrafiltration, in hemodialysis (hemofiltration), 236–237, 236t–238t
Ultrasonography, 18–19, 19t
  in chronic renal failure, 86
  in glomerulonephritis, 37
  in hypertension, 196
  in nephrotic syndrome, 33
  in polycystic kidney disease, 178
  in renal graft rejection, 261–262
  in renal stone disease, 154
  in urinary tract infection, 164t
Urea
  blood (*see* Blood urea nitrogen)
  removal, in peritoneal dialysis, 241–242, 243t
  retention, in chronic renal failure, 85

Uremia
  acidosis in, treatment, 125
  in acute tubular necrosis, 77
  in chronic renal failure, 84–85
  drug absorption in, 278
  drug distribution in, 279–280
  hemodialysis initiation in, 228
Uremic pericarditis, in hemodialysis, 235
Uric acid
  deposition, acute tubular necrosis in, 75
  stones, 153f, 155t, 156–157, 159–160
Urinalysis, 13–16, 16t
Urinary tract infection, 161–167 (*see also* Pyelonephritis)
  acute urethral syndrome, 163
  asymptomatic bacteriuria, 163
  bacteriologic evaluation in, 162–163
  catheter-related, 166
  in chronic renal insufficiency, 167
  complicated, 164t
  computed tomography in, 164t
  cystitis, 162, 165–166, 165t
  in diabetes mellitus, 67
  in dialysis, 167
  etiology, 161
  hematuria in, 28
  incidence, 161
  intravenous pyelography in, 164t
  in medullary sponge kidney, 180
  pathophysiology, 162
  in pregnancy, 162
  prostatitis, 166–167
  radiography in, 163, 164t
  recurrent, 161
  relapse in, 161
  in renal stone disease, 153
  in renal transplantation, from immunosuppressive therapy, 264–265

struvite stone formation in, 156–157
types, 161
ultrasonography in, 164t
Urine
alkalinization, in renal stone disease, 159–160
blood in (*see* Hematuria)
color, 13
culture, in urinary tract infection, 162, 166
dipstick tests, 14–15
for hematuria, 25
for infection, 162
for proteinuria, 33
erythrocytes in, 25 (*see also* Hematuria)
glucose in, 14
hemoglobin in, 14
leukocyte esterase in, 14
microscopic analysis, in nephrotic syndrome, 33
nitrites in, 14
osmolality, 95
paraproteins in, 31–32
pH, 14
phosphorus in, 146–147
protein in (*see* Proteinuria)
sediment
casts in (*see* Casts)
examination, 15–16
in glomerulonephritis, 36–37
in tubulointerstitial nephritis, 172
specific gravity, 14
supersaturation, stone formation in, 152
twenty-four-hour collection
in nephrotic syndrome, 33
in renal stone disease, 154–155
Urine output, in chronic stone disease, 158
Urinoma, in renal graft rejection, 260, 262–263
Uropathy, obstructive (*see* Obstructive uropathy)

Vascular access
for hemodialysis, 229–231
acute, 229–230
assessment, 230
chronic, 230–231
complications, 230
failure of, 244
for hemofiltration, 237
Vasculitis (*see also specific disease*)
vs. acute renal failure, 78–79
glomerulonephritis in, rapidly progressive, 41
hematuria in, 27
renal involvement in, 49–54
Vasoconstriction, acute renal failure in, 70
Vasodilatation, acute renal failure in, 70
Vasodilators
in hypertension, 217–218, 217t
pharmacokinetics, 288t
Vasopressin (*see* Antidiuretic hormone)
Venography, 21
Venous sampling
in hyperaldosteronism, 206
in pheochromocytoma, 204
Verapamil, in hypertension, 220t
Vincristine, in multiple myeloma, 59
Visceral epithelial cells, glomerular, 4, 5f
Vitamin(s), requirements, in renal failure, 271
Vitamin D
deficiency, hypocalcemia in, 145
intoxication with, hypercalcemia in, 141
Volume depletion
acute renal failure in, 70
in metabolic alkalosis, 132
Volume overload, in acute tubular necrosis, 76–77
Volume replacement
in acute renal failure, 71–72
in renal graft rejection, 261
in rhabdomyolysis, 75

Vomiting, in chronic renal failure, 92

Water
  loss, hypernatremia in, 103–104
  restriction, in hyponatremia, 101–102
Water balance
  in chronic renal failure, 89
  disorders (*see* Hypernatremia; Hyponatremia)
  excretion in, 96
  factors affecting, 94
  normal, 94–95

Wegener's granulomatosis
  clinical features, 50
  hematuria in, 27
  management, 50–51
  prognosis for, 50–51
  renal involvement in, 50
Weight, monitoring
  in chronic renal failure, 89
  in hyponatremia, 96
World Health Organization, lupus nephritis classification, 47–49, 48t–49t

Zinc supplementation, in renal failure, 272